DATE DUE

	JAN 0 2 2009	
	APR 1 2 2012	

GAYLORD   #3523PI   Printed in USA

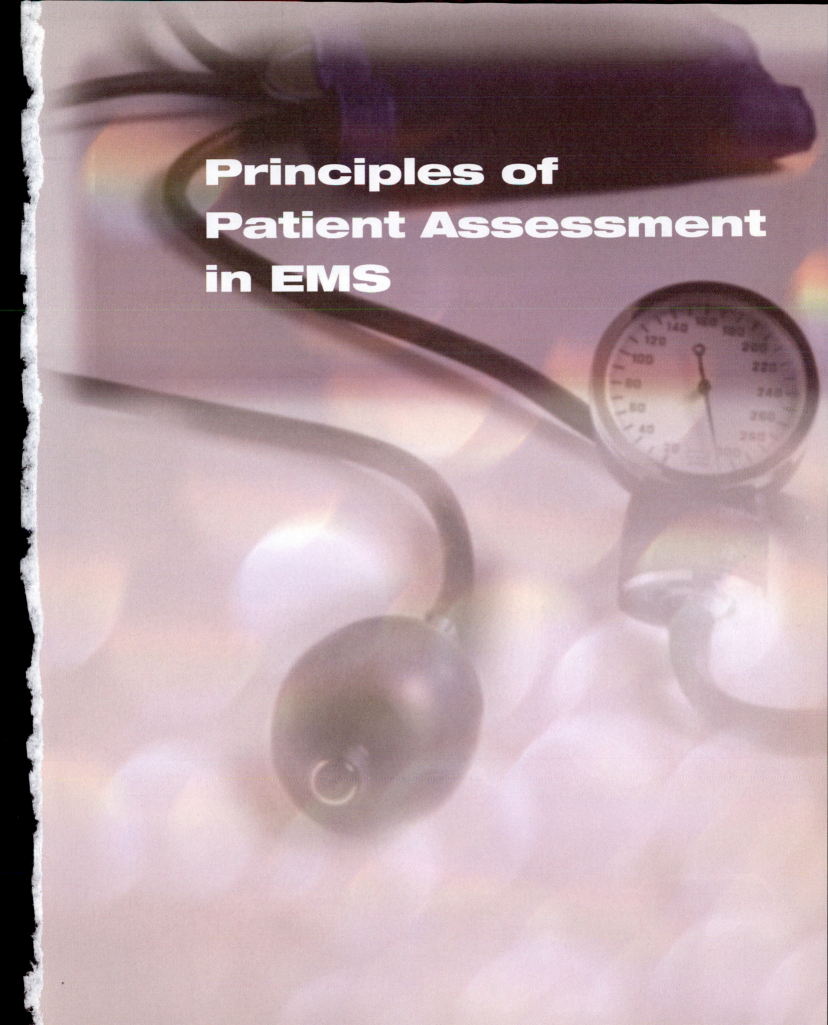

Principles of
Patient Assessment
in EMS

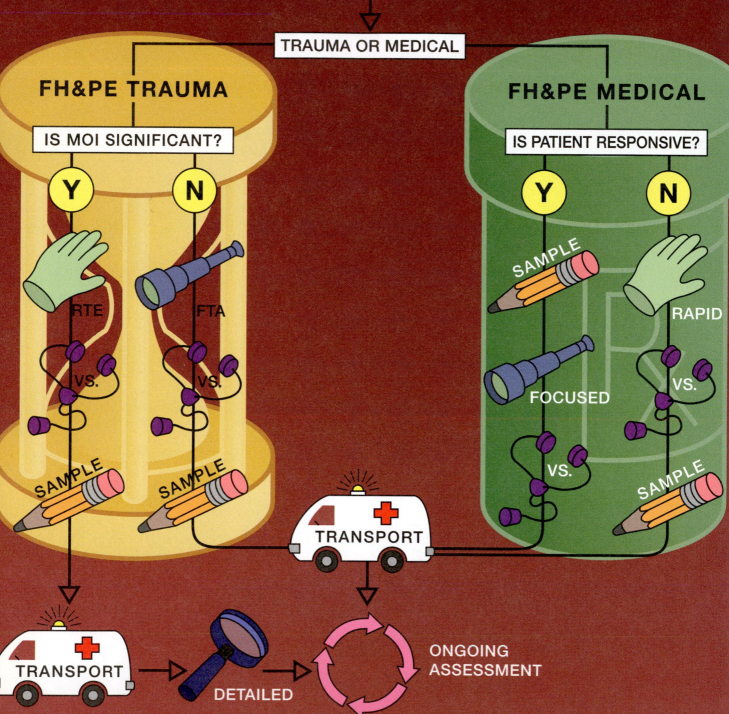

Principles of
Patient Assessment
in EMS

Bob Elling, MPA, REMT-P
Kirsten M. Elling, BS, REMT-P

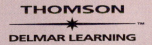

THOMSON

DELMAR LEARNING™

Australia   Canada   Mexico   Singapore   Spain   United Kingdom   United States

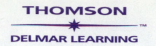

THOMSON
DELMAR LEARNING

Principles of Patient Assessment in EMS
by Bob Elling and Kirsten Elling

Executive Director, Health Care Business Unit:
William Brottmiller

Executive Editor:
Cathy L. Esperti

Acquisitions Editor:
Maureen Rosener

Developmental Editor:
Darcy M. Scelsi

Executive Marketing Manager:
Dawn F. Gerrain

Channel Manager:
Jennifer McAvey

Marketing Coordinator:
Kimberly Lourinia

Editorial Assistant:
Matthew Thouin

Art and Design Coordinator:
Robert Plante

Project Editor:
David Buddle

Production Coordinator:
Nina Lontrato/James Zayicek

For permission to use material from this text or product, contact us by
Tel (800) 730-2214
Fax (800) 730-2215
www.thomsonrights.com

Library of Congress Cataloging-in-Publication Data
Elling, Bob.
  Principles of patient assessment in EMS / Bob Elling, Kirsten Elling.
      p. ; cm.
Includes bibliographical references and index.
  ISBN 0-7668-3899-4
 1. Medical emergencies. 2. Diagnosis. 3. Medical personnel and patient.
  [DNLM: 1. Emergency Medical Services—methods. 2. Diagnostic Techniques and Procedures. WX 215 E46p 2003] I. Elling, Kirsten M. II. Title.
  RC86.7 .E435 2003
  616.02'5—dc21
                                                      2002013368

NOTICE TO THE READER

This work is dedicated to Kirsten and my daughters, Laura and Caitlin. May you always maintain humility as your accomplishments meet the stars!

—BE

This work is dedicated to my husband, Bob, whose support and inspiration continue to drive me to improve patient care in the field.

—KE

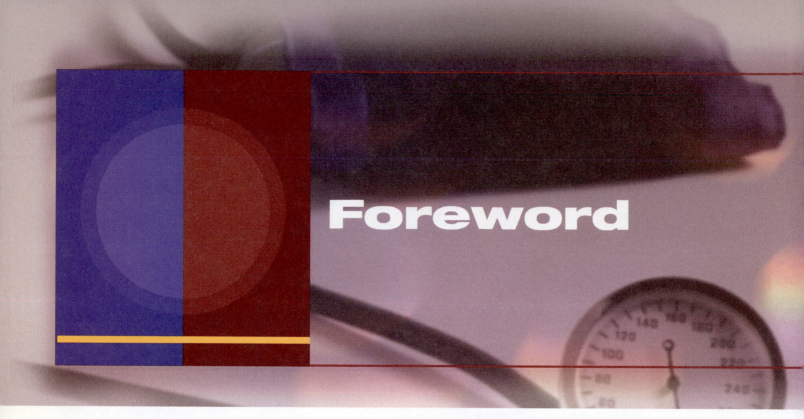

Foreword

Patient assessment is crucial to proper out-of-hospital care for all EMS providers.

This importance is emphasized clearly in the current Department of Transportation (DOT) standardized curricula. Though "traditional" EMS texts provide the necessary basic information; detailed and highly relevant guidelines, recommendations, and helpful hints are hard to find. This void is met head-on by Kirt and Bob Elling's book *Principles of Patient Assessment in EMS*. This wonderful text provides one-stop-shopping for all levels of EMS providers who wish to acquire and maintain superb patient assessment skills.

Principles of Patient Assessment in EMS is organized to follow the DOT patient assessment algorithm. It covers proper assessment for patients of all ages. The book is well organized and easy to follow. In addition, it provides interesting and necessary background information on various, specific patient presentations (e.g., assessment of the neurological patient, assessment of the patient with behavioral problems). Without this knowledge, the EMS provider is simply an automaton, rather than a thinking professional.

Kirt and Bob combine together numerous years of EMS experience involving not only teaching, but administration and many hours of clinical practice too. Both are well-known authors and educators in the EMS community. To me, they are highly respected and loved colleagues and personal friends.

If you really want to give the best possible patient care, become an expert in patient assessment. *Principles of Patient Assessment in EMS* will help you every step of the way.

Mikel A. Rothenberg, M.D.
Emergency Care Educator
Professor of EMS, American College of
    Prehospital Care
North Olmsted, Ohio

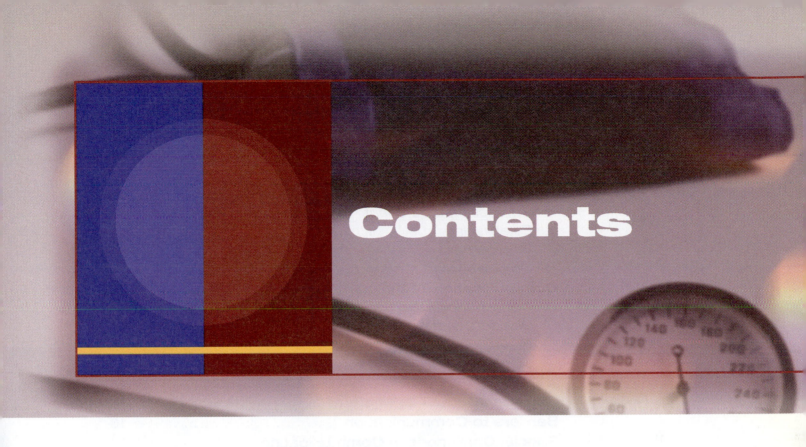

Contents

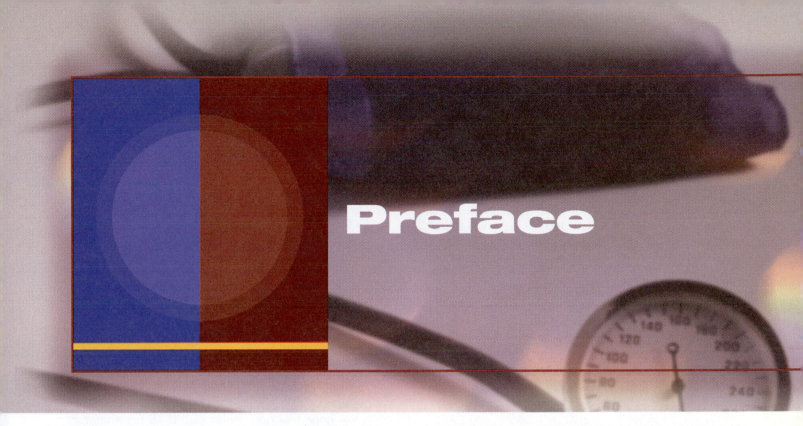

Preface

Before we explain how to use this book, it would be helpful to first understand *why* to use this book. Assessment has always been one of the most complex skills taught to health care providers. The newer trend to move Department of Transportation training curricula to assessment-based has been helpful in affording additional course time to this key skill, yet somewhat misleading. Older curricula were traditionally diagnosis-based. Unless your patients showed up with a diagnosis tattooed on their forehead, such as "I'm a CVA," "Rule out MI," or "Fractured right tibia," someone somewhere had to arrive at a presumptive diagnosis.

Arriving at a presumptive diagnosis has always required assessment and probably always will to some degree. Thus any move toward more assessment practice in the training curricula is clearly a positive one in our view. After all, probably the biggest difference between a clinician and a technician is in their assessment skills.

Have you ever noticed how difficult it is to teach someone how to start an IV, apply a splint, or pass an ET tube? It frankly is not that difficult. Having kids who hung around the college during labs and worked as victims in the lab stations or practical, I used to think it was amazing that my 12-year-old daughter could pass an ET tube or apply a splint just as well as our EMT-B and paramedic students! Of course my children don't always know when to apply the skill, as that involves assessment. Aside from being the greatest kids in the world (because they are mine—aren't yours?), they are nothing special. They just watched closely many times and through repetition have the manual dexterity skills to apply the appropriate steps in the proper sequence. Fortunately, most of the skills of an EMS provider are acquired like that and that is why they are easy to teach and easy to learn.

Assessment is different from all the other EMS skills and is thought by some to be one of the toughest skills to teach. Yet clearly it is the most important skill, as the decision to proceed with most other skills is predicated on assessment. That is because assessment is a complex skill involving critical thinking and your ability to make priority decisions and compare your observations to your knowledge base.

Some great authors have contributed to the prehospital EMS bookshelf, yet we find that very few of these books strictly cover assessment for the EMS provider. One might say there has been a void in books that speak specifically on the topic of prehospital assessment. It is that void that *Principles of Patient Assessment in EMS* fills for the EMS provider and EMS instructor. We have written this book to cover all aspects of prehospital assessment. The format for assessment was updated in the 1999 DOT paramedic curriculum. We have illustrated that format using the assessment algorithm, which we weave throughout this book.

As the training curricula have changed, it has been clear to us in our teaching, travels, and interactions with other EMS educators that some have embraced the changes and moved forward while others continue to hold on to their tried-and-true methods. Unfortunately, continuing to use terminology and techniques of the past tends to confuse students, who now read textbooks updated to the latest format and terminology.

In this book we follow and enrich the 1999 DOT paramedic training curricula. Although history is relevant in the discussion of assessment, current approaches will help move us all forward as we all learn more about the assessment process. To become comfortable with the skill of patient assessment in the field, you must first understand this is a dynamic process and be comfortable with change.

In our more than 41 years combined involvement in EMS, we both have learned that as EMS providers you should never "nail down your tent," as this is an evolving field and we are constantly being asked to pick up and reposition. Change is guaranteed in EMS, as it is in assessment, and you must learn to be flexible and adaptable and willing to go with what is new, even when it seems to contradict previous beliefs. Those who resist or fear change do not do well over the long term and ultimately follow the path to extinction along with the low-top Cadillac ambulance, rotating tourniquets, and lengthy field fluid resuscitation of trauma patients. Today these things, which were popular in their time, are merely milestones in the history of our field.

HOW TO USE THIS BOOK

Although we certainly cover all the assessment skills of the paramedic—because we do not spend a lot of time discussing treatment and medical protocols—the book can be just as valuable to the EMT-Basic who wants to learn more about assessment. Be sure to begin by reading these chapters in order: Chapter 1: Overview of Patient Assessment, Chapter 3: Sizing Up the Scene, Chapter 4: The Initial Assessment, and Chapter 5: Making a Priority Decision. They will give you the foundation on which the rest of the book sits. The remaining chapters can be read in any order, with Chapter 22: Putting It All Together, being last of course.

As you read each chapter, visualize in your mind a patient in front of you and use the assistance of the assessment algorithm, its symbols and colors, and the icons used throughout the book. Ask yourself, "On my patient, what steps or components of assessment have been done so far and what steps need to be done right now?" It is a good habit to constantly justify in your own mind, to that little voice in your head, "Why am I asking this question or doing this exam right now?" and "Is this in the patient's best interest based on what I have learned so far about the patient's condition?" If you do this, you may find it easier to change your course of action midstream. That is to say, as you learn more about the patient from questioning and examination, the information you now have may help to refocus or reprioritize the assessment, as well as the care. Rather than cast your decisions in concrete as you go, ask yourself, "Based on what I have learned about this patient at this time (not 5 or 15 minutes ago), is this now the most appropriate course of action?" This approach helps you be flexible to change and undoubtedly not nail down your tent!

We hope this book helps pull it all together for you, fill in the voids, and at times challenge you to be a better EMS provider. We will all need EMS either personally or for a loved one at some point in our lives. We think it will be a better experience if the clinicians who respond and take care of us are compassionate and caring, as well as passionate in their ability to assess our condition. After all, isn't that what this dynamic field of EMS is all about? Our thanks to the publishing team at Delmar Learning for its hard work on this book and the instructor's manual. Special thanks to Darcy M. Scelsi, developmental editor, for her expertise.

If after reading this book you have any questions, comments, or concerns, feel free to send us an e-mail at Bobelling@usa.net.

See you in the streets!

Bob and Kirsten

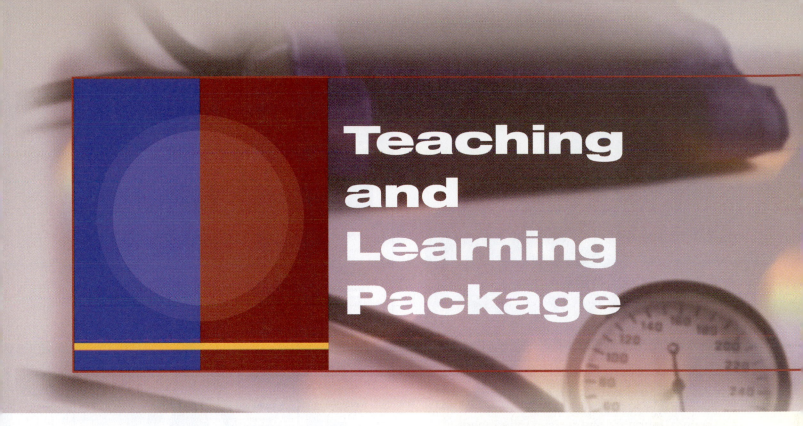

Teaching and Learning Package

Additional resources have been developed for this book to aid the student in additional learning and to aid the instructor in preparing for teaching the content.

INSTRUCTOR'S MANUAL

The *Instructor's Manual* provides tools the instructor can use to develop lecture material and to incorporate activities in the classroom environment to more fully engage the student. The *Instructor's Manual* includes:

- Objectives that mirror those found within the text.
- Suggested Teaching Activities to provide inter-activity in the classroom to further hone the students' problem-solving and communication skills. These skills are critical in patient assessment.
- Teaching Outlines to provide the instructor with a framework for each lecture that corresponds to each chapter in the book.
- Teaching Resources to aid the instructor in finding additional material to use in class and to direct students to more information and further study or course work.
- Case Scenarios to incorporate into classroom discussion or to provide as student assignments.
- Quizzes and Tests to assess the students' knowledge level and comprehension of the course work.
- A correlation guide to the 1999 DOT paramedic curriculum helps incorporate the content of the book within the DOT's framework for assessment.

ON-LINE COMPANION

The on-line companion is a resource for students and instructors alike. It supports the book with additional resources and activities that correlate to each chapter. A PowerPoint presentation is also available for instructor use when developing class materials and for students to use to review and take notes in class. You can access the on-line companion at http://www.delmarhealthcare.com/companions.

LEARNING ENHANCEMENTS

Students will also find value in these additional products from Delmar Learning:

Delmar's Heart and Lung Sounds for the EMS Provider

Order 0-7668-3832-3 (single-user version)

Auscultation is one of the most difficult skills for EMS providers to master. This CD-ROM is an excellent learning tool that helps users identify and interpret both normal and abnormal heart and lung sounds.

Its features include:

- An extensive library of normal and abnormal heart and lung sounds for reference.

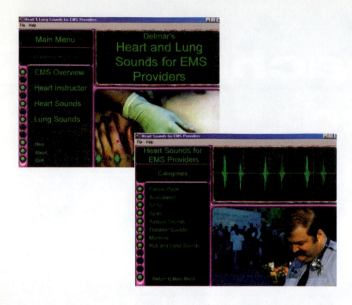

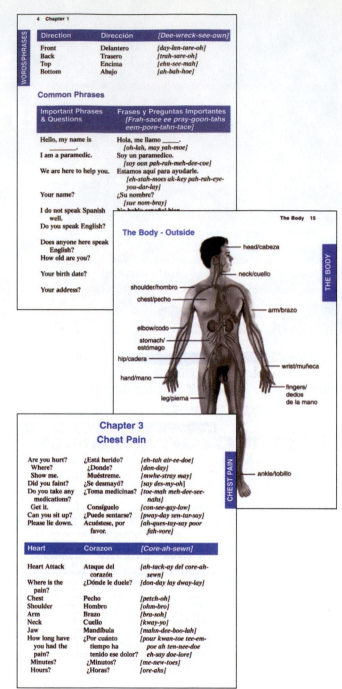

- An eight-part heart sounds module: cardiac cycle, auscultation, S1 S2, splits, systolic sounds, diastolic sounds, murmurs, and rub and valve sounds.
- A five-part lung sounds module: normal, abnormal, adventitious, voice sounds, and auscultation.
- EMS Overview features street sounds normally encountered by EMS providers, testing their ability to recognize heart and lung sounds under these conditions.
- A comprehensive final review.

Emergencia! Emergency Translation Manual

Order 0-7668-3626-6

Emergencia! Emergency Translation Manual is a language reference for English-speaking EMS providers who need to communicate effectively with Spanish-speaking patients. Translations of a wide array of medical emergencies include phonetic pronunciations of words and phrases, diagrams of the human body labeled in Spanish, and pages of commonly used words or phrases to facilitate communication and quicken response times.

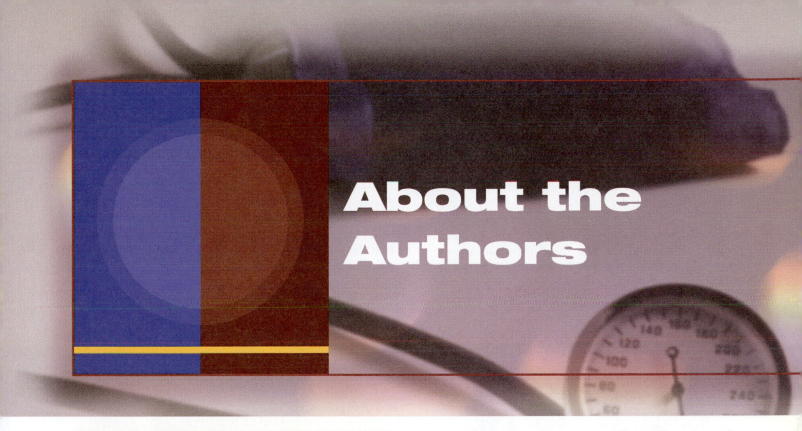

About the Authors

BOB ELLING, MPA, REMT-P

Bob has been involved in EMS since 1975 and is currently a faculty member for the Institute of Prehospital Emergency Medicine at Hudson Valley Community College in Troy, New York. Bob teaches EMT-Basic, Paramedic, and recertification courses. Bob has served as the Institute's program director and was responsible for providing leadership in the expansion of the Institute, accreditation of the paramedic program, as well as the development of the associate degree in applied science for EMT-Paramedic.

Bob is also an active paramedic with the Town of Colonie (NY) EMS Department. Bob is a member of the New York State Department of Health EMS Bureau's Regional Faculty as well as an American Heart Association National Faculty member.

Bob is also a professor of management at the American College of Prehospital Medicine, a distance learning college in Florida. He is a member of the *Journal of Emergency Medical Services* editorial review board; the author of many articles, video scripts, and books, such as *Essentials of Emergency Care, First Responder Exam Preparation and Review, Emergency Care Student Workbook, Pocket Reference for the EMT-Basic and First Responder, Essentials of Emergency Care Instructor's Resource Manual, MedReview for the EMT-Basic*; a coauthor of *Enrichment for the Why Driven EMS Provider* and *The Paramedic Review*; a contributing author for *Paramedic Care: Principles and Practice*; and a coauthor of the current National First Responder, Paramedic and EMT-Intermediate curricula.

Bob has served as a paramedic and lieutenant for New York City EMS, the associate director for New York State EMS, education coordinator for *PULSE: Emergency Medical Update*, evaluation coordinator for the Regional Emergency Medical Organization, and a firefighter-paramedic in Colonie, New York, throughout his 28-year EMS career.

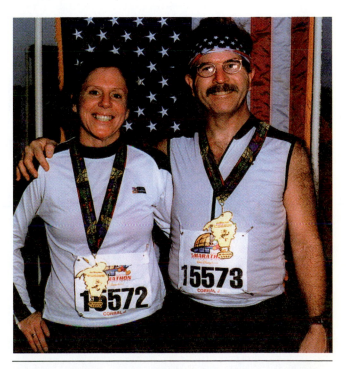

Authors Kirsten and Bob Elling enjoy staying fit by running marathons in their "spare" time. (Photo courtesy of Action Sports International)

KIRSTEN M. ELLING, BS, REMT-P

Kirt Elling is a career paramedic who works in the Town of Colonie in upstate New York. She began work in EMS in 1988 as an EMT/firefighter and has been a National Registered Paramedic since 1991. She has been an EMS educator since 1990 and teaches basic and advanced EMS programs at the Institute of Prehospital Emergency Medicine in Troy, New York. Kirt serves as Regional Faculty for the New York State Department of Health's Bureau of EMS and Regional Faculty for the American Heart Association, Northeast Region. She has written numerous scripts for the EMS training video series *PULSE: Emergency Medical Update*, is a coauthor of *Enrichment for the Why Driven EMS Provider* and *The Paramedic Review*, contributing author of the *Paramedic Lab Manual* for the Institute of Prehospital Emergency Medicine, and an adjunct writer for the revision of the National Highway Traffic Safety Administration, EMT-Paramedic and EMT-Intermediate National Standard Curricula.

A Moment of Silence

This book, *Principles of Patient Assessment in EMS*, was written in the fall of 2001. During that time all members of the emergency services community were forever changed, each in his or her own way, by the horrific attack on America on September 11th. Despite the death that day of 2,823 people, including 8 EMS providers and 341 firefighters and fire officers, the hard work, dedication, and commitment of the rescue workers helped to save thousands of lives in both New York City and at the Pentagon.

While the loss from and full impact of the events of that single tragic day are sure to have an effect on our future practice, how things will change is yet to be determined. Both the authors of this book and its publisher wish to thank those dedicated emergency service providers and the families of those who made the ultimate sacrifice for their kindred human beings. May they never be forgotten!

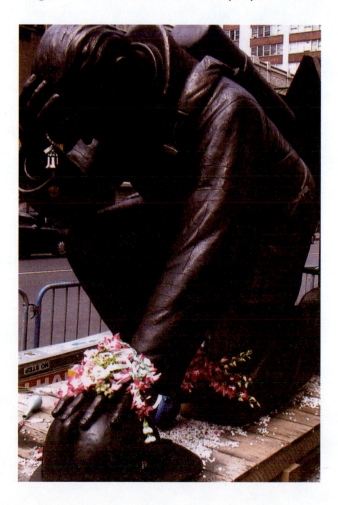

To honor Missouri's fallen firefighters, this bronze firefighter statue was commissioned by the Fire Fighters Association of Missouri from the Pittsburgh-based Matthews International Corp. It was cast in Parma, Italy, and shipped to the United States by way of New York City's Kennedy International Airport. On September 11, 2001, the kneeling firefighter was waiting to clear customs for transport to its final destination of Kingdom City, Missouri. The statue was donated to the City of New York as a tribute to the firefighters killed at the World Trade Center.

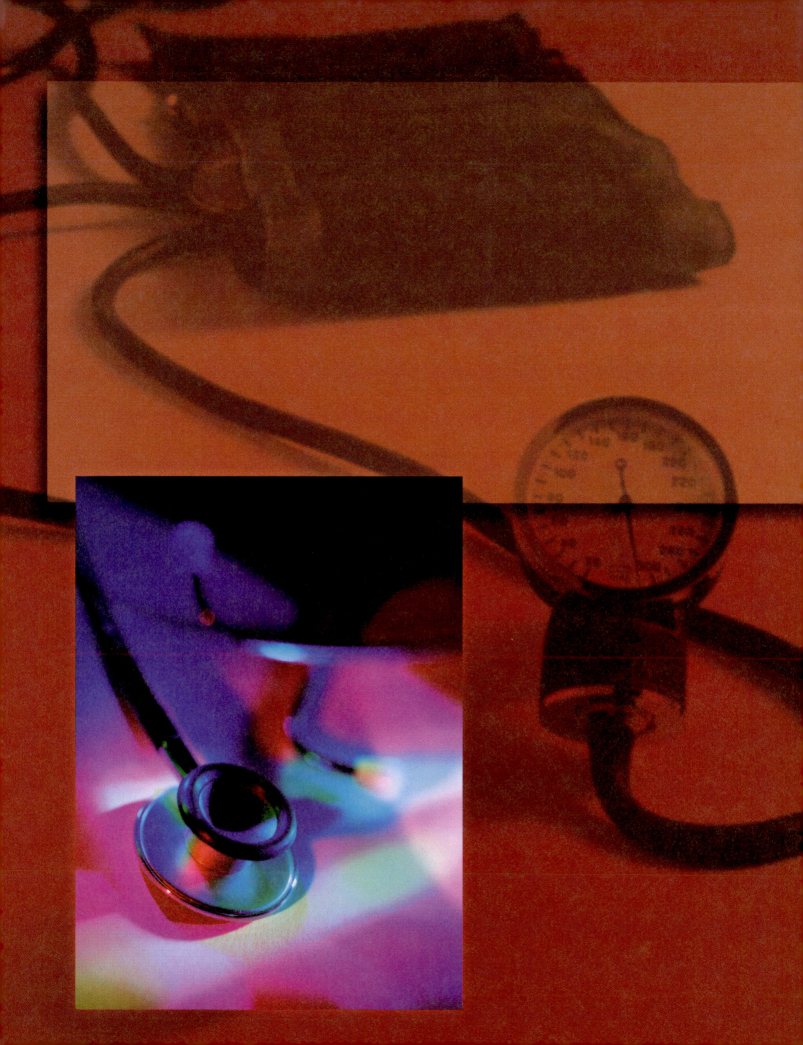

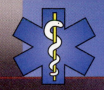

Chapter 1

Overview of Patient Assessment

OBJECTIVES

Upon completion of this chapter, the reader should be able to:

- Describe significant changes in the approach to assessment since the 1980s.
- Discuss the importance of a standardized approach to patient assessment.
- List and describe four key factors to the assessment approach.
- List and describe six components of the standardized approach to patient assessment.

KEY TERMS

detailed physical examination (DPE)
focused history and physical examination (FH&PE)
initial assessment (IA)
mechanism of injury (MOI)
objective information
ongoing assessment (OA)
OPQRST

patient assessment
rapid physical examination (RPE)
rapid trauma examination (RTE)
SAMPLE history
scene size-up
subjective information

INTRODUCTION

This book uses the whole-part-whole strategy of learning. First, an overview and general considerations are provided to enable readers to visualize the entire approach to assessment. Then the individual components are discussed in detail in separate chapters, and, finally, they are brought back together in the last chapter. This chapter provides an overview of patient assessment and introduces the six components of the standardized approach to patient assessment.

The approach to prehospital patient assessment has gone through a series of changes since the 1980s. Some experienced EMS providers have developed an attitude that is best summed up by the statement, "Just when I get it down, they change it on me." The assessment process has evolved from the primary survey, which used an "ABC plan," to the expanded primary survey, with its "ABCDE plan," to the current initial assessment with the "MS-ABC plan." The ABCs (airway, breathing, and circulation) of patient assessment have remained throughout the evolution. However, with the 1994 release of EMT-Basic and the 1998 EMT-Paramedic U.S. Department of Transportation curricula by the National Highway Traffic Safety Administration, assessment was changed to more closely reflect what providers actually do in the field. These curricula were touted as "assessment based" and clearly placed more time and emphasis on the assessment process in training EMS providers.

IMPORTANCE OF A STANDARDIZED APPROACH

When a call comes in for a prehospital emergency, depending on the information that is available to the emergency medical dispatcher (EMD) at the time of dispatch, the initial information can range from very detailed to very sketchy at best. Patients can be found in any of hundreds of combinations of predicaments, such as sudden medical emergencies, sudden exacerbation of a chronic problem, or acute traumatic events. Add to this variety of situations the many positions the patient can be physically found in, from sitting in her living room easy chair to pinned on her bike under a cement mixer's wheels. There are thousands of variations of patient presentations to the EMS provider that need to be assessed.

Even though the patients and the situations they present with are often unique, the EMS provider's approach to patient assessment and physical examination must be similar for each new patient. Imagine trying to learn hundreds of forms of assessment, each unique to a different patient presentation or position the patient is found in. No one would ever become proficient in assessment. The assessment and physical examination need to be standardized for all patients yet must take into consideration four key factors. These factors are the environment the patient is found in, the severity of the patient's condition, whether the patient has an acute illness or an injury, and the level of prehospital care available to the patient in the field.

Environment

Environment is an important factor because some locations simply are not safe for conducting an assessment, for either the patient or the EMS providers. Examples of unsafe environments or scenes would be within the "kill zone" at a hostage situation, in the "hot zone" of a hazmat incident, in a garage filled with carbon monoxide at a potential suicide, or in the middle of a domestic abuse situation. These patients must be moved out of the unstable environment to make it safe for the EMS providers to do their assessment. Some environments are not as obviously dangerous yet contribute to the potential demise of the patient; for example, a very cold or very hot apartment might pose a danger to an elderly patient. In some situations, such as freezing cold or a downpour, it is safest to carefully move the patient into the back of the ambulance and begin assessment there.

Severity

The severity of a patient's condition is a very important factor that takes into consideration the time available before management of the patient's life-threatening illness or injury. A patient from an automobile collision with suspected bleeding from a ruptured spleen cannot be controlled in the field. This patient needs the expertise of surgeons to stabilize her condition, and too much time spent assessing in the field could be counterproductive. Certain medical emergencies, such as hypoxia, hypoglycemia, lengthy seizure, or a rapidly expanding acute myocardial infarction, also need to be dealt with quickly rather than spending a lengthy amount of time on the scene doing a detailed physical examination.

Medical versus Trauma

Whether the patient's problem is an acute medical emergency or a sudden traumatic event is important because the approach to each of these two types of patients is different. The training materials and curricula for EMS providers recognize that the medical patient and the trauma patient are clearly different. In-hospital medical care has traditionally been approached from the medical or surgical perspective, so approaching prehospital patient assessment differently for the medical versus the trauma patient makes sense. Just as trauma patients and medical patients are managed differently, they are also assessed differently in the field depending on their level of responsiveness and the significance of their **mechanism of injury** (**MOI**; the instrument or event that results in harm to the patient). As you will learn later in this book, there is more emphasis on history and prior illness for a medical patient than for an injured patient, whose MOI is a very important consideration.

Level of Care

Any approach to prehospital assessment needs to take into consideration the available level of care for the patient. Some communities have sophisticated response systems and EMS providers who have a wide array of protocols and procedures to manage patients in the field; other communities need to rely on rapid transportation to the local emergency department to provide advanced life support. Many communities use specially trained paramedics (e.g., CCEMT-P, or critical care emergency medical technician–paramedic) and registered nurses in an aeromedical critical care transport service to extend the hospital critical care unit to the scene.

OVERVIEW OF THE SIX COMPONENTS OF PATIENT ASSESSMENT

What is patient assessment? **Patient assessment** is the methodical process by which a patient's condition is evaluated. The assessment is based on the **subjective information**, commonly referred to as symptoms, that is obtained from the patient. Assessment is also based on the **objective information**, which includes clinical signs that can be observed and measured by the examiner such as the pulse, respirations, blood pressure, and oxygen saturation. The degree of detail obtained in an assessment is usually a function of the patient's injury or illness priority.

The standard approach to assessment, based on the National Standard Curriculum, involves six components: (1) the scene size-up, (2) the initial assessment, (3) the focused history and physical examination of a trauma patient, (4) the focused history and physical examination of a medical patient, (5) the detailed physical examination, and (6) the ongoing assessment. Throughout this book, the patient assessment algorithm, shown in Figure 1-1, will be used to illustrate the relationships among these six components for the medical and trauma patient.

The Scene Size-up

The first component, the **scene size-up**, involves determining whether the location, or environment, is safe for the responders, including EMS providers, firefighters, and police, as well as for the patient, family, and bystanders. Ensuring that the appropriate body substance isolation (BSI) precautions are taken and that the responders needed to stabilize the patient and alleviate any hazards at the scene are en route are also part of the scene size-up. Scene size-up is discussed in detail in Chapter 3.

The Initial Assessment

The second component, the **initial assessment (IA)**, is defined as an orderly and sequential examination with correction of life threats and determination of the patient's priority. The initial assessment is actually the first assessment of the patient that is done; thus the name *initial* is appropriate. This assessment involves obtaining a general impression of the patient; determining the chief complaint; assessing the patient's mental status (MS); finding and correcting life threats to the airway, breathing, and circulation (ABC); and determining the patient priority and need for advanced life support (ALS). The initial assessment is the same for both a trauma and a medical patient.

Some patients are so critically ill or injured that it is difficult to know where to start the evaluation. When the patient is bleeding or vomiting profusely, it is a good sense of discipline and priorities that helps the EMS provider through the initial assessment. The last part of the initial assessment involves prioritizing the patient, which will set the pace for the remainder of the assessment steps and determine how much time is appropriate to spend on the scene managing the patient. This key element of assessment is discussed in detail in Chapter 4.

The Focused History and Physical Examination of the Trauma Patient

After the initial assessment has been completed, a **focused history and physical examination (FH&PE)** is done. The third and fourth components of the assessment are generally not conducted on the same patient because they are different for trauma patients than for medical patients. The third component, or FH&PE of the trauma patient, involves determining if the mechanism of injury (MOI) is significant. If the MOI is significant, such as a fall from three times the patient's height, then the plan is to (1) conduct a **rapid trauma examination (RTE)**, (2) obtain a set of baseline vital signs, (3) obtain a **SAMPLE history** (Table 1-1), and (4) transport

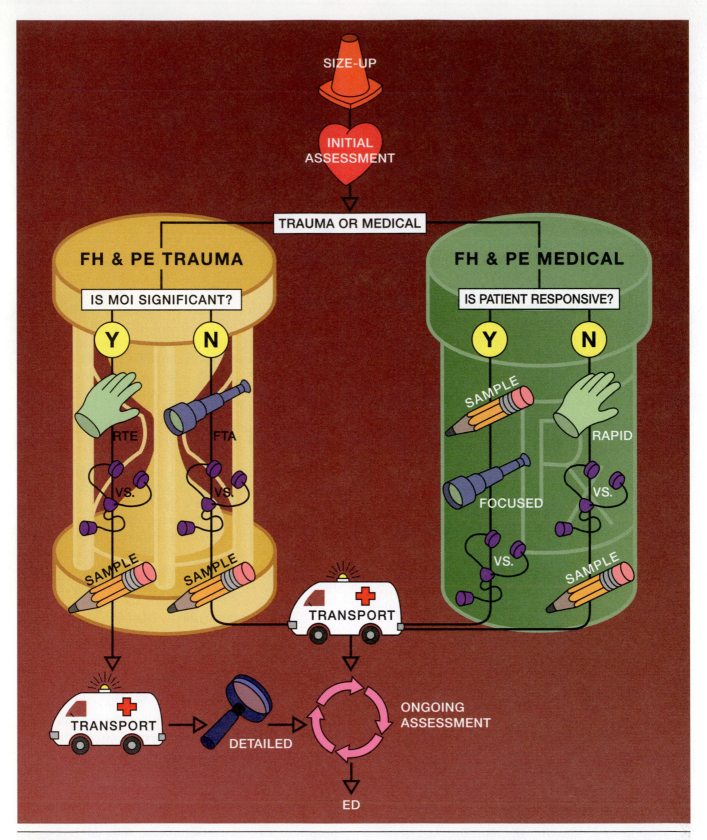

FIGURE 1-1 The patient assessment algorithm is used throughout this book to help illustrate the relationships among the components of assessment for the medical patient and those for the trauma patient.

TABLE 1-1
The SAMPLE History

Signs and symptoms
Allergies
Medications
Pertinent past medical history
Last oral intake
Events leading up to this incident

the patient. (SAMPLE is an acronym for the information needed to assess today's incident.) If the MOI is not significant, such as a twisted ankle without any other trauma or a superficial laceration to an extremity, then the plan is to (1) do an assessment that is focused on the specific injury site, (2) obtain a set of baseline vital signs, (3) obtain a SAMPLE history, and (4) transport the patient as appropriate. The FH&PE of a trauma patient is discussed in more detail in Chapter 7.

The Focused History and Physical Examination of the Medical Patient

The fourth component, or FH&PE of the medical patient, involves an evaluation of the patient's responsiveness. If the patient is responsive, the approach is to (1) obtain a history of the present illness using an abbreviation such as **OPQRST** (see Table 1-2), (2) obtain a SAMPLE history, (3) conduct a focused physical examination based on the patient's chief complaint, (4) obtain baseline vital signs, and (5) transport the patient. If the patient is not responsive, the approach is to (1) do a **rapid physical examination (RPE)**, (2) obtain baseline

TABLE 1-2
For Patients with Pain

Onset
Provocation
Quality
Region, **R**adiation, **R**elief, **R**ecurrence
Severity
Time

vital signs, and then (3) obtain a history of the present illness and a SAMPLE history. Transportation of the patient can be begun either before or after the FH&PE has been completed. The FH&PE of a medical patient is discussed in detail in Chapter 9.

The Detailed Physical Examination

The fifth component, or **detailed physical examination (DPE)**, is designed to be conducted on trauma patients who have a significant MOI. It is to be conducted en route to the hospital and is not to be done on the scene unless the patient is entrapped or transport is delayed for some time. The detailed physical examination is generally not done on patients who do not have a significant MOI. It would not make sense to do a head-to-toe examination on a patient whose only complaint is a twisted ankle or who did not fall or strike her head or injure any other body part. This component of the assessment is discussed in detail in Chapter 11.

The Ongoing Assessment

The sixth and last component of the assessment, called the **ongoing assessment (OA)**, is conducted en route to the hospital. It involves reassessing vital signs, reassessing interventions such as medications administered or treatments applied, repeating the initial assessment as necessary to determine if there are any life threats present, and reprioritizing the patient. Vital signs should be assessed every 15 minutes for stable patients and every 5 minutes for unstable patients. The ongoing assessment is discussed in detail in Chapter 20: The Ongoing Assessment.

CONCLUSION

Assessment is a dynamic process as patients improve or deteriorate while in the care of EMS providers. A standardized approach to assessment that includes the components introduced in this overview will ensure that the patient receives the amount of assessment needed on the basis of the key factors, including the environment, whether the patient has a medical condition or trauma, the severity of the injury or illness, and the level of care the patient will receive in the field. It is essential to continue to reassess the patient throughout the time she is in the care of EMS and to be flexible enough to change the plan of management as the patient's changing condition warrants.

REVIEW QUESTIONS

1. In the evolution of the assessment process for the EMS provider, which of the following "plans" is most current?

   a. ABC

   b. MS-ABC

   c. ABCDE

   d. AMPLE

2. The key factors in the standardized approach to patient assessment must take into consideration all of the following except:

   a. the environment in which the patient is found.

   b. the severity of the patient's condition.

   c. the cost of the care in your community.

   d. whether the patient has an acute illness or an injury.

3. An example of an environmental factor in assessment that may be subtle yet necessary to deal with would be:

   a. a patient in the kill zone during a hostage situation.

   b. an elderly patient found in a cold apartment.

   c. a carbon monoxide–filled garage on the scene of an apparent suicide attempt.

   d. a patient in the hot zone of a chemical spill.

4. The key factor of assessment that takes into consideration the time the patient has available before management of her condition is called:

   a. duration.

   b. elevation.

   c. severity.

   d. provocation.

5. A medical patient and a trauma patient should be:

   a. assessed in the same manner.

   b. assessed in a different manner.

   c. immediately transported in most situations.

   d. completely assessed while on the scene.

6. Of the following, which is not considered an objective finding?

   a. dizziness and nausea

   b. the pulse oximeter reading

   c. the patient's pulse rate

   d. the patient's blood pressure

7. Which is the first component of the standard approach to assessment?

   a. the detailed physical examination

   b. the ongoing assessment

   c. the initial assessment

   d. the scene size-up

8. Of the following, which is not one of the components of the standardized approach to patient assessment discussed in this book?

   a. the focused history and physical examination

   b. the expanded primary survey

   c. the ongoing assessment

   d. the initial assessment

9. The abbreviation used to help the EMS provider elaborate on the chief complaint is:

   a. SAMPLE.

   b. OPQRST.

   c. MOI.

   d. AVPU.

10. The component of the patient assessment that is usually conducted en route to the hospital is called the:

   a. ongoing assessment.

   b. scene size-up.

   c. focused history.

   d. focused physical examination.

CRITICAL THINKING QUESTIONS

1. Explain the rationale for a standardized approach to patient assessment. How will learning a standardized approach help you become a better EMS provider?

2. Think about the consequences that could arise if one step in the assessment process is skipped. What could happen if the EMS provider skipped:

   a. the scene size-up

   b. the initial assessment

   c. the focused history and physical examination of either a trauma or a medical patient

   d. the detailed physical examination

   e. the ongoing assessment

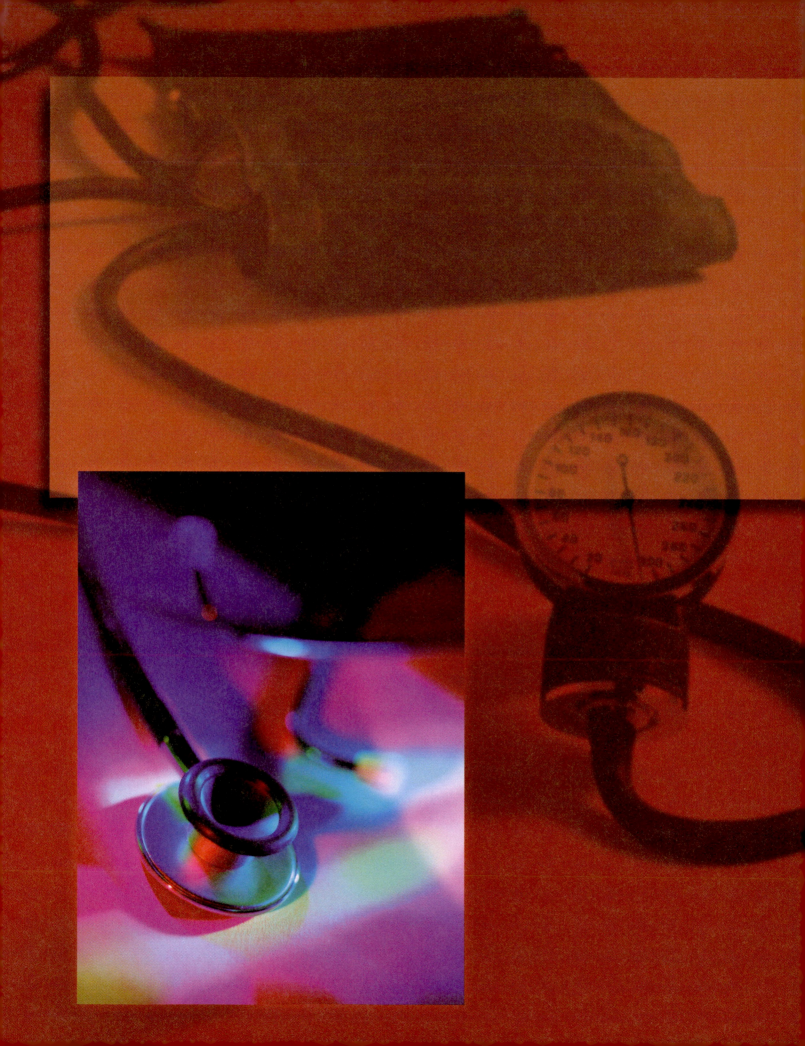

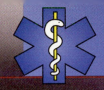

Chapter 2

Listening to Patients

OBJECTIVES

Upon completion of this chapter, the reader should be able to:

- List the major components of the communication process.
- Describe various methods for communicating a message.
- Describe how patient comfort can affect communication.
- Explain why making a proper introduction and identifying the EMS provider's level of training is an important factor for patient communication.
- Provide examples of how the EMS provider can establish trust with a patient.
- Explain the EMS provider's responsibility in maintaining the patient-EMS provider relationship.
- List examples of both positive and negative facilitation.
- Describe the techniques EMS providers may use to encourage feedback from a patient.
- Identify two factors that tend to impede verbal communications.
- Provide examples of special challenges the EMS provider may encounter in communicating with patients and some tips to manage each.
- Describe verbal and nonverbal factors to consider when communicating with a patient with cultural differences.

KEY TERMS

American Sign Language (ASL)
Americans with Disabilities Act (ADA)
clarification
closed question
communication process

cultural diversity
decode
developmentally disabled
empathy
encode

(continues)

INTRODUCTION

Because there is much to ask the patient and often little time to do so, establishing a rapport with the patient and family or caregivers is a significant factor in patient care. Effective communication between the EMS provider and the patient takes a lot of practice and entails being confident, caring, supportive, patient, flexible, and empathetic as well as often becoming a detective in an effort to obtain pertinent and focused information about the patient. Obtaining a good history is often difficult or impossible; for example, the patient may be a poor historian, may have an altered mental status or be unconscious, or may be overwhelmed or nonverbal. Even when a patient is cared for by relatives or a health care facility or resides in an adult residence home, pertinent patient information often is not available. This chapter focuses on interpersonal dynamics and strategies of communication so the EMS provider can communicate well with patients.

COMMUNICATION

A key factor to effective communication is knowing when to talk, when to listen, and how to listen. Communication is a two-way process involving a feedback loop as shown in Figure 2-1. The **communication process** includes a sender, receiver, message, encoding, decoding, and feedback. The sender has a **message** (the point he or she is trying to convey to the receiver) that she **encodes** (decides what terms to use to convey the message) and sends to the receiver, who **decodes** (interprets) the message and then produces **feedback** (a response based on the receiver's interpretation of the original message). The communications process used by the EMS provider is focused around the message (information). A message can be communicated through both verbal and nonverbal methods:

- Verbal. Speaking with the patient and observing feedback is the best way to determine whether the

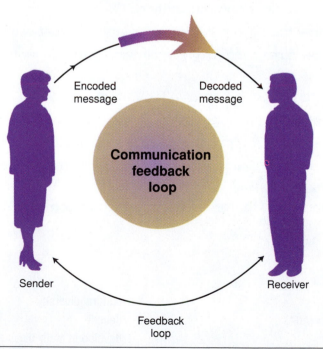

FIGURE 2-1 The communications feedback loop model involves encoding, sending, receiving and decoding, and then sending back a message to ensure the original message was properly understood.

message has been understood. Word content, tone and volume of voice, speed of talking, and inflection all influence the verbal form of communication. Written messages are also considered verbal communication. Written information placed in a note, letter, report, document, or computer is an integral form of communication in the EMS profession. Telecommunication, by means of radio, phone, telemetry, or two-way paging, is also an integral form of communication for EMS providers.

- Nonverbal. Body language and personal space are considered two of the most important forms of nonverbal communication. Physical appearance, dress, personal possessions, posture, body position, and facial expressions are examples of body language, which often can convey much more of the message than verbal language. The personal space theory, developed by anthropologist Edward T. Hall in 1966, suggests that there are four zones of personal distance, measured by physical distance, in the area surrounding an individual. Each zone is characterized by its own type of activities and relationships and conveys certain meanings. Personal space is discussed in the section titled Distance.

Listening

When listening to patients, try to adjust the environment so it is easy to listen. In some cases, this adjustment might involve helping the patient put in or turn up a hearing aid. Or it may involve asking extra rescuers to step outside the room. One partner can move the family members aside, perhaps by asking them a question about what happened or asking them to get the patient's medications. In some cases, the easiest way to create a quiet environment for detailed questioning is to move the patient to the patient compartment of the ambulance.

It is important to listen to what patients have to say about their history and their body. If an EMS provider needs to know where to find the best vein to start an IV on an IV drug abuser, simply ask the drug abuser. He will undoubtedly know where an accessible vein is located better than anyone else would!

The following case illustrates the importance of listening to patients and not judging them, or having **tunnel vision** based on past experiences with a patient. One pair of medic students told us this story. They were assigned to a call for an injured person at a low-income housing project, which consisted of high-rise buildings. As they pulled into the courtyard area of the housing complex, the medics recognized the patient as a drug abuser. Without any additional assessment information, they immediately started to tell the student interns that this person was on the methadone program as a heroin addict and he was a **frequent flyer** (a person who often

uses EMS services for care and treatment). They had picked him up overdosed and intoxicated many, many times before. As they approached the patient, they found him sitting at the base of the building using his arms to prop up his upper body. They called him by name and asked what had happened this time. Unfortunately, when the patient answered in a groggy tone, they did not listen to his response. The student interns said that the patient told them he fell out of the fifth-story window. The crew did not even take a moment to look up. Had they bothered to look up, they would have seen an open window on the fifth story. Well after the team had accused the patient of taking his entire weekend dose of methadone, the patient's level of consciousness continued to diminish. Within a few minutes, the patient was unconscious, so the medics started an IV and administered Narcan, which is a drug that would have been antagonistic to a narcotic overdose such as methadone. The patient did not improve, and within another few minutes he went into cardiac arrest. The medics ran a medical cardiac arrest, with an objective of attempting to stabilize the patient's condition on the scene before transport. In a traumatic arrest, the focus is very different; it is on resuscitating the ABCs (airway, breathing, circulation) and on rapid transportation to the trauma center because true stabilization occurs only in the operating suite. In this case, the medics did not listen to their patient and had tunnel vision based on their prior experiences with this patient. Ultimately, they did transport the patient, and the next morning's autopsy showed that he had massive internal bleeding from a fall from the fifth story of the building. The lesson they all learned the hard way that day was: Always, no matter what prior experiences have arisen with a specific patient, avoid focusing on preconceived notions of what is believed the patient may have and *listen* to the patient.

Nonverbal Cues

Facial expressions, gestures, and posture provide nonverbal cues in both directions of communication. Making eye contact with the patient helps the patient feel the EMS provider is paying attention and is an important way to create rapport and trust. It is important to observe patient gestures, such as clutching the neck or chest, because gestures may indicate the level of distress. The clenched fist of an angry patient shows aggression and may be a warning of a physical attack. How the patient reacts to bystanders and significant others may also provide clues about the patient's mental and behavioral status. Pay close attention to the signals of a potential abuse situation by observing the reaction a child has to a parent or caregiver or an elderly patient has to the family or caregivers. EMS providers need to be aware of their own body language as well as the

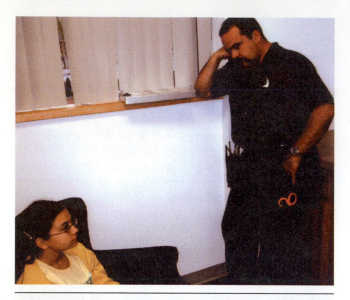

FIGURE 2-2 Be careful not to send the wrong message with your body language and facial expressions.

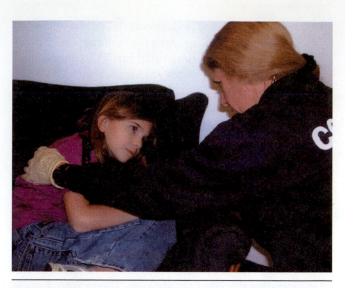

FIGURE 2-3 To improve communications and to be prepared to listen, get down to the patient's level and look her in the eye as she speaks.

patient's body language because, the experts tell us, 65% of communication is transmitted by nonverbal signals. Are you sending a message that you feel superior, bored, tired, or uninterested or that you are judging the patient (Figure 2-2)?

Distance

In some instances, it may be helpful for the EMS provider to position herself at the patient's level as in Figure 2-3. Each individual has a comfort zone for personal space as shown in Table 2-1. The EMS provider frequently occupies this space, which is otherwise reserved for people who are in a close relationship with the patient. Typically, occupying a person's comfort zone is considered an intrusion and can make the person uneasy. The EMS provider should be aware of the effects of distance and should try to minimize invading the personal space of the patient. In addition, the EMS provider should be aware that different cultures have

TABLE 2-1
Personal and Interpersonal Space

Type of Space	Distance	EMS Implications
Intimate	18 inches	Explaining intent Assessing vital signs Performing physical examination Performing invasive procedures
Personal	18 inches to 4 feet	Patient interview and history taking
Social	4 to 12 feet	Interviewing relatives, caretakers, or bystanders Safety considerations
Public	More than 12 feet	Safety considerations

Based on data from Luckmann, J. (2000). *Transcultural communication in health care*. Clifton Park, NY: Delmar Learning.

TABLE 2-2
Cultural Attitudes toward Social Distance

Group	Social Distance
African American	Closeness acceptable
Asian American	Closeness avoided
European American	Close contact often avoided
Hispanic American	Closeness acceptable
Native American	Closeness should be avoided

Based on data from Luckmann, J. (2000). *Transcultural communication in health care.* Clifton Park, NY: Delmar Learning.

different attitudes toward social distances (as illustrated in Table 2-2) and direct eye contact.

MAKING THE PATIENT COMFORTABLE

EMS providers typically find patients in an unusual circumstance and position of discomfort, embarrassment, and distress. One way to facilitate effective communication is to make the patient comfortable by providing emotional, psychological, and physical comfort whenever possible. Making a patient comfortable is often as simple as propping the patient up with a pillow and respectfully addressing the patient using a surname; other situations call for a variety of skills and techniques.

Approach

The EMS provider needs to appreciate the significance of her own body language in an effort to keep from overwhelming a patient. Many times, the patient is not the person who called EMS. The patient may be surprised, scared, or overwhelmed to see the EMS provider. This reaction may be compounded when multiple responders arrive.

During the interview, the body language of the EMS provider is important. Towering over the patient while holding a clipboard and making faces at a partner

as the patient tells his story sends a very different message than sitting on the couch next to the patient while leaning forward and looking into the patient's eyes to show interest and concern.

Introductions

Just as a nurse, physician, banker, or any other professional would do, the EMS provider should make a proper introduction right away. Making a proper introduction to the patient and the family or caretaker is professional and respectful and helps establish trust. The EMS provider needs to introduce herself and identify her level of training; for example, "Hello, my name is Kirsten, and I will be the paramedic taking care of you today." Many EMS providers dress in uniforms that resemble those of other professions (e.g., police, firefighters), so establishing your identity may quickly help to put the patient at ease.

Addressing the Patient

Always use the adult patient's name and the level of formality accepted by the patient. For example, if an EMS provider calls the patient Mr. Jones and the patient says "You can call me Bill," then that level of informality is acceptable because it was established by the patient. It would be inappropriate, however, to start off by calling Mr. Jones by his first name. Never make up names or call people pet names such as Chief, Buddy, Dude, Dolly, Missy, Dear, or Babe. Such terms are disrespectful. Learn the patient's name and use it! Do not refer to the patient by a medical diagnosis (e.g., by telling the emergency department staff this is the rule out MI or here is the fractured left arm).

Establishing Trust

In addition to demonstrating professionalism and respect for a patient and his family, maintaining privacy and showing empathy help establish trust. One of the most important aspects of an interview is to maintain privacy for the patient. The patient who is not providing feedback appropriately may be embarrassed or may not want other people to know certain information. Avoid asking

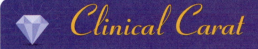

Clinical Carat

- Learning and using the patient's name demonstrates respect for the patient.

personal questions in front of coworkers, or even certain family members.

Showing empathy is a therapeutic communication technique. Learn the difference between empathy and sympathy. **Empathy** involves sensitivity to and an understanding of another person's feelings. **Sympathy** is an expression of sorrow for another's loss, grief, or misfortune; it implies similar or shared feelings and emotions. There is a difference between the two terms. Sympathy is a less effective communication technique and involves actually assuming the patient's pain. Empathy acknowledges the patient's circumstances and their seriousness without the provider's becoming emotionally involved. True empathy is best described in the words of an ancient Native American leader who said you can never have empathy until you have walked a mile in someone else's moccasins. Having empathy in emergency medicine means understanding the feelings, situations, and motives of your patients. It is well to ask, "How would I feel if this were happening to me?" Empathy should be demonstrated to patients, their families, and other health care professionals. Examples of behavior demonstrating empathy include:

- Being supportive and reassuring
- Exhibiting a calm, compassionate, and helpful demeanor
- Being respectful of the patient's and the family's feelings

Another important aspect of establishing trust is to believe your patient. A few patients may have memorized the list of signs and symptoms for a complaint from some first aid book, but most patients call because they are in distress and believe they need emergency assistance, not because of a whim or a desire for attention or excitement. If the patient says he is having chest pain, believe him. If he says it is the worst he has ever had, believe him. The EMS provider may have encountered four other patients who seemed much worse off during today's shift; yet, this is the worst pain this patient has ever experienced, and it needs to be acknowledged appropriately. Do not play down a patient's pain or emotions or send the message that this event is not serious.

Environment

Sensitivity to patients' needs includes consideration not only of medical circumstances but also of physical and emotional effects of the environment. If it is cold at the scene, is the patient cold? Does the patient have the sun in his eyes? Is the patient in a location that may be dangerous, such as a smoke-filled room or a high-noise area? Be aware of the patient's modesty concerns or embarrassment with onlookers at the scene. No patient likes having other people gawk while being undressed to be assessed in a public place.

Confidentiality

Patients have a right to have their medical conditions held in confidence, and breaching that right may cause harm or embarrassment to the patient and the family. Maintaining the patient–EMS provider relationship requires confidentiality regarding patient history, assessment findings, and the treatment rendered. EMS providers are invited into private parts of patients' lives; whatever is observed should be kept in confidence. An exception to this rule is the reporting of observations if required by law, such as a mandated report of suspected child abuse. Any discussion of patient information for quality improvement or for educational purposes that is related to a patient care report should not include the patient's name or specific identifying information.

COMMUNICATION TECHNIQUES

The way the EMS provider responds to a patient's feedback should encourage expression. **Facilitation** is the method in which EMS providers speak and use posture and actions to encourage the patient to say more. Facilitation can be positive or negative. Positive examples include sitting close to the patient and making eye contact and nodding or stating, "I'm listening" or "Please tell me more," or "Continue." Negative examples include standing over a patient barking out rapid-fire questions without waiting for responses and not making eye contact while interviewing. Additional techniques EMS providers may use to encourage feedback from a patient are using open-ended and closed questions, reflecting, clarifying, remaining silent, and explaining.

Open-Ended Questions

An **open-ended question** is one that requires more than a simple yes or no answer and that does not lead the patient to any particular conclusion. Examples of open-ended questions include: "Why did you call EMS today?" "How is the pain different today?" Open-ended questions encourage patients to talk freely and are useful in obtaining descriptive information in a narrative form. They are especially appropriate when the patient's condition is not particularly urgent and there is time to spend with the patient.

Closed Questions

If the time the EMS provider can spend with a patient is limited and the distress the patient is experiencing is severe, the need to get to the point quickly becomes significant. **Closed, or direct, questions** are asked when specific information or facts are required. When a patient is in severe distress, the EMS provider should ask questions that require a one- or two-word response, such as: "Are you having difficulty breathing?" or "When did the pain begin?" It is important not to lead the patient to an answer or to put words in the patient's mouth by the way the question is phrased. For example, instead of asking "Do you have crushing chest paint?" try asking, "Would you describe your pain as sharp, dull, or something different?"

Reflection

Reflection is the repetition or paraphrasing of the patient's words to encourage the flow of conversation without interrupting the patient's concentration. An example of reflection is to state, "You say the chest pain woke you up this morning at 6 A.M." Reflection demonstrates to the patient that the EMS provider is listening.

Clarification

Clarification is used when the patient's responses are confusing or ambiguous. For example, ask the patient to clarify by, "Using your finger, please point to where the pain is." Ask questions to clarify what the patient is saying, but be careful not to dominate the conversation or interrupt the patient. Taking a few notes and summarizing what the patient has said help clarify the patient's response. Ask the patient to confirm the accuracy of the summary.

Silence

Some new EMS providers feel uncomfortable with silence when interviewing their patients. Do not be afraid of or uncomfortable with a little silence. It gives the patient a chance to collect his thoughts, to focus, or, in some instances, to pray. After completing the medical assessment questions, consider asking the patient about one of the following topics: his children or grandchildren, his home or community, his interests or what he does for a living, what he did before he retired. The EMS provider can learn a lot of interesting things, promote trust and rapport, and even help take the patient's mind off the pain.

Explanation

Explanation is necessary to help put a patient at ease and can make the interview, assessment, and entire call go better. Explaining procedures or the steps of a procedure to a patient beforehand lets the patient anticipate and feel informed; for example, "I am going to lift your shirt to listen to your breathing now."

 Clinical Carat

- In some situations, time constraints discourage lengthy verbal exchanges, but they should not prevent proper communication. Many patients react to rapid yes or no questions by simply blurting out an answer to get the process done quickly. Use closed questions when necessary, but not at the risk of preventing the patient from giving you an accurate history.

 Exploring the Web

- Search the Web for additional information on therapeutic communication techniques for use in the prehospital environment. Are there techniques not discussed in the text that you think would be helpful? Check out the links at the Patient Communication and Interview Techniques Directory prepared by Charly D. Miller, paramedic (http://www.angelfire.com/co/CharlyDMiller/ PtCommMain.html). Miller has published many articles on the subject of communicating with patients and has prepared many training and presentation materials.

BARRIERS TO COMMUNICATION

EMS providers should be aware of and avoid the obstructions to communication. Two factors tend to impede verbal communications: semantics and technical terminology. **Semantics** is the study of the meanings in language, whereas **technical terminology** is related more to the jargon of a profession. Select words and phrases with the audience in mind. In conversations with other health care professionals, technical terms can be used, but when talking to a patient or a child, minimize the use of technical terms. Some examples to consider when selecting words are:

- Ask the patient whether he has had problems with his heart or lungs rather than "Is this your first heart attack?"
- Say "I would like to touch your wrist to feel your pulse" instead of "I would like to take your pulse." A child might wonder where you are going to take it and if you are going to give it back.
- When inserting an IV, say "It will hurt for just a second" rather than "It's just a little prick."
- Do not refer to a patient's pulse rate as irregular in front of him.
- Do not use terms such as *bottomed out* or *crashing* in front of the patient.
- Do not refer to pacing as "shocking the patient" in front of him.
- Do not say "Did your water break?" Say, "Has there been a fluid discharge from your vagina?"

SPECIAL CHALLENGES IN COMMUNICATING WITH A PATIENT

There are numerous challenges that may be encountered during the interview process. Some EMS providers will be more comfortable with certain special challenges than others. Therefore, let the person who is most experienced or most comfortable do the interview for that particular patient. This allows other crew members to observe and learn. The following are examples of special challenges the EMS provider may encounter and some tips to manage each.

Hearing Impairment

Hearing impairment is common, and many people with borderline hearing impairment are unaware that they

Clinical Carat

- An easy makeshift hearing amplifier is a stethoscope. Place the earpieces in the patient's ears and speak in a normal tone into the bell of the stethoscope. Be certain the patient can understand what the intent is before using this technique.

have a problem. A hearing deficit is not always made apparent by the use of a hearing aid. Often, patients remove the hearing aid and store it out of sight. Many hearing aids are small and difficult to see. There are, however, other clues to hearing impairment. Patients with a long-term hearing deficit may have poor diction and speech that is difficult to understand. Another clue to hearing impairment is a patient's inability to respond to verbal communication until the EMS provider makes eye contact.

Check to see whether the patient owns a hearing aid; ask the patient to use it; and bring it to the hospital. Speak in a normal tone while facing the patient or write out messages. Avoid shouting because a great percentage of hearing deficit is related to the inability to hear high-pitched sounds, which are exaggerated by shouting and speaking loudly. Use low-pitched sound directly into the ear canal. There are several commercially available ear amplifiers for the hearing impaired.

Many deaf people are able to read lips. Make eye contact with the patient and ask, "Can you read lips?" If the patient can, continue to make eye contact and speak slowly, but do not exaggerate lip movements; lip readers are trained to read normal lip movement. If the patient can sign, use **American Sign Language (ASL)** only if trained. Attempts to communicate with only a few signs may result in improper information being received or given to the patient. Attempt to provide a translator as soon as possible. Notify the receiving facility as early as possible if an ASL interpreter is needed. Federal regulations specific to the **Americans with Disabilities Act (ADA)** require that an interpreter be present within 30 minutes of the patient's arrival at the hospital.

Writing messages to the patient and allowing him to answer verbally is effective. There are several types of picture books available that illustrate basic needs or procedures. These books also work well with non-English-speaking patients.

Visual Impairment

Visual impairments are not always obvious. When a patient fails to make eye contact when speaking, ask the patient whether he is able to see clearly. Patients who are completely blind often fail to make eye contact when speaking; other patients have obvious abnormalities of the eyes. Announce to the patient who you are and why you are there, and explain as much as possible. If the patient uses glasses, encourage the patient to wear them. Ask permission before touching the patient, and describe any procedures performed such as taking a blood pressure or placing an oxygen mask. If the patient is ambulatory, the EMS provider may lead by directing the patient to take her arm while walking. People who are chronically visually impaired expect to be led. Do not hesitate to ask a patient the best way to help him navigate. When the patient has a guide dog (Seeing Eye dog), allow the animal to remain at the patient's side during the entire encounter, including transportation to the hospital. Dog guides are working dogs; the EMS provider should not allow bystanders to play with the animal or to distract it in any way unless the patient initiates the interaction.

Speech Impairment

When the EMS provider detects speech impairment, it is necessary to determine whether this is a new or a pre-existing condition. Allow the patient time to respond to questions, and provide any aids (e.g., a writing tablet) necessary. Remember that the patient is aware of the problem and is likely to be frustrated by the inability to communicate.

Foreign Language

For a non-English-speaking patient, obtain a reliable interpreter as soon as possible. Sometimes phrase books (e.g., Medical Spanish) may be helpful, but do not expect to become an instant interpreter with these. Use these as guides and notify the receiving facility of the need for an interpreter as soon as possible, especially if the patient's native language is not spoken commonly in the receiving area. Consider using the AT&T Language Line if no interpreter is immediately available and the need is urgent. Always obtain permission to treat when possible. A calm and professional manner goes far to overcome many cultural differences.

Developmental Disability

Developmentally disabled refers to an individual with impaired or insufficient development of the brain, resulting in an inability to learn at the usual rate. Many individuals with developmental disabilities may not be legally capable of making informed decisions, so follow local protocols. It is important for the EMS provider to act in a gentle and calm manner and to explain everything beforehand. Attempt to get the history from the patient first, but also use information from bystanders, relatives, and other caregivers. In general, no other special accommodations are necessary.

Terminal Illness

A patient's physical appearance is often a poor guide to the presence of a terminal condition. The information an EMS provider receives about a terminal illness is often obtained from the patient, a relative, or a caregiver. If a patient tells the EMS provider, "I have end-stage cancer," that information should not alter the care of that patient. The most important consideration is a clear understanding of the patient's end-of-life decisions. Always offer the patient compassion, keeping in mind that EMS medical priorities may differ radically from the patient's end-of-life priorities. Whenever possible, follow the patient's wishes, following local protocols and consulting with medical control when necessary.

Pain control is a major issue for patients with a terminal illness such as cancer. The EMS provider can attempt to make the patient as comfortable as possible while following local protocols. Death with dignity should be a goal of all health care providers for their patients.

Clinical Carat

- Take an inventory of the languages, including ASL, spoken by the personnel with whom you routinely work (e.g., crew members, police, firefighters) to use as a resource when needed.

Hostility

A patient's anger and hostility are often misdirected at the caregiver. Do not get angry in return because doing so can easily escalate the event. The EMS provider should watch the patient's body language and should not turn her back on the patient. It is also important for EMS providers to maintain an escape route and not allow access to the escape to be blocked. Do not hesitate to back away and get backup from the police before it is actually needed. Remember that nearly anything can be used as a weapon, so be very careful with hostile patients. Technically, EMS providers are not allowed to search a patient. However, EMS providers often do a patdown during the patient assessment and act with caution, assuming that a weapon could always be present.

Anxiety

The EMS provider should be sensitive and alert to nonverbal clues of anxiety in any patient. Reassurance, an explanation, or a distraction often helps reduce a patient's anxiety. Keep in mind that an emergency situation for the patient is disconcerting and may induce patients to act in an unpredictable manner.

Abuse

Abuse comes in many forms, and often the patient will decide whom he wants to talk to, if he talks at all. For example, a rape victim may not be comfortable with an EMS provider of the same gender as the attacker. An abused patient may benefit from the attention of the more experienced member of the EMS team, but allow the patient a choice if requested. Provide supportive psychological care, and always ask permission before touching the patient.

Multiple Symptoms

The patient with multiple symptoms can be a real challenge for the new EMS provider. Sorting through the multiple symptoms to discover and prioritize the complaints takes practice. Consider using the most experienced EMS provider to perform the interview, allowing other crew members to observe and learn.

Lack of Symptoms

The patient with no complaints can also be a challenge, especially when it has been confirmed that the patient has just experienced a significant medical or traumatic event such as a seizure, fainting, or a significant MOI (mechanism of injury). Use the most experienced crew member (the best detective) to ask any questions the initial interviewer may have omitted.

Overtalkativeness

The excessive talker can be a challenge when there is limited time for interview and care. It is easy to become impatient or frustrated with this type of patient. The general approach with this patient is to employ patience, use direct questions requiring yes or no answers, summarize frequently, and do not expect to obtain a great deal of relevant information.

COMMUNICATING WITH CHILDREN

The sick or injured child presents many challenges for the EMS provider. Young children may not understand what is happening to them and may not be able to tell adults what they are feeling. Children may also be fearful of a stranger in a uniform. Parents of sick or injured children may be difficult to communicate with because of their fears for their child. They may overreact to a situation or become very protective of the child. There are specific techniques the EMS provider can use to communicate with distraught children or their parents.

The Child

The EMS provider's approach to the child is to establish trust with the child and the family. Communication with a child varies and needs to be age appropriate. Gearing the approach to the age of the patient is key to obtaining an accurate patient assessment and providing the appropriate medical care. The EMS provider should consider that the chronological age of some pediatric patients will not match the emotional age and should modify techniques accordingly. See Chapter 17 for a description of the approach to each pediatric age group.

The Parent or Caregiver

The parent or caregiver is often considered a patient who may require emotional support. The EMS provider must be calm and must reassure the parents that everything possible is being done to help their child. Keeping the patient and parents calm is vital to both an accurate assessment and preventing the child from agitating the condition, especially with young children. Encourage the parents to perform as many tasks as possible in the care of the child.

COMMUNICATING WITH THE ELDERLY

The number of people age 85 and older is steadily increasing. As a general rule, body systems become less effective with advancing age. The aging rate varies widely among people, as does the development of impairments in cognitive and physical functions that may hinder communication. Many of the special challenges that affect communication, such as hearing and vision impairment, are associated with the aging process. Communicating with the elderly, in general, however, is the same as communicating with other patients. Make the patient comfortable; demonstrate respect, patience, and compassion; and acknowledge the patient's concerns in an effort to establish trust and open communication. The EMS provider should speak directly to the patient, first giving the patient the opportunity to discuss the current illness or injury and medical history. When the patient is recognized as being a poor historian, unreliable with information, or simply not capable of effectively communicating, the EMS provider should attempt to validate patient information with a relative or caregiver.

CULTURAL CONSIDERATIONS AFFECTING COMMUNICATION

The EMS provider can recognize the non-English-speaking patient as someone who is culturally different. Clothing, physical characteristics, or immediate surroundings can also make the EMS provider aware of **cultural diversity**. However, certain differences, such as religious belief systems, may emerge only during treatment. A patient's culturally based preferences may conflict with the learned medical practice of the EMS provider. Language barriers often compound cultural differences. Always obtain permission to treat when possible. A calm and professional manner goes far to overcome many cultural differences. Do not assume that because a person is culturally different his needs, wants, aspirations, or desires are different. Be aware of cultural differences but not to the point of limiting thinking about the other person. Consider verbal and nonverbal factors when communicating with a patient with cultural differences.

Verbal Factors

Messages in either English or another language convey meaning through tone, volume, speed, and inflection; these are called **paraverbal cues**. Shouting or hissing paraverbal cues convey anger, whereas singing or laughing cues convey happiness even with any language barrier.

Nonverbal Factors

Universally, eye movement, including pupils, lids, and eyebrows, provides clues to a person's feelings, including shock, sadness, fear, anger, pleasure, flirtation, excite-

ment, and displeasure. Cultures have different attitudes about eye contact. Many Americans believe that eye contact is positive, whereas looking away is discourteous, devious, or inattentive. Some Asians and Native Americans consider prolonged eye contact as impolite and an invasion of privacy. Muslim females may avoid eye contact as a show of modesty. Appalachians believe that eye contact expresses hostility and aggressiveness. In India, social status dictates the amount of eye contact permitted.

Certain emotions, such as fear, anger, happiness, and surprise, are reflected in facial expressions that are the result of natural biological programming and do not have to be learned. These facial expressions, such as a frown and a smile, are universal and convey the same meaning in almost all cultures.

Unlike facial expressions, body movements used to communicate an idea, emotion, or attitude vary widely from culture to culture. For example, in the United States shaking the head from side to side indicates no, but the Malayan Negritos say no by looking downward.

The effects of personal space vary from person to person as well as from culture to culture. Many Americans, Canadians, and British prefer to reserve intimate space for people who are in close relationships and may react with withdrawal or anger when a person they do not know well gets too close. Africans, Arabs, African Americans, French, and Indonesians prefer to stand close when holding a conversation.

Cultures have specific beliefs about times, locations, and situations in which it is acceptable to touch others. Obtain permission to touch, and touch only when touching is known to be acceptable. Many Americans and Hispanics are comfortable with supportive touch. Vietnamese, Cambodians, and Thais disapprove of touching on the head. Southeast Asians fear bodily intrusion, while Filipinos, Chinese, and Japanese consider touching the hand or tapping the shoulder appropriate supportive touch.

Posture (the way the body or limbs are positioned) is often not given much thought, but it can convey a lot about how a person feels. Posture can convey information

Exploring the Web

- Search the Web for information on cultural diversity. What resources are available to help you better understand the cultural groups in your service area? Are there any tools available that may help you when working with patients for whom English is not their primary language?

that may not have been intended to be divulged. Examples of postures that indicate feelings include:

- Pain: tensed muscles and flexed body
- Like or interest: leaning toward another
- Dislike or offense: leaning away from another
- Standing tall: positive self-image
- Standing slumped: negative self-image
- Standing with crossed arms tight to body: non-acceptance

CONCLUSION

Listening to patients is an essential skill that the EMS provider needs to practice frequently. The most proficient provider who has poor communications skills will have difficulty obtaining a good history and gaining patient confidence and trust. Remember that no patient wants to be judged. The patient wants quality emergency care and kindness. An understanding of basic communication principles, sensitivity to others' needs and emotions, as well as compassion and empathy can go a long way in improving the EMS provider's ability to assess patients. Basically, remember to always treat patients as you would expect other EMS providers to treat your loved ones in their time of need.

REVIEW QUESTIONS

1. Effective communications between the EMS provider and the patient entails the provider's being:
   a. confident.
   b. empathetic.
   c. supportive.
   d. all of the above.

2. For a verbal message sent by the EMS provider to be clearly understood by the patient, there should be a:
   a. third party listening.
   b. visual cue.
   c. feedback loop.
   d. all of the above.

3. Making eye contact is _____ that creates rapport and trust.
   a. a verbal cue
   b. a subliminal cue
   c. a nonverbal cue
   d. an avoidance behavior

4. An example of a patient's nonverbal cue that could warn the EMS provider of a potential safety hazard would be:
   a. a bored facial expression.
   b. a clenched fist.
   c. a statement that he is angry.
   d. an uninterested tone of voice.

5. In general, _____ Americans prefer a social distance that is close.
   a. Native
   b. Asian
   c. European
   d. African

6. When speaking to the patient, the EMS provider should use:
   a. the patient's last name only.
   b. Sir or Madam to refer to the patient.
   c. the level of formality accepted by the patient.
   d. the patient's first name if he is under 65.

7. Examples of behaviors demonstrating empathy include all of the following except:
   a. accompanying the patient into surgery to make sure the physicians know the MOI.
   b. demonstrating respect for the patient and his family.
   c. being supportive of and reassuring to the patient.
   d. exhibiting a calm, compassionate demeanor.

8. A communications technique that involves repeating or paraphrasing the patient's words is called:
   a. explanation.
   b. reflection.
   c. clarification.
   d. silence.

9. A patient with an impairment or insufficient development of the brain is referred to as:
   a. developmentally disabled.
   b. crippled.
   c. handicapped.
   d. retarded.

10. Prolonged eye contact is impolite and considered an invasion of privacy for which group of people?
    a. African Americans
    b. Native Americans
    c. Muslims
    d. Italians

CRITICAL THINKING QUESTIONS

1. What cultural groups do you commonly encounter in your service area? What key cultural influences should you be aware of to improve communications with members of these cultural groups? What can be done to improve rapport between your EMS service and these cultural groups? What tools would be beneficial to have available on calls?

2. Reflect on a call you experienced recently in which communication was key to the successful outcome of the patient encounter and patient care. What factors presented hindrances to the communication between you and the patient? What techniques did you employ to improve communication between you and the patient? What could you improve about your communication skills in future patient encounters?

3. What concerns would you have if you encountered a patient with one of the following difficulties, and how would you respond to these difficulties?

   a. a hearing impairment

   b. blindness

   c. a developmental disability

   d. hostility

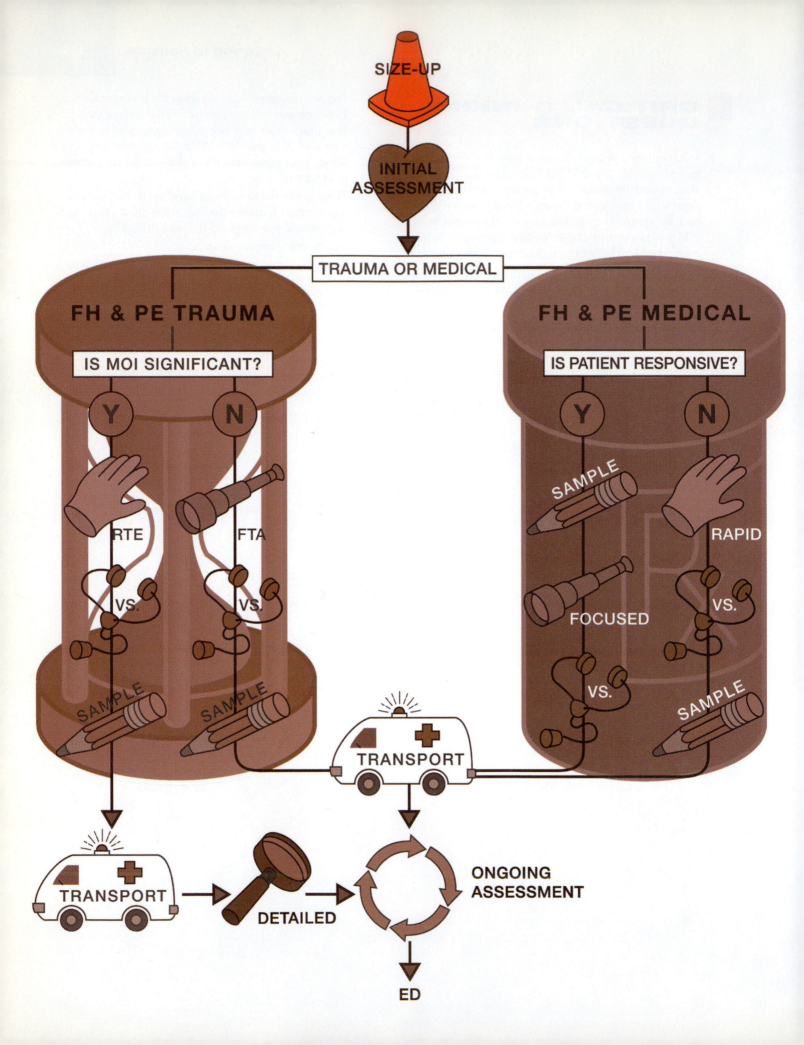

Chapter 3

3

Sizing Up the Scene

OBJECTIVES

Upon completion of this chapter, the reader should be able to:

● List the components of the scene size-up.

● List nine areas of hazards the EMS provider may encounter and provide an example of each.

● Name the two primary agencies that recommend what type of personal protective equipment is appropriate for the EMS provider.

● Describe the appropriate personal protective equipment for given mechanisms of injury and illnesses.

● Describe the laws of motion that apply to the mechanism of injury and how understanding these laws can help the EMS provider recognize predictable injury patterns.

● Describe why the nature of present illness is often more difficult to determine than the mechanism of injury during the scene size-up.

● List examples of additional resources that might be considered by the EMS provider during the scene size-up.

KEY TERMS

coup-contrecoup
first responder awareness level
first responder operations level
hazardous material (hazmat)
Incident Management System (IMS)

loaded bumper
North American Emergency Response Guidebook (NAERG)
personal protective equipment (PPE)
rubberneckers

INTRODUCTION

All of the other chapters in this book prepare the EMS provider for assessing patients. This chapter focuses on the very first assessment that must be conducted on all calls. This first assessment involves more than just the patient; it also involves an evaluation (size-up) of the scene. No matter how simple or complex the incident may be, the size-up should never be skipped. When asked, "What is the first priority?" many EMS providers will automatically say, "Patient care comes first." This is one of those medical misconceptions, or, better yet, a public relations statement, that simply is not true. The patient does not come first. Although the patient is undoubtedly a high priority, *the safety of the rescuers must always come first*! An EMS provider who is injured or killed while responding to or arriving at the scene cannot help the patient.

The concept of dealing with scene hazards before dealing with the patient is not new, but the term *size-up* did not appear in the earlier versions of EMS curricula. It is a term taken from the fire service. The components of the scene size-up include an assessment of the hazards, body substance isolation precautions, the mechanism of injury or the nature of present illness, the number of patients, and the resources that may be needed.

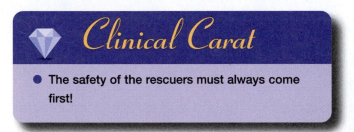

Clinical Carat

● The safety of the rescuers must always come first!

HAZARDS ON THE SCENE

Upon arrival at the scene, the EMS providers must do a quick size-up to determine whether there are any hazards that may be a threat to themselves, the patient, or bystanders. In some instances, the management of hazards may be simple and require steps such as deploying flares, positioning the emergency vehicle to protect the scene (as shown in Figure 3-1), positioning a crew member to direct traffic, or calling for police to take over the traffic flow responsibility. In other instances, such as an overturned leaking tanker truck, the management may involve contacting the fire department and the hazmat team while beginning to establish a perimeter (Figure 3-2) and keeping the crowd back from the scene.

EMS providers should assess for, size up, and know the dangers of the hazards present on the scene of each incident. The EMS provider may not always be trained at the operations level in dealing with specific hazards, but he should always be trained at the awareness level and know who to call for additional help. At the **first responder awareness level**, the responder is trained to recognize a **hazardous material** (**hazmat**; any substance that can cause injury or death) incident, back off, and call for help. Many EMS providers and fire personnel are trained to the **first responder operations level**. At this level, the responder can perform risk assessment procedures; select and don appropriate **personal protective equipment (PPE)** such as disposable gloves, eye shields or goggles, masks, and gowns; carry out basic control, containment, and confinement operations; and carry out basic decontamination procedures.

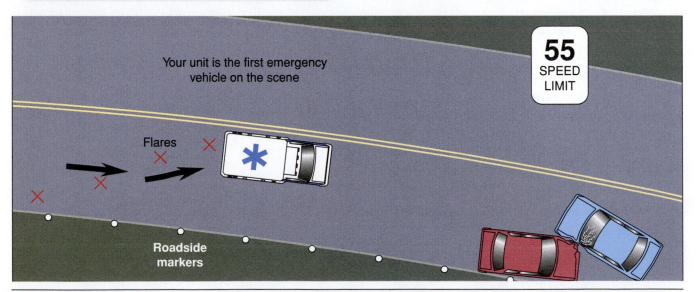

FIGURE 3-1 The EMS vehicle should be at least at least 100 feet away from the collision, and flares should be properly placed on a controlled-access highway if EMS arrives before the police come to control the traffic.

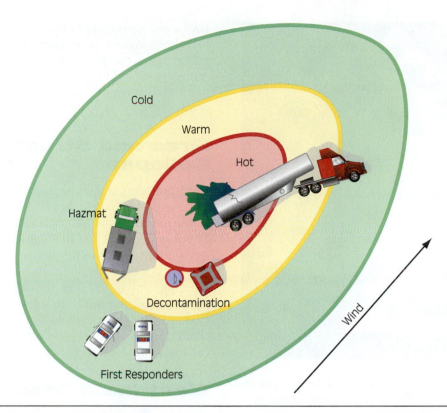

Cold

Warm

Hot

Hazmat

Decontamination

First Responders

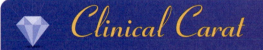

Wind

FIGURE 3-2 A perimeter; placement of the response vehicles on the upwind, uphill side of the scene; and hot, warm, and cold zones need to be established as soon as possible to minimize the hazards to the responders and the public.

Typically, hazards at the scene fall into the following categories:

- Traffic
- Vehicular damage
- Violence
- Fires and structural collapse
- Electrical hazards
- Weather-related hazards
- Hazardous materials
- Animals
- Crime scenes

Traffic

Traffic hazards include the dangers of responding to the scene, traffic still operating at the scene, poor weather conditions (e.g., snow, fog), poor visibility of the rescuers and their vehicles, intoxicated or drugged drivers, "**rubberneckers**" (curious onlookers who pose a hazard), and other emergency vehicles responding to or working at the scene. The number one potential hazard to the EMS provider is traffic, and it is essential to wear highly visible outer clothing or a safety vest with retroreflective

Clinical Carat

- The number one potential hazard to the EMS provider is traffic.

tape. It is just as important to stay keenly aware of the ongoing hazard of traffic. Rescuers have been killed by intoxicated drivers who drove into them at the collision site. Always stay alert to the traffic around you!

Vehicular Damage

Vehicular damage can include a **loaded bumper** (a shock-absorbing bumper that has been compressed and can release suddenly without warning), hot undercarriage parts (e.g., catalytic converter), truck tires that can explode, unstable vehicles, undeployed airbags, glass, fire hazards, leaking fluids, batteries, and sharp metal. EMS providers should always dress properly for the incident. PPE for a collision should include goggles or an eye shield, a helmet, a heavy coat or turnout gear, and light leather gloves (Figure 3-3).

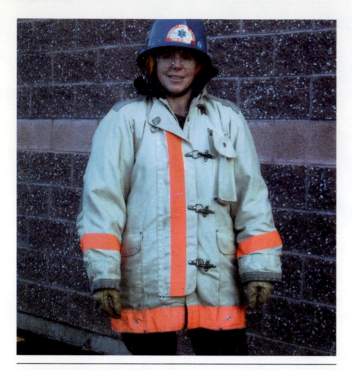

FIGURE 3-3 The EMS provider who works in the hot zone at a vehicular rescue should be dressed in this manner.

Violence

Violence encountered at the scene includes domestic violence (which is one of the biggest threats to emergency service personnel); the activity of gangs, angry crowds, and snipers; drive-by shootings; bombings; and acts of terrorism (Figure 3-4). In the wake of the attack on the United States on September 11, 2001, rescuers have a new sensitivity to threats to their lives. Terrorists have been known to set secondary bombs designed to kill or injure the responding rescue workers. All EMS providers should learn about weapons of mass destruction and their communities' preparations for response to terrorist acts.

Fires and Structural Collapse

EMS providers should be aware of the dangers of fires and should be trained to call for the fire department, usher the public to safety, and take the proper steps to put out a small fire that can be handled with a fire extinguisher after the fire department has been called. EMS providers should also be aware of the dangers of buildings collapsing and should stay out of areas of potential collapse until the scene is made safe to enter. Collapse is not limited to buildings; trenches, mine shafts, tunnels, bridges, and other structures could also collapse during a rescue.

Electrical Hazards

Occasionally, EMS providers are dispatched to an incident involving a patient who has been injured by electricity. In these cases, it is essential to ensure that the power has been turned off and will not come back on while the patient is being removed from the scene. Some electrical hazards are more subtle and may involve downed wires (Figure 3-5) at the scene of a collision. Be especially careful for vehicles that may be in contact with ground-level transformers found in newer residential communities.

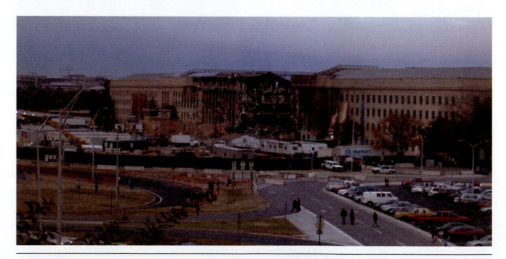

FIGURE 3-4 Americans eyes opened to the threat to homeland security on September 11, 2001, when a Boeing 757 taken over by terrorists crashed into the west side of the Pentagon, setting off a fire and killing 189 people.

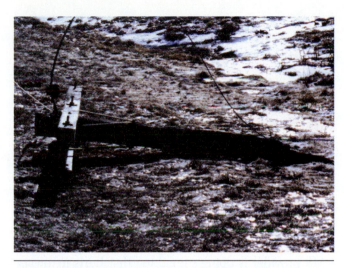

FIGURE 3-5 Downed power lines can pose a serious threat to EMS providers.

Weather-Related Hazards

Although extremes of weather, such as tornadoes and hurricanes, can cause devastation, the EMS provider needs to be prepared to handle more ordinary environmental hazards. Heavy weather conditions (e.g., heat wave, flood, drought) can contribute to the death and injury toll. They can also make it difficult to reach patients; for example, a snowstorm in Buffalo, New York, dumped 7 feet of snow in 2 days. EMS providers should be trained to cope with the weather hazards that typically occur in their community and should know who to call for additional rescue expertise (e.g., ice, swift-water, confined-space, rough-terrain, and high- or low-angle rescue).

Hazardous Materials

All EMS providers should be trained to be aware of the indicators that there may be a hazardous material involved in the incident. In some communities, depending on the levels of responsibility, emergency personnel are trained to the operations or technician's level of hazmat training. EMS providers should be familiar with the most current edition of the **North American Emergency Response Guidebook (NAERG)** (Figure 3-6) as well as with the clues for identifying hazardous substances (e.g., placards, types of containers, types of locations, and labels). It is wise to carry a pair of binoculars so the placards can be read from a safe distance (Figure 3-7). Although trauma incidents often involve multiple patients (e.g., multiple-car collision, collapsed bleacher, explosion, fires), it is unusual to have multiple patients with medical complaints at the same incident (e.g., headache, dizziness, chest pain, respiratory distress, watery eyes, coughing).

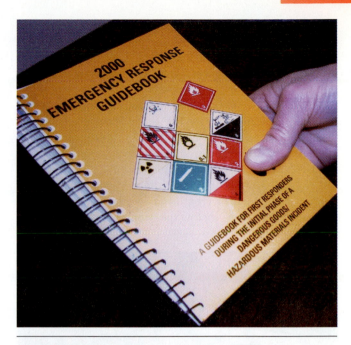

FIGURE 3-6 The most current *North American Emergency Response Guidebook* should be carried in every response vehicle, and all rescuers should be well practiced in its use.

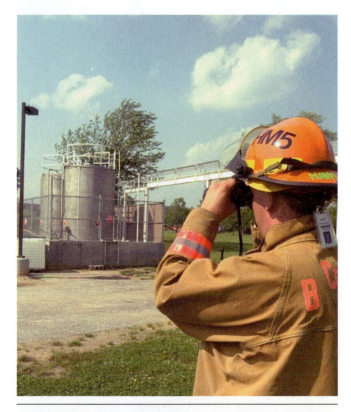

FIGURE 3-7 All EMS vehicles should have a set of binoculars that can aid in identifying placards from a safe distance.

Be especially wary of the multiple-patient medical complaint call, which often is caused by subtle hazardous material exposure such as exposure to carbon monoxide or other gases. An EMS provider who suspects that the patients have been exposed to something in the air should not go inside without the proper respiratory protection. Notify the fire department, whose members can don self-contained breathing apparatus (Figure 3-8) and remove the patients to a safer location for EMS to treat them. Hazardous environments with low oxygen content are often found in confined spaces, storage tanks, water treatment facilities, and rescues that are below grade (below the ground). EMS providers should also know who to call and what initial steps to take to prevent additional rescuers and bystanders from being exposed to biological (e.g., anthrax-laced envelopes) and radiological (e.g., medical testing labs and hospital facilities) hazards.

Animals

It is important to be aware of the potential hazards of animals at the scene. It may be necessary to contact the animal control division of the police department or town government to help secure the patient's pet. Large dogs might be assumed to be a potential threat to the EMS provider (Figure 3-9), but even a small dog that may seem harmless can become aggressive when it thinks the EMS provider is doing something that hurts its owner (e.g., starting an IV, applying a splint). Make it a practice to have someone secure the pet in another room to avoid any problems. Also be aware of the hazards of reptiles, snakes, and nontraditional pets.

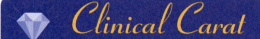

Clinical Carat

● Approach all scenes cautiously. Someone at the scene might be dangerous.

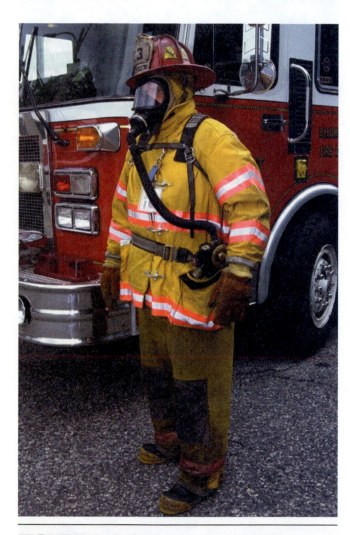

FIGURE 3-8 Self-contained breathing apparatus is needed if the EMS providers suspect that the patient is in a toxic environment. Depending on the nature of the hazardous substance, the rescue personnel may have to wear more sophisticated protection such as an encapsulated suit.

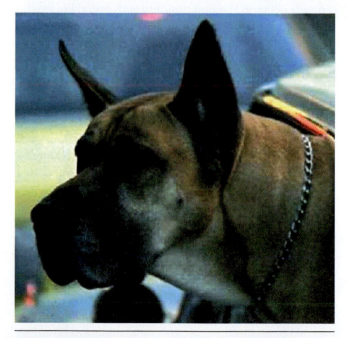

FIGURE 3-9 Be careful when treating patients who have pets present because they can be a serious threat to rescuers.

Crime Scenes

Crime scenes can present a serious hazard to the EMS provider. A perpetrator may still be hiding on the scene, or there may be weapons present. Do not look just for typical weapons such as guns or knives; be aware that many objects, such as a baseball bat, ash tray, statue, or razor blade, can be used as a weapon. Approach all crime scenes cautiously, keeping in mind that there could be someone at the scene who is dangerous. Watch for signs that violence has occurred or still is occurring, such as hearing screaming upon approach, the presence of an intoxicated patient or bystanders, or broken glass. Many EMS providers routinely respond with a police backup. When there is known violent activity at the scene, they are told to stage (remain in place) until the police have secured the scene. If an EMS provider

finds himself in the middle of a violent or unsafe scene, he should withdraw to a safe position and wait for the police to arrive. Learning the concepts of cover and concealment will help the EMS provider stay out of harm's way.

BODY SUBSTANCE ISOLATION

Body substances can be hazardous to the EMS provider's health. Communicable conditions such as hepatitis B and C, human immunodeficiency virus (HIV) infection, meningitis, pneumonia, mumps, tuberculosis (TB), chicken pox, staphylococcal skin infection, and pertussis can be spread to EMS providers who do not properly isolate themselves from body substances. Many of these conditions can be spread to the EMS provider who is exposed to blood, respiratory secretions, airborne droplets, saliva, or oral or nasal secretions.

In the early years of EMT and paramedic training, having the blood of a rescued patient all over one's hands and clothing was sometimes thought of as a badge of courage. That attitude changed radically after the AIDS crisis served to heighten awareness of infectious diseases and routes of exposure and transmission. Today, an EMS provider seen with blood on his hands might be ridiculed or disciplined and certainly would be quickly shuffled away for handwashing and the appropriate follow-up.

The Centers for Disease Control and Prevention (CDC) and the Occupational Safety and Health Administration (OSHA) recommend that the EMS provider wear disposable gloves, an eye shield or goggles (Figure 3-10), and a mask and consider the use of a gown in situations where blood might be splashed. Other body substances, such as airborne droplets, may require the use of specialized masks such as an N-95 or a high-efficiency particulate air (HEPA) respirator (Figure 3-11) to prevent the spread of tuberculosis or other airborne diseases.

OSHA regulations (CFR 1910.1030) specify requirements for EMS agencies: employee vaccination, the availability of personal protective equipment (PPE), annual training, and the existence of an exposure control plan that defines work practices and engineering controls regarding the spread of pathogens. Although the terminology has changed somewhat over the years—from universal precautions to body substance isolation (BSI) precautions and standard precautions—the concept has not. EMS providers need to protect themselves from pathogens they might come into contact with. It is important to become familiar with the laws and regulations regarding body substance isolation and precautions

Exploring the Web

The following Web sites have information and tips on dealing with specific safety issues on the scene:

- Emergency Rescue Guidelines for Air Bag Equipped Vehicles

  http://www.nhtsa.dot.gov/people/injury/ems/airbag

- Disconnect Vehicle Batteries Safely

  http://www.nhtsa.dot.gov/people/injury/ems/disconne.htm

- Approaching Alternative-Fueled Vehicle Crashes

  http://www.nhtsa.dot.gov/people/injury/enforce/pub/altfuel.pdf

- Guidelines for the Role of EMS Personnel in Domestic Violence

  http://www.acep.org/1,4613,0.html

- Highway Incident Safety for Emergency Responders

  http://www.lionvillefire.org/hwy_safety/sld001.htm

Search the Web for additional informational sources on scene safety. Bookmark these resources for future reference and share with your classmates and colleagues additional resources you find.

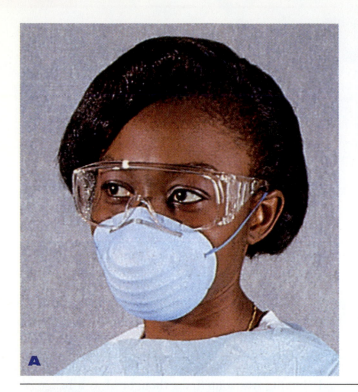

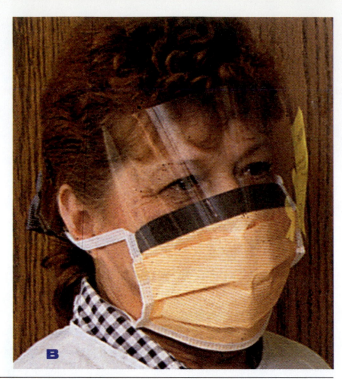

FIGURE 3-10 Goggles with a mask (**A**) or an eye shield that has a mask attached (**B**) should be worn if splattering of body fluids is possible.

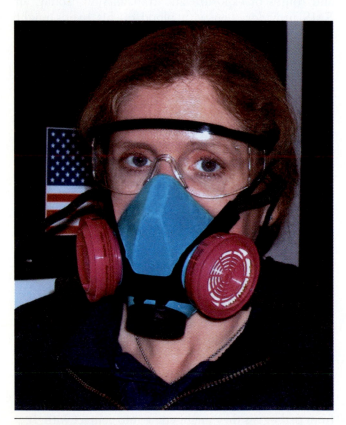

FIGURE 3-11 A fitted HEPA mask is appropriate to wear if you suspect the patient has tuberculosis.

against occupational hazards, which are summarized in Table 3-1.

The prevention of the spread of diseases boils down to responsibility. The responsibility lies with the EMS agency, the EMS provider, the patient's physician, and the patient to comply with the physician's instructions. It is the responsibility of every EMS provider to learn and follow his agency's exposure control plan and use the appropriate PPE that is provided for him. The agency is responsible for annual training, providing employee physicals and immunizations, and staying alert to advances in PPE, work practices, and engineering controls to limit exposure. It is also the agency's responsibility to provide for the appropriate, medically driven follow-up and confidential counseling should an employee suffer an exposure to a communicable disease. The patient's health care provider, such as the physician who is treating the condition, should take responsibility for educating the patient about the disease and measures that should be taken to limit the spread of the disease. Although many patients are certainly forthcoming with their medical history, not all patients will tell the EMS provider that they have a communicable disease. Many patients are embarrassed by their medical conditions or do not even know that they have a communicable disease. Consider all patients to be potential carriers of communicable diseases.

PPE should be within reach when the EMS provider is caring for a patient, and the appropriate type of

TABLE 3-1
Safety Laws and Regulations

Occupational Safety and Health Administration (OSHA)

- Code of Federal Regulations (CFR) 1910.120: establishes the training levels for first responders to hazardous materials incidents

- CFR 1910.1200: the "right to know law," which requires employers to inform their employees about the hazards of exposure to chemicals in the workplace and to train them in relevant safety procedures

- CFR 1910.1030: the regulation that applies to all circumstances in which occupational exposure to blood or other potentially infectious materials is possible; establishes the requirement for employers to have a written exposure control plan designed to eliminate or minimize employee exposure

Centers for Disease Control and Prevention (CDC)

- Ryan White Comprehensive AIDS Resources Emergency Act: the federal mandate that established procedures for emergency response employees (EREs) to determine whether they have been exposed to an infectious disease while providing patient care; establishes that every employer of EREs must designate an officer who will be responsible for gathering information about the exposure incident and communicating with the medical facility to ensure that the appropriate follow-up plan is in place for the ERE

- Guidelines for Preventing the Transmission of *Mycobacterium Tuberculosis* in Health-Care Facilities, 1994: document that provides guidance to hospital personnel that is also applicable to prehospital agencies

National Fire Protection Association (NFPA)

- 471: the standard that defines the recommended practice for responding to hazardous materials incidents

- 472: the standard that establishes professional competencies required of responders to hazardous materials incidents

- 473: the standard that establishes professional competencies required of EMS personnel responding to hazardous materials incidents

- 1500: the standard that established fire department occupational safety and health programs

- 1710: the standard for the organization and deployment of fire suppression operations, emergency medical operations, and special operations to the public by career departments

- 1720: the standard for the organization and deployment of fire suppression operations, emergency medical operations, and special operations to the public by volunteer departments

PPE should be used. When arriving on the scene and beginning the size-up, determine what type of PPE is needed to take BSI precautions. Remember, handwashing is probably the most important part in prevention of disease. Hands should be washed after every call. The following examples provide some guidance as to the appropriate PPE for certain situations:

- Trauma patient with no significant MOI and no obvious bleeding seen. Disposable gloves should be worn.

- Trauma patient with significant MOI sitting in the front seat of a car and bleeding from a head wound. Disposable gloves should be worn. Light leather gloves may also be appropriate if there is glass on the seat or patient. If the wound is still bleeding, goggles or an eye shield and mask may be appropriate. If the patient is still bleeding profusely or there is a lot of blood present, it would be appropriate to consider a gown to protect the uniform.

- Medical patient who is responsive and complaining of chest pain. Disposable gloves should be worn. If the patient has a productive cough or feels warm to the touch, use goggles or a face shield and a mask. If the patient has a history of TB, don an N-95 or a HEPA respirator mask.

- Medical patient who is in her third trimester and birth is imminent. Disposable gloves, mask, goggles or an eye shield, and a gown are all appropriate owing to the potential for blood splattering.

- Any patient with an altered level of consciousness who may vomit. Always wear disposable gloves and goggles or an eye shield and a mask to protect against exposure to oral secretions and splattering vomitus. If available, a bag-valve-mask (BVM) with a one-way valve is preferred over the use of a pocket mask should the patient need ventilatory assistance.

- A patient who has been unattended for considerable time in an extremely dirty environment and who is lying in urine or fecal material. Consider using all BSI precautions as well as a disposable Tyvek jumpsuit (Figure 3-12) as protection from fleas, lice, ticks, and other critters.

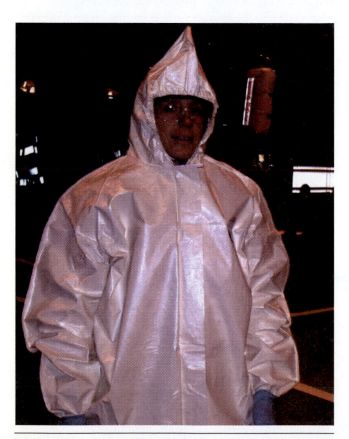

FIGURE 3-12 EMS providers may need to don a Tyvek jumpsuit to protect themselves from fleas and lice and situations in which the patient is covered with body fluids.

MECHANISM OF INJURY OR NATURE OF ILLNESS

Before touching the patient, during the scene size-up, the EMS provider should develop a sense of the mechanism of injury (MOI; the instrument or event that caused the injury) or the **nature of illness** (**NOI**; the condition or chief complaint of the patient). One reason EMS providers should not run right up to the patient upon arrival on the scene is that they might miss important clues about the MOI and scene safety. For example, it is not enough to simply say the MOI was a car crash. The following are questions to consider at the scene of a car crash:

- How many cars are involved?
- Is there a spider web crack on the windshield (Figure 3-13) that was probably caused by the patient's head striking the windshield?
- Is there damage or intrusion into the passenger compartment of the vehicle? Are the doors crushed in? Is there any entrapment?
- On the basis of the collision scene and the type of roadway, was this collision a high-, moderate-, or low-speed collision?
- What type of collision was this: frontal or head-on (Figure 3-14); rear-end, lateral, or side-impact (broadside) (Figure 3-15); or rollover (Figure 3-16)?

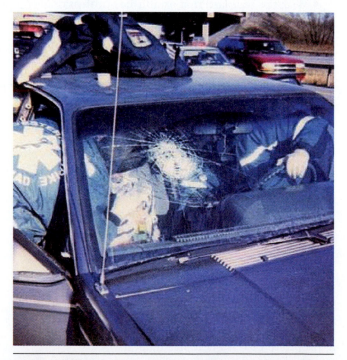

FIGURE 3-13 A spider web crack on the windshield indicates that a head struck the windshield with great force. (Courtesy of Deborah Funk, MD, Albany Medical Center, Albany, NY)

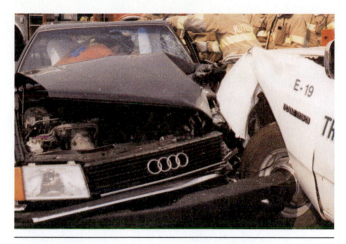

FIGURE 3-14 In a frontal collision, the speed and force of each vehicle combine to cause significant damage. (Courtesy of David J. Reimer Sr.)

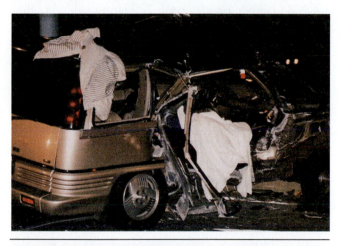

FIGURE 3-15 Side-impact collisions can be very serious if there is intrusion into the passenger compartment. (Courtesy of Craig Smith)

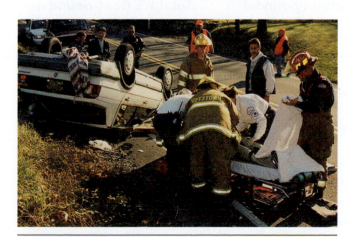

FIGURE 3-16 Rollover collisions frequently involve ejections from the vehicle. (Courtesy of David J. Reimer Sr.)

An understanding of the collision type can help predict specific injury patterns (see Table 3-2).

An understanding of certain laws of physics can help the EMS provider appreciate the impact of physical trauma on the patient's body. The physical laws that apply to MOI are as follows:

- Newton's first law of motion (inertia). An object in motion tends to stay in motion, and an object at rest tends to stay at rest, unless the object is acted upon by an outside force.

TABLE 3-2
Types of Automobile Collisions and Mechanisms of Injury

Frontal (head-on). The unrestrained driver and occupant may sustain injuries whose pattern depends on their route of travel in relationship to the dashboard:

- Up and over the dashboard: often involves head injury and lacerations, cervical spine injuries, and chest and upper abdomen injuries
- Down and under the dashboard: usually involves the knees, femurs, hips, and lower spine

Rear-end. This type of collision typically causes whiplash injuries to the cervical spine as well as the above injuries, depending on the occupants' course of travel in relationship to the dashboard.

Lateral or side-impact (broadside). The injury on the side of the impact is more serious than that on the opposite side, especially if there is more than 12 inches of vehicular intrusion. Expect to see fractures to the humerus, ribs, pelvis, and femur on the side of the impact. Other severe internal injuries may include ruptured spleen and aortic tears.

Rollover. These collisions involve considerable, and hard-to-predict, injury to the unrestrained occupant. They frequently involve ejections or partial ejections. It is estimated that the chances of a spinal injury increase up to 1,300 times and the chance of death increases 25 times when ejection from the vehicle occurs. Partial ejections involve crushing of the patient's head, arms, or legs as the vehicle rolls over her.

- Conservation of energy. The energy of interacting bodies or objects cannot be created or destroyed, only transferred or exchanged.

- Kinetic energy (KE). This is the form of energy an object has by reason of its motion. The more speed (motion) there is, the more kinetic energy there is. The formula for kinetic energy is $KE = (m/2)v^2$, where m is mass and v is velocity. Speed contributes considerably to KE because velocity is squared and only half the value of the mass is used. Because velocity is squared, it contributes considerably. Notice in Table 3-3 that an increase of 50 pounds yields an increase of 22,500 foot-pounds (kinetic energy), while an increase of 10 miles per hour yields an increase of 52,500 foot-pounds.

- Newton's second law of motion. The force acting on a body is equal to the mass of the body (m) times its acceleration (a) (or deceleration): $F = m \times a$.

If the EMS provider is responding to a call for a patient who fell, questions to consider upon approaching the scene include:

- From what height did the patient fall? It has been estimated that patients who fall from a height that is three or more times their own height will likely sustain a spinal injury, as well as other multiple injuries.

- Did anything break the fall, and what type of surface did the patient fall onto (e.g., cement, trees, a fence, into water, grass)?

- Which body part struck first? Was it the head, as in a pool diving incident, or was it the outstretched arms as in a fall down a few steps, or did the patient land on her legs? The experts tell us that patients who fall landing on their feet, suffering open fractures of the legs or ankles, have absorbed enough energy into the spine that they have also injured the spine.

EMS providers should also be aware that velocity has a significant impact on the patient suffering from gunshot wounds. Even a slow-moving penetrating object, such as a knife or an ice pick, that strikes a vital organ or vessel can be life threatening. Yet, the faster the muzzle velocity, or speed with which the bullet leaves the weapon, the greater the diameter of the temporary and permanent injury tract in the patient. If a patient has sustained a penetrating injury, consider the following questions:

- What is the caliber of the weapon (e.g., .22, .38, .44 caliber, or a 9 mm)? The larger calibers often cause more damage. However, even a .22 can be deadly at close range because once the bullet enters the skull, it bounces around like a "BB in a boxcar," tearing the brain apart rather than simply exiting the opposite side of the skull.

- What was the profile (shape) of the bullet? Was it a solid-nosed or a hollow-point bullet or a shotgun shell? What was the muzzle velocity (see Table 3-4)?

- Were there powder burns from a close-range (point blank) shooting?

- Was an exit wound found?

TABLE 3-3
The Impact of Velocity on Kinetic Energy (KE): "Speed Kills"

Velocity (miles per hour)	Mass (patient weight in pounds)	Total KE (foot-pounds)
30	150	67,500
40	150	120,000
30	200	90,000
40	200	160,000

An increase of 50 pounds at 30 miles per hour increases kinetic energy by 22,500 foot-pounds, whereas an increase of 10 miles per hour at 150 pounds yields an increase of 52,500 foot-pounds. An increase of 50 pounds at 40 miles per hour increases kinetic energy by 40,000 foot-pounds, and an increase of 10 miles per hour at 200 pounds increases it by 70,000 foot-pounds.

TABLE 3-4
Penetrating Injury and Mechanisms of Injury

For penetration from high-velocity projectiles (more than 200 feet per second), consider these factors:

- Tumble. The bullet tumbles or rolls through space (see Figure 3-17) with the potential that the side of the bullet, rather than the point, may enter the patient's skin.

- Fragmentation. The projectile bursts into many smaller pieces, and each causes its own injury path.

- Profile. Does the bullet have a solid or a soft hollow nose? The solid ones penetrate farther and often exit. The soft-nosed bullets mushroom out, causing a very large temporary space, sometimes 20 times the diameter of the bullet, and a large permanent injury tract.

- Cavitation. This is the momentary acceleration of tissue laterally away from the projectile tract, similar to the ripple effect of a rock dropped into a pond. These waves of tissue can cause damage and explain why a bullet near the spine can injure the spine. Cavitation also explains why the exit wound is usually larger than the entrance wound (Figure 3-18).

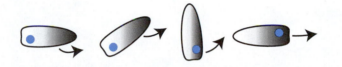

FIGURE 3-17 Tumbling bullet.

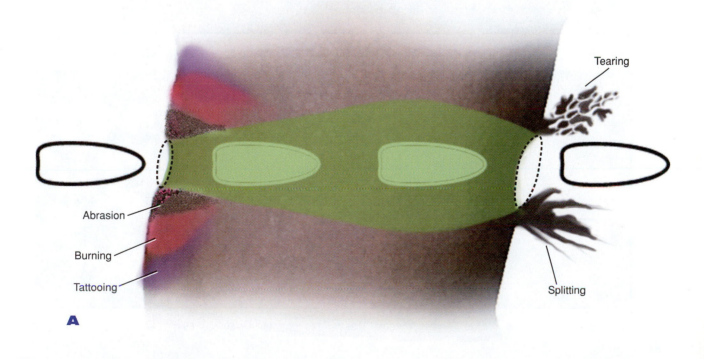

FIGURE 3-18 Cavitation. (**A**) The exit wound is often larger than the entrance wound.

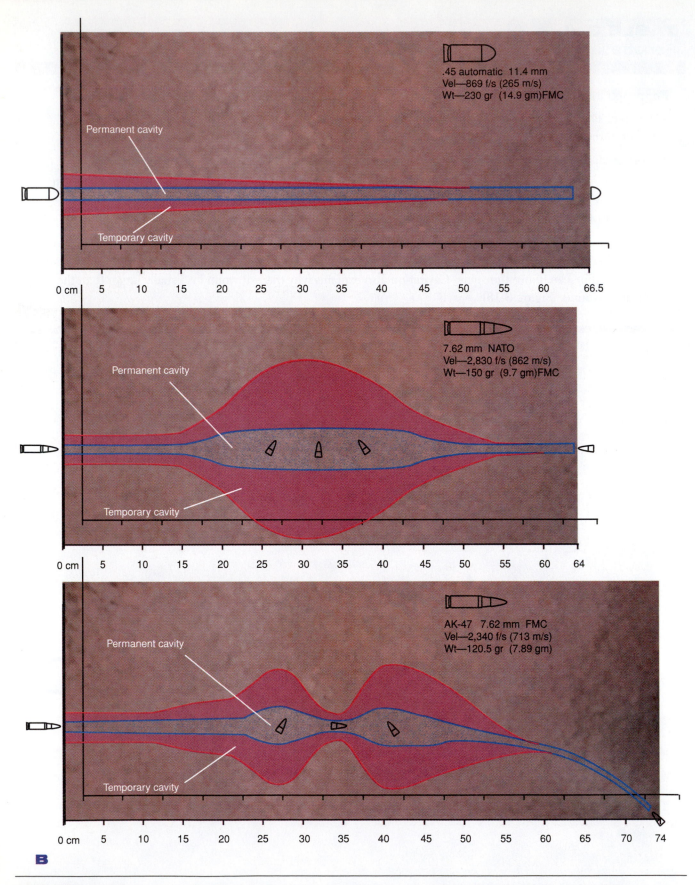

.45 automatic 11.4 mm
Vel—869 f/s (265 m/s)
Wt—230 gr (14.9 gm)FMC

Permanent cavity

Temporary cavity

0 cm   5   10   15   20   25   30   35   40   45   50   55   60   66.5

7.62 mm NATO
Vel—2,830 f/s (862 m/s)
Wt—150 gr (9.7 gm)FMC

Permanent cavity

Temporary cavity

0 cm   5   10   15   20   25   30   35   40   45   50   55   60   64

AK-47   7.62 mm FMC
Vel—2,340 f/s (713 m/s)
Wt—120.5 gr (7.89 gm)

Permanent cavity

Temporary cavity

0 cm   5   10   15   20   25   30   35   40   45   50   55   60   65   70   74

B

FIGURE 3-18 *(continued)* **(B)** A bullet can cause permanent and temporary cavitation.

Other MOIs for the EMS provider to consider in the trauma patient include rapid deceleration and its impact on the internal organs and vessels, stabbings, blunt trauma to the chest or abdomen, blast injuries in confined places, **coup-contrecoup** head injury, and electrical injuries. A coup-contrecoup head injury occurs when a patient strikes one side of the head and the blow causes blunt trauma to the brain in the area that was struck as well as to the opposite area of the brain. Striking the temple (the side of the head above the ears) area of the skull with a blunt object may cause the middle meningeal artery to bleed, and an epidural hematoma develops. Baseball players wear a batter's helmet to protect the side of the head.

Abuse injuries should also be considered. They are usually found in areas that are not often injured (e.g., upper arms, upper back) or in unusual patterns (e.g., dipping burn lines, cigarette burns, or rope burns from being restrained). Motorcycle collisions often cause road rash (serious abrasions). Bilateral femur fractures may occur when the biker stops suddenly and is propelled over the handlebars. Crushing injuries are also common from sideswiping another vehicle or laying the bike down because most large motorcycles are very heavy (e.g., a Harley 1,200 cc Heritage weighs 710 pounds).

It is also important to note that not all patients are experiencing only trauma or only a medical complaint. Some patients present with both medical and traumatic complaints. The EMS provider should ask, "Could a medical incident have caused the injury?" For example, syncope (fainting) could have resulted in the fractured hip of an elderly patient, or syncope could have caused a driver to strike the bridge abutment and crush her chest. Also consider, "Could the stress from the traumatic incident be the cause of the chest pain the patient is complaining of?"

The nature of present illness (NOI) of medical patients may be a little more difficult to determine during the scene size-up than is the MOI. Yet, upon approaching the scene, the EMS provider should watch for clues:

- Can you hear a patient wheezing, coughing, or sounding as if she is having respiratory distress?
- Is there erratic behavior, yelling, screaming, arguing, or intoxicants at the scene? These may indicate the need for police backup.
- Is the patient clutching her chest or neck or sitting in the tripod position (Figure 3-19) to ease the struggle to breathe?
- Does the house smell of vomit, urine, diarrhea, or acetone? (The smell of acetone might indicate diabetic coma.)
- Is the patient lying in a bed unconscious with a pillow behind the neck, as opposed to behind the shoulders, to assist in opening the airway?

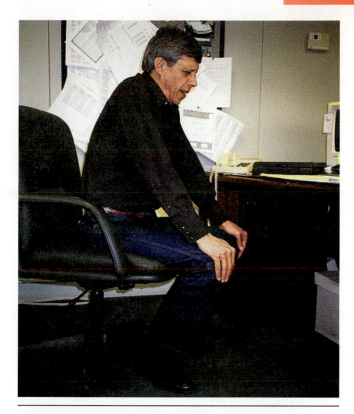

FIGURE 3-19 Patients with significant respiratory distress may be found in the tripod position.

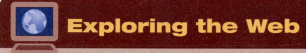

Exploring the Web

- For statistical information regarding mechanism of injury, visit the Web site of the National Trauma Data Bank (http://www.facs.org/dept/trauma/ntdb.html). View the 2001 report. What does this information tell you about traumatic events? After reviewing the report, consider what your expectations are regarding emergency care. What information does the Web site provide to help you be better prepared for your job?

- Is the third-trimester pregnant woman in the bathroom with the urge to bear down?

Be sure to consider the MOI and the NOI as a part of the scene size-up. Of course, this is just an initial impression of the MOI or NOI, and the EMS provider will reevaluate them again later in the assessment of the patient as more information is obtained from the scene, patient, and bystanders.

THE RESOURCES NEEDED AND THE NUMBER OF PATIENTS

The final and yet important component of the scene size-up is to determine additional resources that may be needed and the number of patients involved. Most of the calls will be for a single patient, and the additional resources might be an advanced life support (ALS) unit or the police. If there are hazards on the scene, often the awareness and size-up of the hazards will determine the additional resources that may be needed. Examples of additional resources include:

- Police. Police may be needed for investigation and documentation of a "breach of the peace," securing the scene, protecting the EMS providers, dealing with a crime, and controlling traffic.

- Fire department. Although many fire departments provide EMS first response, ALS, or ambulance service (or any combination thereof), the traditional role of the fire service is to control and extinguish fires and potential fire hazards. Some EMS agencies have a standard operating procedure that the fire department is to be dispatched to all vehicular collisions owing to the potential for a fire and need for a washdown.

- Rescue company. Depending on what the resources are in the community, specialty rescue units are developed to provide services such as vehicle rescue, confined-space rescue, hazardous materials response, water rescue, ice rescue, off-the-road rescue, low-angle rescue, trench rescue, and high-angle rescue. The agency that provides these services is often a component of the local community resources and may be placed in the police, fire, or EMS service.

- Helicopter. Med-Evac air transport or specialty helicopter assistance in search and rescue activities may be available. Become familiar with the types of calls the regional Med-Evac program will respond to, how to alert it to respond, and how to assist it in setting up a landing zone.

- Utilities company. If there is an electrical hazard or gas leak, it will be important to have the utilities respond to the scene.

In instances in which there are multiple patients, aid and cooperation from neighboring communities may be necessary. All EMS providers should be aware of the community's **Incident Management System** (IMS) and the resources that are available to deal with a major incident involving multiple patients. The IMS is a system of organization and administration involving all emergency service providers that focuses on three critical components of large-incident management: command, control, and communications. When the EMS provider is confronted with multiple patients, skills in establishing divisions of responsibility (sectors), making triage decisions, and utilizing the IMS will be very important. All EMS providers should review their service's plan and participate in practicing the plan in many ways as often as possible. Review and practice ensure that the plan can be revised as needed and that it will be familiar to all responders when incidents occur.

It is clear that once the EMS provider has determined the number of patients and the additional resources that are needed at the scene, the additional resources should be called for as soon as possible. Often, the additional units take time to respond, and waiting to call for them will just delay their arrival further. As the saying goes, "Don't undersell overkill!" The EMS provider can always cancel their response if they are not needed at the scene.

CONCLUSION

The scene size-up is a very important step that should not be skipped at any call. The components of the scene size-up include assessing the potential for hazards, determining the type of personal protective equipment (PPE) to be used, the mechanism of injury (MOI) or the nature of present illness (NOI), the number of patients, and the need for any additional resources. Awareness of the MOI of the trauma patient can help the EMS provider predict injury patterns to better formulate a management plan. The NOI of a medical patient is not always as obvious as the MOI, but the observant EMS provider can obtain clues during the scene size-up. Information gathered during the scene size-up may save the life of the EMS provider or that of the patient, other crew members, and bystanders.

REVIEW QUESTIONS

1. The components of the scene size-up include an assessment of each of the following except the:
   a. hazards.
   b. BSI precautions.
   c. extent of a burn injury.
   d. mechanism of injury.

2. Hazards that the EMS provider may find at the scene of an incident fall into which of the following categories?
   a. traffic
   b. animals

c. crime scenes

d. all of the above

3. The number one potential hazard to the EMS provider is:

  a. fires and structural collapse.

  b. hazardous materials.

  c. traffic.

  d. vehicular damage.

4. One of the biggest threats to the EMS provider from violence is due to:

  a. terrorist bombings.

  b. domestic disputes.

  c. drive-by shootings.

  d. angry crowds.

5. An example of a subtle electrical hazard is:

  a. a car in contact with a ground-level transformer.

  b. wires arcing at the scene of the collision.

  c. a patient who is lying across a train's third rail.

  d. a patient who was injured while installing an outlet.

6. Situations that may require additional specialty rescue teams include:

  a. swift water.

  b. confined space.

  c. high-angle situations.

  d. all of the above.

7. To assist at a potential hazardous materials incident, all emergency vehicles should carry a copy of the:

  a. *Physician's Desk Reference.*

  b. *North American Emergency Response Guidebook.*

  c. paramedic curriculum.

  d. NFPA standards.

8. If there is known violence at the scene of an incident, the EMS providers should:

  a. remain staged nearby until police secure the scene.

  b. carry a portable radio when entering the scene.

  c. be prepared to fight their way out of the incident.

  d. cancel the response because it will be unsafe.

9. If upon scene size-up the EMS provider suspects the patient could have TB, it is recommended that:

  a. the response be canceled because it will be unsafe.

  b. a HEPA mask be worn and a surgical mask placed on the patient.

  c. gloves be worn as the only precaution.

  d. no special precautions be taken because TB is not communicable.

10. If your patient is a trauma patient with a significant MOI, the recommended PPE will include:

  a. disposable gloves.

  b. goggles or eye shield.

  c. a gown if there is spurting blood.

  d. all of the above.

CRITICAL THINKING QUESTIONS

1. You are dispatched to an apartment building from which a call came in that a man was found unconscious on the sidewalk in front of the building. You arrive before the police and can see the man on the sidewalk from a block away. The apartment building is dark, and there are no other people in sight. It is eerily quiet. What are the dangers on this scene? What actions should you take?

2. You respond to a call for a man who is having respiratory difficulties. You are met at the door by the man's wife. As you follow her into the home, you can hear a fit of productive coughing. What personal protective equipment should you be wearing before beginning care of the patient? Are there any other precautions that should be taken in caring for this patient? What are the risks involved in caring for this patient?

3. It has been snowing all day, and there is an accumulation of about 5 inches of snow on the ground. You have already put in a full shift but are asked to stay for backup. There has been a multiple car pileup on Highway 9. Another EMS unit is already on scene and is requesting additional support. They are reporting six patients with injuries. You are dispatched to the scene. What hazards are present at this scene? What actions should you take?

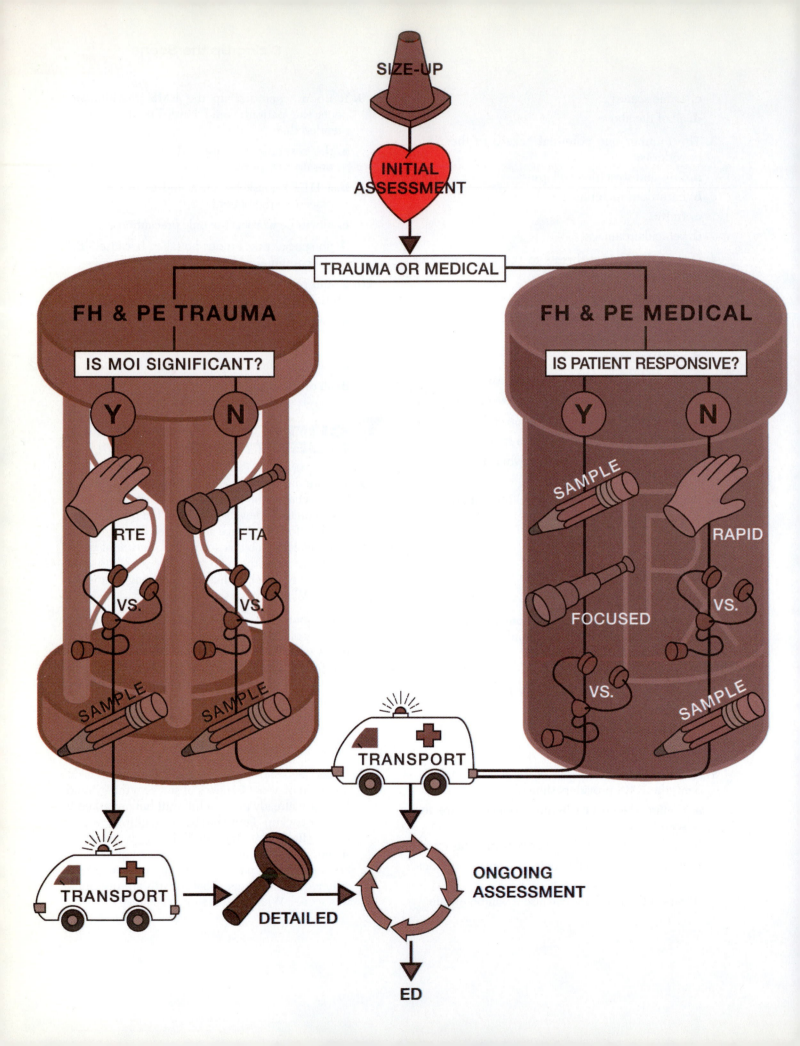

The Initial Assessment

OBJECTIVES

Upon completion of this chapter, the reader should be able to:

- Describe the importance of obtaining the chief complaint in the patient's own words and list examples of chief complaints.
- Define AVPU and discuss how it is used to assess a patient's mental status.
- List the three key questions the EMS provider needs to ask when assessing the airway of any patient.
- Describe how to assess a patient's breathing.
- List three key questions the EMS provider must keep in mind when assessing circulatory status.
- Describe how to assess a patient's skin and list several abnormal skin conditions.
- Describe the last step of the initial assessment and how it is used to make a transportation decision.

KEY TERMS

aspirate	flail segment
AVPU	general impression
chief complaint (CC)	mental status
decerebrate	perfusion
decorticate	piloerection
diagnosis	skin color, temperature, and condition (CTC)
dyspnea	tenting

INTRODUCTION

The goal of the initial assessment is to *find the life threats first*! After the appropriate body substance isolation (BSI) precautions have been taken and the scene is safe for the crew and the patient, it is time to prepare for the initial assessment (IA) of the patient. An evaluation of the mechanism of injury (MOI) or the nature of the illness (NOI) is helpful in preparing to conduct the initial assessment. The number of patients and available resources should have been factored in during the scene size-up. This discussion assumes that the scene is safe; there is only one patient to be evaluated; and there is an adequate number of trained EMS providers for the situation.

The purpose of the initial assessment is to identify any life threats and quickly attempt to manage those threats. In essence, the initial assessment is the one area of the approach to evaluating a patient in which the EMS provider actually treats the patient while conducting the assessment. All patients in the prehospital environment should receive an initial assessment; very few of the patients seen in the field (approximately 10%) actually have a life threat requiring immediate management.

FIRST IMPRESSIONS

For many years clinicians have been taught to form a general impression of the patient as they approach the patient for the first time. Forming this first impression has been referred to as the "look test," a "gut reaction," or "assessment from the doorway." The latest editions of training curricula have standardized the term to be the **general impression**. Whatever term is used, the concept is the same; the EMS provider is getting a first impression of the patient to determine the priority of care, taking into consideration the environment and the patient's chief complaint. A **chief complaint (CC)** is the reason why the EMS unit was called. Whenever possible, it is best to put the chief complaint in the patient's words. It is important for the patient to describe what he is experiencing. Using the patient's words will help others who will be involved with the patient to have a sense of how the patient responded to the experience. Patients cannot always speak for themselves, and in such cases the EMS provider's observations are recorded. Examples of chief complaints are:

- "I passed out."
- "I fell."
- "I crushed my leg."
- "I can't catch my breath."
- "I was involved in a car crash."
- "I feel dizzy."

Pediatric Pearl

- It is especially useful to form a general impression of small children from the doorway because the presence of EMS providers may change the situation. Note whether the child is crying, playing, or concentrating on his breathing too much to be concerned with anything going on

A chief complaint usually does not include a **diagnosis**, which is the identification of a specific disease or condition. The diagnosis is made after the medical team has evaluated the entire situation.

The general impression includes a quick size-up of the patient to include the mechanism of injury (MOI) or the nature of the illness (NOI) and the approximate age, sex, and degree of distress of the patient. Examples of general impressions made of patients include:

- "I have a middle-aged male patient at the bottom of a ladder who appears to be in severe distress."
- "I have a young female patient of child-bearing age clutching her abdomen at the scene of a collision."
- "I have an elderly male patient unconscious on the floor in a nursing home cafeteria."

There are key points to notice in the general impression of the MOI or NOI, such as the crack in the windshield where the patient was sitting in the crashed vehicle (Figure 4-1) or the home oxygen and inhalers in the patient's living room. Once a general impression has been made, the EMS provider continues to approach the patient and begins to assess whether there are any

Clinical Carat

- At the scene of a collision, it is helpful to approach from in front of the patient rather than from the side so the patient is less likely to move his neck. One EMS provider should instruct the patient not to move while another rescuer gets into the vehicle to manually stabilize the cervical spine.

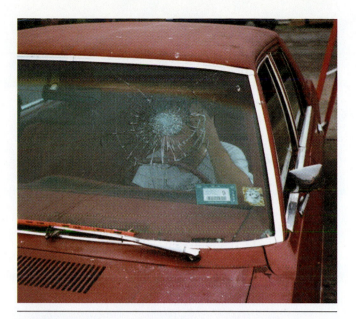

FIGURE 4-1 Recognizing a cracked windshield as the potential MOI for head and neck injury should alert the EMS provider to approach the patient from the front of the vehicle.

life threats. If a life-threatening condition is found, it is dealt with immediately. For example, if, while doing the initial assessment, the EMS provider finds that the patient's airway is not open, she will immediately proceed to manually open the airway using the head tilt-chin lift or the jaw thrust maneuver if cervical spinal trauma is suspected. If the MOI dictates the need for spinal immobilization, be cautious not to startle the patient because startling him may cause him to move his neck.

MENTAL STATUS

If a patient is conscious, the EMS provider begins to talk to the patient to determine the patient's **mental status (MS)**. The EMS provider should speak directly to the patient and introduce herself, specifying her training level and explaining that she is here to help. For example, "Hi, I'm Maria and I am a paramedic. What is your name and how can I assist you?" Ask the patient his name and use it. Writing down the patient's name helps to remember it. Many EMS providers forget to use their patient's name and arrive at the emergency department referring to their patient as a "fractured leg" or "an AMI." As the famous educator and author Dale Carnegie taught us, one of the most pleasant sounds to anyone's ears is his own name—so use it! The credibility of all the information received from the patient is often determined by whether the patient is "alert and oriented." Information obtained from a verbally responsive patient

who does not appear to be oriented is often questioned by EMS providers because of the patient's confusion, which may be a result of hypoxia, hypoglycemia, or intoxication.

If the patient is unconscious, then a "CPR quick check" should be done before the mental status evaluation. Most patients do not need the CPR quick check, but this does help to tie the initial assessment into previous CPR training. Table 4-1 reviews the steps in the CPR quick check.

To quantify a patient's mental status on a "yardstick," the EMS provider will need to use the right tool. The right tool for this mini-neurological exam should be easy to use, have increments or steps that are easily understood by all users, and allow multiple EMS providers to repeat assessments without significant variance due to the user of the tool. The tool also needs to have increments that will detect the relevant subtleties of the patient's changing condition (e.g., a developing hematoma in the brain or lack of sugar to the brain). Because terms such as *obtunded*, *comatose*, *lethargic*, *stuporous*, and *semiconscious* do not meet those criteria, they are no longer used to describe the patient's mental status in a prehospital assessment.

The tool used to measure the mental status is called **AVPU**, which is an abbreviation for *a*lert, *v*erbally responsive, *p*ainful response, and *u*nresponsive (no response).

TABLE 4-1
CPR Quick Check

- Check responsiveness
- Open the airway appropriately
- Look, listen, and feel for breaths
- Administer ventilations
- Check circulation
- Administer chest compressions

Alert

The mental status assessment begins with the EMS provider's first observation of the patient and continues with the first words of introduction to the patient. The EMS provider should note whether the patient seems aware of her presence and makes eye contact with her as she begins to speak to the patient. Consider adding two other quick questions to the introduction. Simply ask the patient whether he knows where he is and the day of the week. Although these questions might seem awkward at first, they do help the EMS provider to determine right away whether the patient is alert. An alert patient is able to tell you his name, roughly where he is, and the day of the week. Ask about the day of the week, not the date, because most people have to check their watch for the correct date!

The phrase "alert times three" has crept into the EMS provider's language. This was intended to mean the patient is alert and oriented to person, place, and day. Basically, saying a patient is alert times three and saying a patient is alert are the same, so just say "Alert." Some EMS providers have tried to describe a patient's mental status as "alert times one or two," meaning the patient knows the correct answer to only one or two of the questions. This phrase is no longer used. The correct description is to say the patient is verbally responsive and state whether the responses are appropriate. The new training curricula use the term *alert* to signify a patient who knows his name, where he is, and the day of the week.

Verbally Responsive

A patient who responds to verbal stimuli but is not alert is classified as V for verbal. This classification includes known inappropriate responses such as a patient who is asked his name and responds with someone else's name. It is helpful to note what the patient can answer in order to quantify a subtle change in his mental status as his condition progresses. For example, the patient may ini-

tially not recall the day of the week but know his name and roughly where he is located. As the call proceeds, the EMS provider, upon reassessment of mental status, may find the patient no longer has any idea where he is located. Noting this subtle change in the mental status helps to measure changes in the patient's condition before the patient's condition deteriorates further.

Painful Response

The next category of AVPU is P, responsive to painful stimuli, and is reserved for patients who do not respond to verbal stimuli but do respond to painful stimuli. Whenever applying painful stimuli to a patient, the EMS provider should remember that the bystanders might not fully understand what is being done and may think the EMS provider is being abusive. Examples of painful stimuli include:

- Applying a sternal rub as shown in Figure 4-2
- Pinching the muscle that lies above the clavicle
- Squeezing your pen between the knuckles of two of the patient's fingers
- Attempting to insert an oropharyngeal or naso-pharyngeal airway
- Thumping a finger on the bottom of an infant's foot

How the patient reacts to painful stimuli is important. Using AVPU, we classify the patient as a P for any reaction to pain. To further break down the response to pain from the highest level of brain function to the lowest level of brain function, simply observe what the reaction to the pain is. Think of it this way: If your hand is on the burner and the burner is turned on, the smartest response is to pull your hand away from the

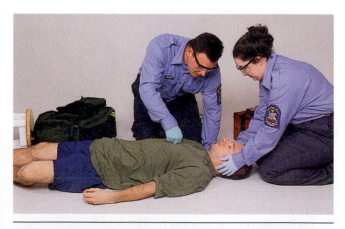

FIGURE 4-2 If a painful stimulus is needed to determine the patient's mental status, a sternal rub can be used.

Geriatric Gem

- It is often difficult to determine whether an Alzheimer's patient is alert. In this case, it is better to ask a caregiver whether this patient's mental status is normal or diminished with today's presenting problems. Using examples of what the patient is able to recognize is often helpful.

source of pain. A lower level of response would be to push into the painful stimulus, and an even lower level would be to show a form of neurological posturing. Two commonly referred to forms of neurological posturing are decorticate and decerebrate posturing. The first level, **decorticate**, involves the patient's flexing the upper extremities to the torso, or core of the body, while extending the lower extremities. The next and lower level of the two neurological postures is **decerebrate**, in which the patient stiffly extends both the arms and legs and retracts the head. The lowest level of response is no response at all. Table 4-2 summarizes patient response to pain.

Unresponsive

The total lack of response to painful stimuli is the last classification on the AVPU scale, which is U for unresponsive. Do not confuse U with unconscious; an unconscious patient may be responsive to verbal or painful stimuli that the EMS provider has yet to apply.

TABLE 4-2
Response to Pain

- Purposeful response
  - Localizes pain
  - Withdraws from pain

- Nonpurposeful response (neurological posturing). Flexion-extension posturing occurs in a progressive and predictable pattern with brain herniation and other severe brain injuries. Decorticate posturing may appear followed by decerebrate posturing.
  - Decorticate posturing, or flexion: characterized by muscle rigidity with arms and fists flexed and held tightly to the chest and legs extended and internally rotated
  - Decerebrate posturing, or extension: characterized by muscle rigidity, clenched jaw, extended neck and head, extended arms with the forearms turned out and wrists and fingers flexed; the legs are extended with the feet plantar flexed

---

- No response to pain

AIRWAY STATUS

The next step in the initial assessment is one of the most important steps: assessment of the patient's airway status. There is usually little control of the airway, gag reflex, and swallow reflex of an unresponsive patient; thus, the patient is likely to **aspirate** (inhale vomitus, blood, or other secretions into the lungs) unless the rescuers pay close attention to the airway. It is the responsibility of one rescuer to manually position the airway and ensure that it stays open and clear. Keeping the airway open can become a lot of work if the patient has copious secretions, is vomiting, or has a suspected spinal injury.

Assessing the airway status may be easier on the responsive patient, but do not be lulled into a false sense of security. A baby's crying is usually a good sign of an airway that is open, but it does not mean the airway will stay open. A patient who is responsive to verbal stimuli or even alert may still have serious compromising airway problems. Suppose the patient was in a bar fight and has a head wound, a broken jaw, and a broken nose. The combination of the bleeding into the airway from the nose with the inability of the patient to move his jaw could be a life-threatening airway injury, especially in the supine patient. When assessing the airway of all patients, the EMS provider needs to ask three key questions:

- Is the airway open?
- Will the airway stay open?
- Does anything endanger the airway?

If the airway is not open, the EMS provider must immediately open it using the head tilt–chin lift technique. If the EMS provider suspects that the patient has sustained a high-energy impact above the clavicles, then the jaw thrust technique should be used instead of the head tilt–chin lift. Any patient who requires manual positioning of the airway will have to have one rescuer assigned to the airway for the duration of the patient contact. If the airway is open, the next priority is to ensure that it will stay open on its own. If there is any

---

Pediatric Pearl

- Pediatricians may say that the initial assessment steps for children should be renamed from MS-ABC to AAA (airway, airway, airway) because assessing the airway is so important in young patients.

doubt about the patency of the airway, the EMS provider must continue to check the airway status or assign a rescuer to the airway to keep it open by manual positioning. If the patient's airway is closed and completely obstructed, as in Figure 4-3, the EMS provider must immediately manage the obstructed airway using the procedures learned in basic life support training (i.e., abdominal thrusts for adults and children and chest thrusts for infants, obese patients, and obviously pregnant patients). If an advanced provider who is appropriately trained is on the scene, she can look in the airway to determine whether there is a chunk of food or an object such as a balloon that can be removed with the laryngoscope and Magill forceps. If removal of the obstruction fails, it may be necessary to perform a surgical airway technique—provided the EMS provider is appropriately trained. If the patient's airway is completely obstructed, all efforts will turn from completing the initial assessment to keeping the airway clear and immediately transporting the patient.

The airways of many patients, both responsive and unresponsive, are partially obstructed owing to vomitus, blood, or secretions that have collected in their mouth

 Clinical Carat

● The airway must be cleared, or there will be no patient to assess!

and nose. If the patient has a medical problem or trauma that does not include a potential injury to the spine, roll the patient on his side. If a possible spinal injury is suspected, the roll is a bit more complicated but just as urgent. This will require a combination of proper positioning of the neck using a jaw thrust and in-line manual stabilization, as shown in Figure 4-4. If the EMS provider cannot keep up with the volume of secretions or vomitus, a controlled logroll may be necessary, with additional rescuers all working together to position the patient on his side. Once the patient is on his side, quickly suction the mouth using a rigid-tipped Yankauer attached to a suction unit. Remember to suction on the way out of the mouth, and always keep sight of the end of the rigid tip. In some instances, especially if the vomitus contains large chunks of the last meal, it will be necessary to sweep out the mouth using a tongue blade or the Yankauer or even the wide-bore suction tubing before suctioning. All this needs to happen very fast because the patient with a partially obstructed airway is not breathing well and the suctioning is removing oxygen from the respiratory tract.

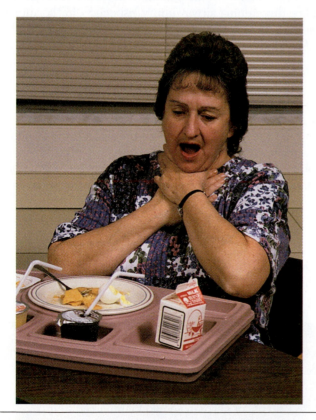

FIGURE 4-3 A completely obstructed airway, as in a patient choking on food who is unable to speak, must be managed immediately.

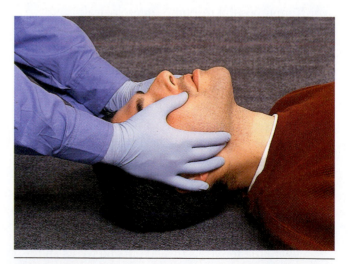

FIGURE 4-4 To do a jaw thrust maneuver, place the middle and index fingers on the angles of the patient's jaw and the thumbs on the cheekbones while avoiding any movement of the neck.

Clinical Carat

- Performing a finger sweep in adults continues to be recommended by the American Heart Association (AHA). However, most providers do not actually do finger sweeps for fear of exposing even a gloved finger to oral secretions and blood from a bite.

Complex Life-Threatening Airway Obstructions

Some patients have mechanical or anatomical obstructions to their airway caused by trauma or swelling. Consider the patient who has an object, such as a knife or a bullet, embedded in the neck. It could be partially occluding the airway or causing bleeding into the airway (see Figure 4-5 for an example of major facial trauma). Some patients who attempt suicide with a rifle under the chin move the head back at the last moment and blow the chin and jaw off. These patients have grotesque soft-tissue trauma, and sometimes the only way to locate the trachea is to look for the bubbles as the patient exhales. This patient's airway will require a great deal of attention to ensure he is well oxygenated. Another complex problem that may be found in the field is a rapidly swelling airway from airway burns, inhalation of superheated gases, a severe allergic reaction, or direct blunt injury to the throat. A fractured larynx might initially

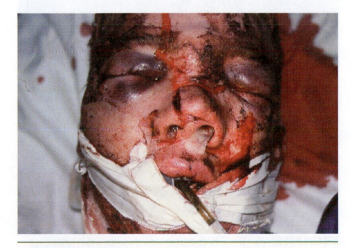

FIGURE 4-5 Major facial trauma can cause life-threatening airway complications that must be managed right away. (Courtesy of Kevin Reilly, MD, Albany Medical Center, Albany, NY)

show up as a very low-volume raspy voice subsequent to a car crash in which the patient struck his anterior neck on the steering wheel. Over time, this patient's neck and its structures can easily swell and partially occlude the airway.

BREATHING

The next step in the initial assessment, after ensuring the patient has a patent airway, is to assess the patient's breathing. There are six questions the EMS provider will need to keep in mind about the patient's breathing:

- Is the patient breathing?
- What is the respiratory rate?
- Is the rate adequate?
- Does anything endanger breathing?
- Can the patient take a deep breath?
- Is the patient having trouble breathing (**dyspnea**)?

The CPR quick check is used to determine whether an unconscious patient is breathing. The EMS provider should look, listen, and feel for breathing by placing her ear near the patient's mouth and nose to listen and feel for breathing while looking at the patient's chest and abdomen for movement. If the EMS provider is unsure whether the patient is breathing, the assumption is made that the patient is not and ventilations are begun. If the patient is not breathing, proceed with artificial ventilations and insert an oropharyngeal airway. Once advanced providers are on the scene, this patient will need to have an endotracheal tube inserted.

If the patient is breathing quickly, count the rate to see whether it is within normal range for the patient's age (see Table 4-3). Is breathing labored or shallow? Determine whether the patient has any trauma or medical condition that may endanger breathing. Some impediments to breathing are obvious, as when a patient pinned under a concrete slab is having difficulty expanding his chest. Other conditions are subtle; for instance, the pain caused by a few broken ribs sustained in a motor vehicle crash may be limiting the patient's willingness to expand his chest. A patient who has sustained a penetrating injury to the chest wall, such as a bullet wound or stabbing, will have difficulty breathing that continues to worsen over time unless managed appropriately with an occlusive dressing and ventilation. The asthmatic patient having bronchoconstriction and thick mucus in the lower airways may exhibit life-threatening breathing difficulty.

Dyspnea, or difficulty breathing, is not always obvious to the evaluator because it is a subjective finding. Always ask the patient whether he is having any

TABLE 4-3
Normal Respiratory Rates

Patient Age (yr)	Breaths/Minute
Newborn	30–50
Infant (birth–1)	25–40
Toddler (1–3)	20–30
Preschooler (3–5)	20–30
School-ager (6–10)	15–30
Adolescent (11–14)	12–20
Adult (15+)	12–20

difficulty breathing or chest pain. If the patient says yes to either of those questions, the EMS provider must apply oxygen and follow up in the focused history and physical examination. If the patient denies having difficulty breathing yet appears to be in some form of distress, such as presenting in the tripod position in Figure 4-6, try using other words (e.g., "Are you short of breath?" or "Is it hard for you to take a deep breath?")

If breathing is adequate and the patient is responsive, oxygen may be indicated depending on the condition exhibited and the respiratory rate. Many regional protocols suggest that patients breathing at rates of more than 24 breaths per minute or less than 8 breaths per minute should receive high-flow oxygen at 15 liters per minute through a non-rebreather mask. Some of these patients may also need ventilatory assistance, especially if the rate stays at less than 8 breaths per minute. Always follow your local protocols. During the initial assessment, the EMS provider should not assume that a rapidly breathing (hyperventilating) patient is having an anxiety or behavioral problem. You may decide later in the patient's evaluation that this is the situation, but at this point assume that the rapid, shallow respiratory rate is due to a medical cause such as hypoxia.

If the patient is unresponsive and the breathing is adequate, with an airway that is open and maintained, provide high-concentration oxygen by non-rebreather mask. If the breathing of an unresponsive patient is inadequate, the EMS provider must open and manually maintain the airway. Next, assist the patient's breathing with a bag-valve-mask (BVM) hooked up to an oxygen reservoir system, using two rescuers as shown in Figure 4-7, or a pocket mask with a one-way valve and supplemental oxygen if there is only one rescuer to commit to the airway. Either way, insert an oropharyngeal or nasopharyngeal airway if the patient does not have a gag reflex. A nasopharyngeal airway may be used when the gag reflex is intact. Be sure to continue to maintain in-line manual stabilization and a jaw thrust maneuver if trauma to the neck is suspected. When advanced

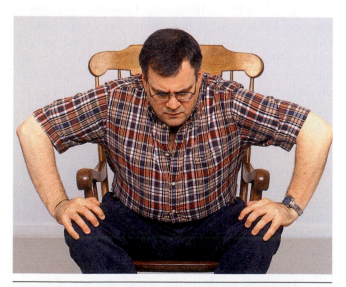

FIGURE 4-6 Pay attention to the patient's position. This patient is in the tripod position because of his respiratory distress.

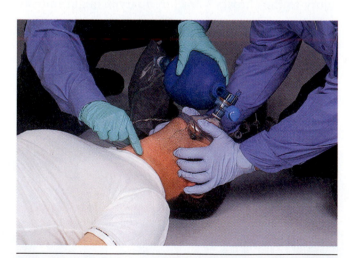

FIGURE 4-7 Two rescuers are ventilating this patient. One rescuer maintains the jaw thrust, mask seal, and in-line stabilization, while the other rescuer squeezes the BVM and applies cricoid pressure as necessary to prevent regurgitation.

providers are available, this patient will need to have an endotracheal or nasotracheal tube inserted.

If the patient is breathing, the EMS provider will need to inspect the chest. Look for symmetry from side to side as the patient expands the lungs. If the patient is having difficulty breathing, take a close look to see whether there are any holes in the chest wall that need to be sealed with an occlusive dressing or flail segments that need to be stabilized with a bulky dressing or tape. A **flail segment**, also called flail chest, is an injured portion of the chest wall where two or more ribs are fractured in two or more places, thereby creating a free-floating segment that moves in the opposite direction of the rest of the chest wall. This paradoxical motion can dramatically reduce the lung expansion. Sandbags are no longer used to stabilize a flail segment of the chest. Placing a 5-pound sandbag on the patient's chest will just make it more difficult to breathe. Also, taping circumferentially around the chest may be counterproductive and restrict chest expansion. If the patient is having difficulty breathing or is unresponsive, palpate the chest to determine whether there is equal expansion from side to side. Using a stethoscope, auscultate the breath sounds for the presence of lung expansion on both sides of the chest by listening to the anterior chest either in the area of the second rib midclavicular line or in the anterior axillary line at the nipple level. A more detailed chest assessment will be done later in the physical examination of the patient if it is appropriate to the problem.

Check to see whether there are any objects embedded in the chest that need to be stabilized. If the patient is responsive and talking, take a moment and listen to the effort of how he is talking. Patients who are having life-threatening breathing difficulty cannot talk in long sentences. They usually talk in short, choppy sentences, as would a person who is out of breath. Ask the responsive patient to take a deep breath; if he can easily and painlessly do so, he probably does not have life-threatening breathing difficulty.

CIRCULATORY STATUS

After evaluating the mental status, airway, and breathing, the EMS provider moves on to assessing the patient's circulation. There are three key questions to keep in mind when assessing circulatory status:

- Does the patient have a pulse?
- What is the quality of the pulse?
- Is there any major bleeding that needs to be controlled?

The presence of a pulse in an unconscious patient is determined during the CPR quick check. Take another

opportunity to palpate the pulse, this time a distal pulse. If the patient does not have a radial pulse, recheck the carotid, and, if there is no pulse, begin CPR and prepare to use the automated external defibrillator (AED). The immediate priority for a medical patient is to apply the AED, whereas the immediate priority for a trauma patient is to begin CPR and then apply the AED. This difference is a function of the typical initial cardiac rhythms of patients in cardiac arrest. Medical patients often go into ventricular fibrillation or pulseless ventricular tachycardia, which are treatable with defibrillation. Trauma patients usually go into asystole, or "flatline," or a pulseless electrical activity, for which defibrillation is not indicated (no shock advised). Studies continue to show that the most effective piece of equipment carried in an emergency vehicle is the AED (Figure 4-8). Every emergency vehicle should be carrying some type of defibrillator.

Assessing the radial pulse is more useful in the initial assessment than a carotid pulse because it gives insight into the effectiveness of the distal circulation. In certain shock states, a patient may have a palpable carotid pulse but a distal circulation that is so poor the

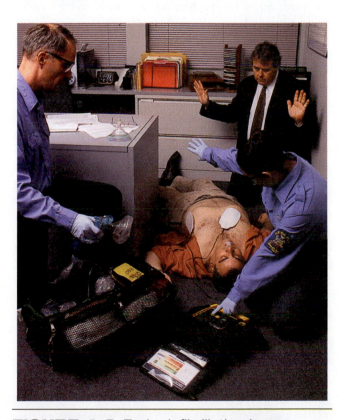

FIGURE 4-8 Early defibrillation is one of the most effective treatments EMS providers can offer the cardiac arrest patient. Many communities and businesses have established public access defibrillation programs to help save lives.

radial pulse cannot be felt. Assessing the radial pulse helps to estimate the systolic blood pressure without applying a blood pressure cuff. Approximately 80 mm Hg pressure is needed for the radial pulse to be palpated. A femoral pulse takes about 70 mm Hg, and a carotid pulse takes approximately 60 mm Hg of systolic pressure. So, if the patient has a carotid but no radial pulse, provided there is no obstruction to the circulation in the arm on which the EMS provider is taking the pulse, the blood pressure could be estimated as between 60 and 80. The lack of distal pulses is of great significance because it demonstrates that the patient may already be in decompensated shock.

Next, the EMS provider will need to examine the patient for major external hemorrhaging. This is not a head-to-toe examination but rather an observation for pools of blood around the patient or in the patient's clothing. If bleeding is present, control bleeding using direct pressure, elevation (provided there is no obvious fracture), a pressure bandage, a pressure point if necessary, or only as the last resort, a tourniquet. Although life-threatening external bleeding is rare, when found, it must be controlled immediately or the patient can bleed to death.

Assessing for life-threatening internal hemorrhaging is more difficult. The EMS provider must rely on signs, symptoms, and the mechanism of injury. The patient who was involved in a motor vehicle collision who has no signs of external bleeding yet is presenting

with signs of shock may have sustained an injury in the upper abdomen, such as a ruptured spleen. This is the reason he is presenting with no external bleeding. The theory is that any patient with an unexplained presentation of shock can be assumed to have internal bleeding until proved otherwise in the hospital.

Assess the patient's **perfusion** (blood flow) by evaluating **skin color, temperature, and condition (CTC)**. The normal skin of Caucasians is pink, warm, and dry (depending on the surrounding weather conditions). The patient's skin color can be assessed by looking at the nail beds, lips, and eyes. Abnormal skin colors include:

- Pale: indicating constricted blood vessels, possibly resulting from blood loss, shock, hypotension, hypothermia, or emotional distress
- Cyanotic (blue): indicating a lack of oxygen resulting from inadequate breathing or heart function
- Flushed (red): indicating heat exposure, hypertension, or emotional excitement
- Jaundiced (yellow): indicating possible abnormalities of the liver, such as hepatitis or liver failure
- For patients of color, consider looking for cyanosis of the lips, eyelids, or nail beds.

Capillary refill is a useful indicator for assessing the distal perfusion of a pediatric patient. Recent training curricula have downplayed the use of capillary refill in adults because many unreliable factors interfere, such as heavy smoking history, skin color, normal poor distal circulation, and skin temperature. To assess the capillary refill of a pediatric patient, press gently for a moment on a fingertip, the palm, or bottom of an infant's foot or the skin on an extremity, as shown in Figure 4-9. Upon release, the blanched skin should return to its normal color within 2 seconds or the amount of time it takes to

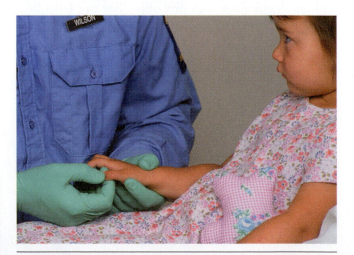

FIGURE 4-9 Capillary refill is a dependable indicator of distal perfusion in pediatric patients.

Clinical Carat

- It is possible to have poor skin turgor because of increased tension or a connective tissue disease. Elderly people commonly have poor skin turgor owing to a loss of connective tissue.

Exploring the Web

Search the Web for additional information on the following topics:

- Assessing mental status
- Assessing the airway
- Assessing breathing
- Assessing circulation

Are there additional tools available to help in these assessments? Create index cards that will help you practice the appropriate steps associated with each of these assessments. List questions that can be asked to guide your assessment, signs and symptoms that indicate the presence of life threats, and management techniques that may be used to control the life threats.

say "capillary refill." Taking longer than 2 seconds is referred to as delayed capillary refill.

To assess the patient's skin temperature and condition, place the back of the hand on the patient's forehead and then on one of the patient's forearms. Normal skin should be warm and dry, although the temperature may vary a little with the surrounding environment. Abnormal skin temperatures and conditions include:

- Cool and moist (clammy): indicating shock
- Cold and moist: indicating the body is losing heat
- Cold and dry: indicating an exposure to cold, hypothermia, poor peripheral circulation
- Hot and dry or moist: indicating high fever or heat exposure
- **Piloerection**, or "goose pimples," with shivering, chattering teeth, blue lips, and pale skin: indicating chills, exposure to cold, communicable disease, pain, or fever
- **Tenting** of the skin: indicating dehydration (tented skin stays up when pinched and does not return to its original shape quickly)

If life-threatening internal or external bleeding is suspected, the EMS provider should begin to support the patient's circulation by laying the patient down and raising the legs, as long as they do not appear to be broken. Apply high-concentration oxygen; keep the patient warm; and prepare for immediate transport with advanced life support monitoring and IV fluid replacement en route to the hospital.

PRIORITY

The next step in the initial assessment, prioritizing, is important because it determines procedures for the rest of the patient contact. Various formats are used to make a priority decision. Prioritizing is discussed in detail in Chapter 5. The following conditions may be indications of critical or unstable patients who need immediate transport to the hospital:

- Poor general impression

- Unresponsive, no gag or cough reflex
- Responsive but not following commands
- Difficulty breathing
- Shock (hypoperfusion)
- Complicated childbirth
- Chest pain with systolic blood pressure of less than 100 mm Hg
- Uncontrolled bleeding
- Severe pain anywhere

Patient priority determines the need for transport and advanced life support (ALS) intervention. The EMS provider may have already begun to remove the patient from the scene; this would be the case for a patient whose life-threatening condition, such as a blocked airway or major external bleeding, cannot be controlled in the field. If, however, the EMS provider has completed the initial assessment, she then needs to decide whether the patient should be transported right away or whether the focused history and physical examination should be continued on the scene.

If your community does not routinely send paramedics to the scene, part of the initial assessment is to determine the need for ALS support. Indications for ALS may be found in later parts of the patient assessment, but any life-threatening situation found in the initial assessment warrants an ALS response to the scene or, at the minimum, a rendezvous en route to the hospital. The key is to call early to be sure ALS will be there when the patient needs its assistance.

CONCLUSION

The initial assessment is an important part of every patient's evaluation; the focus of this assessment is to quickly identify the patients who would not live long without rapid interventions. It is during the initial assessment that life threats are identified and their management begun. The initial assessment is also the stage during which patients are prioritized and decisions are made regarding transport and the need for additional resources. To help remember the key steps of the initial assessment, keep MS-ABC (mental status–airway, breathing, circulation) in mind and learn the questions posed in this chapter. They will help you ascertain the most important information and will help you make a patient priority and transportation decision. To see how the entire assessment process flows, refer to the patient assessment algorithm (Figure 1-1) and the Practical Evaluation Skill Sheets in Appendix D.

REVIEW QUESTIONS

1. A patient's statement such as, "I can't catch my breath" is referred to as the:

    a. general impression.

    b. field diagnosis.

    c. chief complaint.

    d. scene size-up.

2. The general impression is a quick assessment of all of the following factors except:

    a. MOI or NOI.

    b. approximate age of the patient.

    c. degree of distress.

    d. the need for a detailed examination.

3. The tool used to measure the mental status is called:

    a. GSC.

    b. AVPU.

    c. CUPS.

    d. SAMPLE.

4. For an adult patient to be described as alert, he should be capable of telling you all of the following except:

    a. his name.

    b. the day of the week.

    c. the date of the month.

    d. approximately where he is.

5. The mental status of a patient who is confused about his name and the day of the week but complains of pain in the head should be noted as:

    a. A.

    b. V.

    c. P.

    d. U.

6. When evaluating a patient's breathing during the initial assessment, the EMS provider should seek to answer all of the following questions except:

    a. What is the respiratory rate?

    b. What is the quality of the breath sounds?

    c. Does anything endanger the breathing?

    d. Can the patient take a deep breath?

7. An injured portion of the chest wall involving two or more rib fractures in two or more places is called:

    a. an embedded object.

    b. a crushed chest syndrome.

    c. a flail segment.

    d. a cardiac contusion.

8. If an adult patient who has sustained a serious injury involving internal bleeding has a weak radial pulse, the systolic blood pressure can be estimated as at least:

    a. 50 mm Hg.

    b. 60 mm Hg.

    c. 70 mm Hg.

    d. 80 mm Hg.

9. When assessing the patient's skin, the EMS provider should use the abbreviation:

    a. CTC.

    b. AVPU.

    c. CUPS.

    d. RSI.

10. Of the following patients, which would not be initially considered as a critical or unstable patient or a top-priority patient?

    a. an unresponsive patient

    b. a patient with difficulty breathing

    c. a patient who had chest pain that was relieved by nitroglycerin

    d. a patient who is in shock from blood loss

CRITICAL THINKING QUESTIONS

1. Reflect on the importance of a patient's airway, breathing, and circulatory status in regard to the patient's overall health. What are the effects of an ineffective airway, ineffective breathing, or poor circulation? What makes each of these three things so critical to a person's well-being? Support the argument that this may be the most important assessment the EMS provider can make in caring for a patient.

2. It is a sunny summer day, and you are called to a residence for a woman who is having problems breathing. Upon your arrival, the woman's husband meets you in front of the house and directs you to the backyard. As he walks back with you, he explains that his wife was out gardening when he left to go to the grocery store. When he got back, he found his wife in the backyard having extreme difficulty breathing. She was unable to tell him what happened because she could not speak in full sentences. What is your initial assessment of this patient? What do you suspect is the problem? What challenges might you encounter in caring for this patient? What priority might this patient be?

3. You are dispatched to the scene of an accident in which a person riding a bicycle was struck by a car. The cyclist is unconscious but was wearing a helmet. The driver of the car said she was making a left-hand turn and did not see the cyclist. The cyclist hit the front of her car and went flying over the hood of the car onto the pavement. What is your initial assessment of this patient? What challenges might you encounter in caring for this patient? What priority might this patient be?

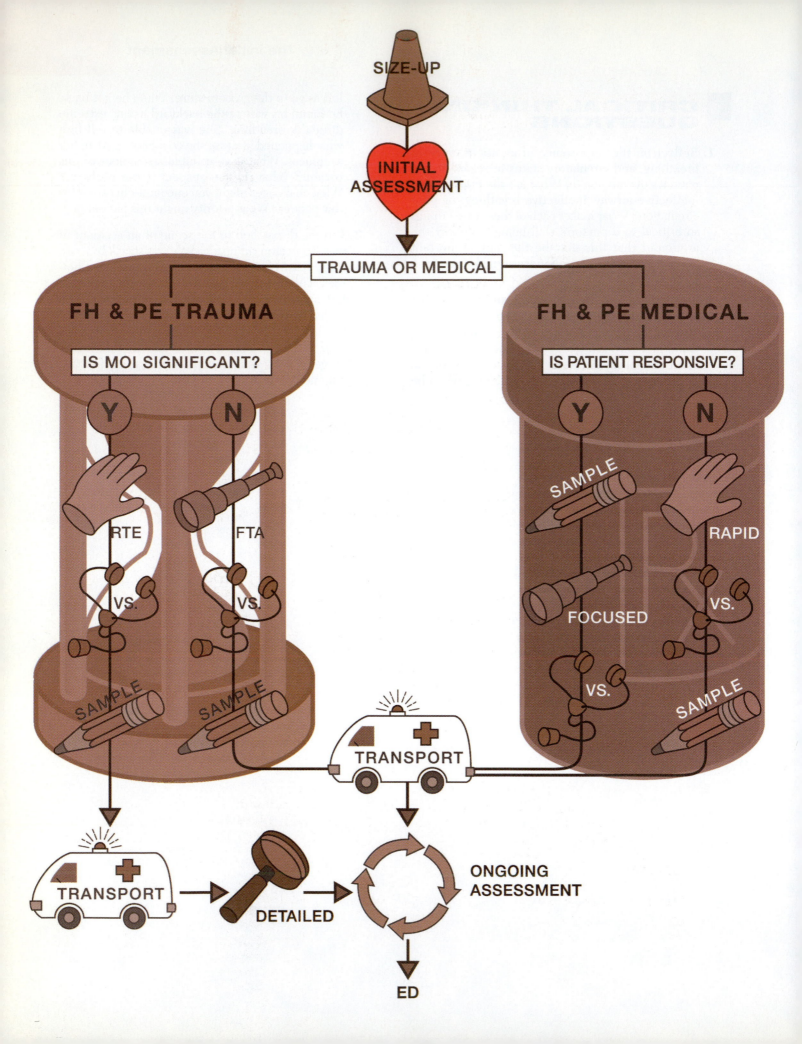

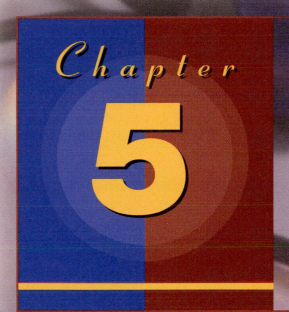

Chapter

5

Making a
Priority Decision

OBJECTIVES

Upon completion of this chapter, the reader should be able to:

- Describe how the priority decision affects the care of the patient.
- Define *up triaging* and explain how it applies to patient care.
- List four types of systems the EMS provider can use to make the priority decision.
- List and describe two trauma-scoring tools used for triage and for making priority decisions.
- List the three common classifications of burn severity and describe examples of each.
- Define the START system and describe how EMS providers can use this system in a multiple-casualty incident.
- Describe how EMS providers use triage tags during a multiple-casualty incident.
- Describe the four levels of trauma center and how a facility's level is determined.
- Provide examples of the types of patients who would be transported to a level I trauma center.

KEY TERMS

body surface area (BSA)
CUPS
escharotomy
Glasgow Coma Scale (GCS)
golden hour
platinum 10 minutes

revised trauma score (RTS)
START
trauma center
trauma score
triage
up triaging

INTRODUCTION

The final step in the initial assessment involves making a priority decision. This important decision determines the course of the rest of the patient's assessment, management, and transportation, and, in some cases, it determines the patient's destination. There are many opportunities for reassessment and updating the patient's priority throughout the assessment process. This chapter discusses several systems that are used for prioritizing patients and triage.

Triage is a French word that means "to sort." All emergency departments have a triage desk, where a nurse or other qualified health care professional asks a few key questions of all patients to determine their priority for treatment. In the emergency department, patients may appear to be treated in a first-come first-served order, but a patient who arrives with a condition more severe than that of any other patient will be moved to the top of the list.

THE PRIORITY DECISION

Most EMS calls involve a single patient who would not suffer deleterious effects if an EMS provider had trouble making a decision on the patient's priority. On the other hand, the remaining small percentage of patients have a condition that could change rapidly; these patients can suffer serious consequences if the EMS provider cannot make a priority decision. They are the patients who have only a **golden hour** (an optimum limit of 1 hour between time of injury and surgery) or merely a **platinum 10 minutes** (an optimum of 10 minutes at the scene) for the EMS provider to assess and manage them before transportation. These could be heart patients who are potentially losing cardiac cells (to a cardiologist, "time is muscle") or stroke patients losing brain cells or patients with bleeding that can be stopped only by surgery. Learning to quickly decide on a patient's priority is essential for all levels of EMS provider because failure to make a priority decision could have life-threatening implications for the patient.

Up triaging is a concept used in medicine that means that if the patient's presenting problem could be either more or less serious, the patient should be managed as having the more serious of the two possibilities until the patient's condition has been absolutely determined. For example, a patient with a twisted ankle may have only sprained her ankle, but this injury could be a fracture. Because an x-ray is not available in the field, it is necessary to immobilize the ankle as for a fracture instead of wrapping the joint as for a sprain. Another example is to treat a patient who could be suffering from either angina or acute myocardial infarction for the more serious condition, myocardial infarction (oxygen, position of comfort, 12-lead electrocardiogram and vital sign monitoring, precautionary IV line, baby aspirins, nitroglycerin, and consultation with medical control for morphine if the pain is still present), because it is difficult to distinguish between the two conditions in the field.

SYSTEMS OF PRIORITIZING

In the initial assessment (IA), the EMS provider can use any of several systems to make a priority decision. The U.S. Department of Transportation curriculum is flexible in that it emphasizes the need for a priority system rather than specifying one particular system over another. The patient may be classified as C, U, P, or S; hot or cold; high or low; severe, moderate, or minor; P-1, P-2, or P-3; red, yellow, or green; or other categories. No matter which system is used, it is imperative that all the EMS providers in the region know the same system and be familiar with types of patients who would fit into each category. Table 5-1 shows a comparison of six systems that the EMS provider can use to make a priority decision.

CUPS

One system used to prioritize patients is the **CUPS** format. This system was originally introduced in the basic trauma life support (BTLS) course and has been adopted for use in several states. The CUPS format is used on the prehospital care report (see Figure 5-1) in a number of regions. CUPS is an acronym that stands for *c*ritical, *u*nstable, *p*otentially unstable, and *s*table. In the last part of the initial assessment, patients are classified into one of the four CUPS categories.

The critical category includes actual or impending cardiorespiratory arrest, respiratory failure, decompensated shock or hypoperfusion, rising intracranial pressure, and severe upper airway difficulties. Basically, any patient who requires the use of the bag-valve-mask (BVM) to assist ventilations is considered a C, or critical, patient. The management should include circulatory and ventilatory assistance, CPR (as necessary), bag-valve-mask (BVM), oxygen administration, and volume resuscitation. This is considered a high-priority patient.

The unstable category includes cardiorespiratory instability; respiratory distress; compensated shock or hypoperfusion; two or more long-bone fractures; trauma associated with burns; amputation proximal to the wrist

TABLE 5-1
Systems of Prioritizing

	System Designation					Examples of Injury or Illness
Critical	Hot	High	Severe	Priority-1	Red	Cardiorespiratory arrest, respiratory failure, decompensated shock (hypoperfusion, or inadequate circulation), rising intracranial pressure, severe burns, open chest or abdominal wounds, severe head injuries
Unstable	Hot	High	Severe	Priority-1	Red	Cardiorespiratory instability, respiratory distress, compensated shock (hypoperfusion), burns, multiple fractures, spinal injuries, uncomplicated head injury
Potentially unstable	Cold	Low	Moderate	Priority-2	Yellow	Minor fractures and wounds, burns on more than 10% of the body surface area, psychological emergencies, uncomplicated childbirth
Stable	Cold	Low	Minor	Priority-3	Green	Minor illness, minor isolated injury

or ankle; penetrating injury to the head, neck, chest, abdomen, or pelvis; uncontrollable external bleeding; chest pain with a systolic blood pressure of more than 100 mm Hg; severe pain; poor general impression; unresponsive patients; or responsive patients who do not follow commands. The management should include supplemental oxygen. This is considered a high-priority patient.

The potentially unstable category includes cardiorespiratory instability, a mechanism of injury (MOI) indicating a possible hidden injury, a major isolated injury, general medical illness, or an uncomplicated childbirth. The management should include careful monitoring of the patient. An adult in this category is considered a low-priority patient; an infant or a child is considered a high-priority patient.

The stable category includes patients with a low potential for cardiorespiratory instability, low-grade fever, minor illness, minor isolated injury, or an uncomplicated extremity injury. The management should include continued observation. This is considered a low-priority patient.

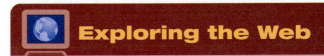

Exploring the Web

● What system is used in your service area to prioritize patients? Search the Web for other prioritization systems used in other states. A good place to start may be the state EMS Web site. Compare and contrast the various methods you find.

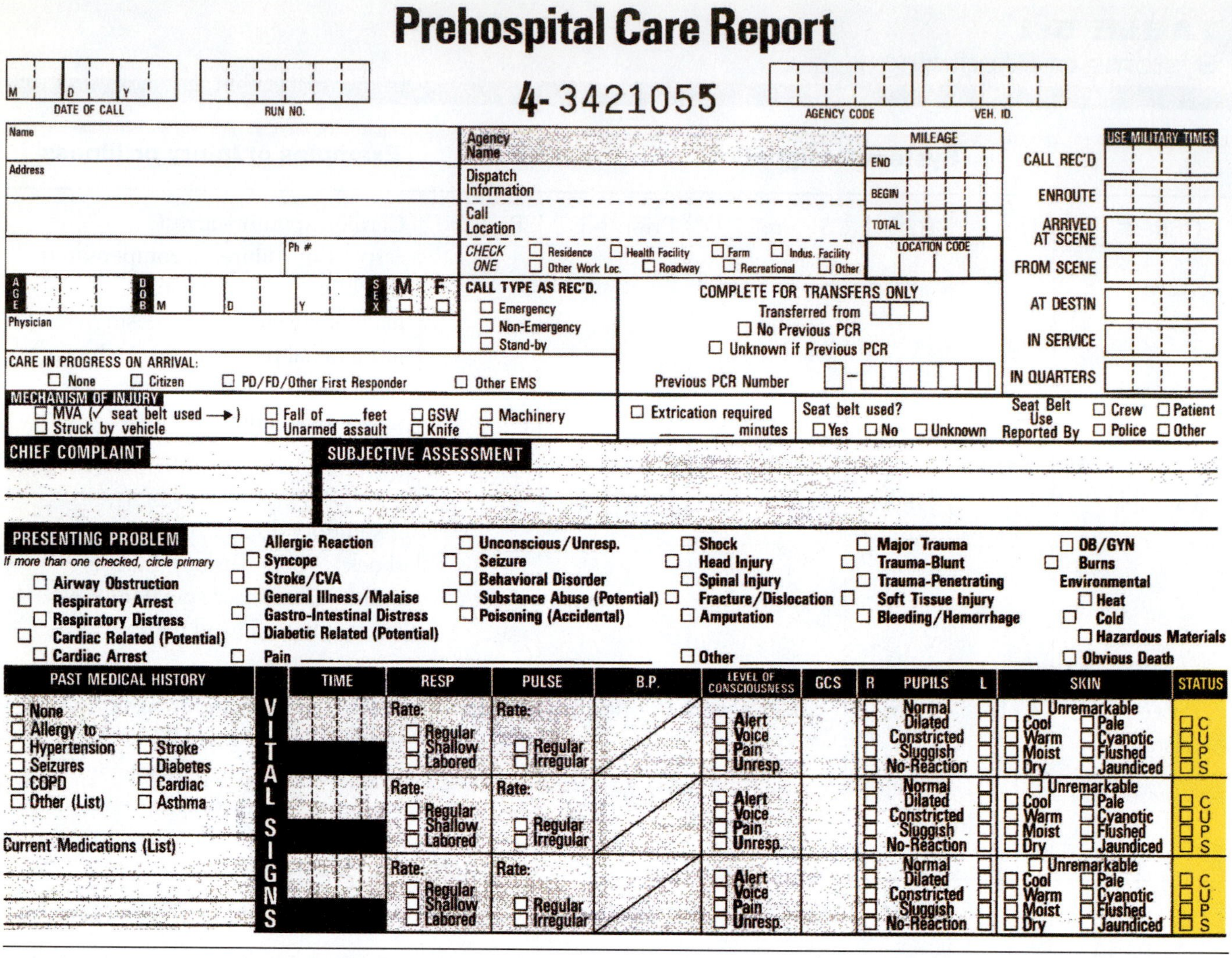

Prehospital Care Report

M D Y DATE OF CALL | RUN NO. | 4-3421055 | AGENCY CODE | VEH. ID.

Name | Agency Name | MILEAGE END / BEGIN / TOTAL | USE MILITARY TIMES CALL REC'D

Address | Dispatch Information | ENROUTE

Call Location | ARRIVED AT SCENE

Ph # | CHECK ONE ☐ Residence ☐ Health Facility ☐ Farm ☐ Indus. Facility ☐ Other Work Loc. ☐ Roadway ☐ Recreational ☐ Other | LOCATION CODE | FROM SCENE

AGE | DOB M D Y | SEX M F | CALL TYPE AS REC'D. ☐ Emergency ☐ Non-Emergency ☐ Stand-by | COMPLETE FOR TRANSFERS ONLY Transferred from ☐ No Previous PCR ☐ Unknown if Previous PCR | AT DESTIN | IN SERVICE

Physician

CARE IN PROGRESS ON ARRIVAL: ☐ None ☐ Citizen ☐ PD/FD/Other First Responder ☐ Other EMS | Previous PCR Number | IN QUARTERS

MECHANISM OF INJURY ☐ MVA (✓ seat belt used →) ☐ Struck by vehicle ☐ Fall of ____ feet ☐ Unarmed assault ☐ GSW ☐ Knife ☐ Machinery ☐ | ☐ Extrication required ____ minutes | Seat belt used? ☐ Yes ☐ No ☐ Unknown | Seat Belt Use Reported By ☐ Crew ☐ Police ☐ Patient ☐ Other

CHIEF COMPLAINT | SUBJECTIVE ASSESSMENT

PRESENTING PROBLEM *If more than one checked, circle primary*
☐ Airway Obstruction ☐ Respiratory Arrest ☐ Respiratory Distress ☐ Cardiac Related (Potential) ☐ Cardiac Arrest
☐ Allergic Reaction ☐ Syncope ☐ Stroke/CVA ☐ General Illness/Malaise ☐ Gastro-Intestinal Distress ☐ Diabetic Related (Potential) ☐ Pain
☐ Unconscious/Unresp. ☐ Seizure ☐ Behavioral Disorder ☐ Substance Abuse (Potential) ☐ Poisoning (Accidental)
☐ Shock ☐ Head Injury ☐ Spinal Injury ☐ Fracture/Dislocation ☐ Amputation ☐ Other
☐ Major Trauma ☐ Trauma-Blunt ☐ Trauma-Penetrating ☐ Soft Tissue Injury ☐ Bleeding/Hemorrhage
☐ OB/GYN ☐ Burns Environmental ☐ Heat ☐ Cold ☐ Hazardous Materials ☐ Obvious Death

PAST MEDICAL HISTORY ☐ None ☐ Allergy to ☐ Hypertension ☐ Seizures ☐ COPD ☐ Other (List) ☐ Stroke ☐ Diabetes ☐ Cardiac ☐ Asthma
Current Medications (List)

VITAL SIGNS | TIME | RESP Rate: ☐ Regular ☐ Shallow ☐ Labored | PULSE Rate: ☐ Regular ☐ Irregular | B.P. | LEVEL OF CONSCIOUSNESS ☐ Alert ☐ Voice ☐ Pain ☐ Unresp. | GCS | R PUPILS L ☐ Normal ☐ Dilated ☐ Constricted ☐ Sluggish ☐ No-Reaction | SKIN ☐ Unremarkable ☐ Cool ☐ Warm ☐ Moist ☐ Dry ☐ Pale ☐ Cyanotic ☐ Flushed ☐ Jaundiced | STATUS ☐ C ☐ U ☐ P ☐ S

FIGURE 5-1 The CUPS format is used in this prehospital care report (bottom of form not shown). (Reprinted with permission of the New York State Department of Health)

TOOLS USED TO DETERMINE PRIORITY

Many EMS systems use tools such as the Glasgow Coma Scale (GCS), trauma score, and revised trauma score (RTS) to triage, determine priority, and make transportation decisions. These tools were developed to logically examine, evaluate, and rate the severity of a trauma patient's assessment findings using a numerical grading system. Although the GCS was developed for the trauma patient, it is routinely used on medical patients in many systems.

The Glasgow Coma Scale

The **Glasgow Coma Scale (GCS)** is used to determine the severity of head trauma. In some systems, it is used in conjunction with other measurements to form the trauma score or the revised trauma score, as discussed later. The GCS is an objective measure of eye opening, verbal response, and motor response. The patient's best responses are given a numerical score (Table 5-2). A patient with a mild head injury would have a GCS score of 13 to 15. A patient with a moderate head injury would have a GCS score of 8 to 12, and one with a severe head injury would have a score of less than 8, or, as they say in the field, "less than 8, intubate."

The Trauma Score and the Revised Trauma Score

Some systems use the trauma score as a means of triaging patients. Usually, the **trauma score** is determined later in the care of the patient than is the GCS score; for

TABLE 5-2
Glasgow Coma Scale (GCS)

Eye opening response:	Spontaneous	4
	To voice	3
	To pain	2
	None	1
Best verbal response:	Oriented	5
	Confused	4
	Inappropriate words	3
	Incomprehensible sounds	2
	None	1
Best motor response:	Obeys commands	6
	Localizes pain	5
	Withdraws from pain	4
	Flexes on pain	3
	Extends on pain	2
	None	1

TABLE 5-3
Original Trauma Score

Respirations/minute	>36	2
	25–35	3
	10–24	4
	1–9	1
	None	0
Respiratory Expansion	Normal	1
	Shallow	0
	Retractive	0
Systolic blood pressure (mm Hg)	>90	4
	70–89	3
	50–69	2
	0–49	1
	No pulse	0
Capillary return	Normal	2
	Delayed	1
	None	0
Glasgow Coma Scale contribution	14–15	5
	11–13	4
	8–10	3
	5–7	2
	3–4	1

Total trauma score 1–16

example, it might be used to help decide whether to transfer a patient from a local hospital to a regional trauma center. The trauma score was developed in 1980 to be used for triage and to predict patient outcomes. Howard Champion is the physician responsible for the latest version of the trauma score, referred to as the **revised trauma score (RTS)**. This is a numerical grading system that combines the Glasgow Coma Scale and measurements of cardiopulmonary function as a gauge of the severity of injury and a predictor of survival after blunt injury to the head. Each parameter is given a number with high being normal and low being impaired or absent function.

In the original trauma score (Table 5-3), the severity of injury is determined by summing the numbers for the following categories: respiratory rate, respiratory expansion, systolic blood pressure, pulse, capillary refill, and a conversion scale for the GCS, as shown in Table 5-4. The trauma score has a value from zero to 16, with 1 being the score of a patient who has virtually no chance of survival; 8 indicates a 26% chance of survival, 12 an 87% chance of survival, and 16 a 99% chance of survival.

TRIAGING AND PRIORITIZING THE BURN PATIENT

A burn's severity is determined by the source type (i.e., thermal, chemical, electrical, lightning, or radiation) and the **body surface area (BSA)** affected. The rule of nines has been taught to EMS providers for many years (see Figure 5-2A) and has been adapted to the child and infant to take into account the proportionately shorter legs and larger head of children and infants (Figure 5-2B, C). An alternative is to use the surface area of the

TABLE 5-4
Revised Trauma Score with Glasgow Coma Scale Conversion

Respirations/minute	
10–29	4
>29	3
6–9	2
1–5	1
None	0

Systolic blood pressure (mm Hg)	
>89	4
76–89	3
50–75	2
1–49	1
No pulse	0

GCS total points	Apply to the trauma score
14–15	5
11–13	4
8–10	3
5–7	2
3–4	1

Total revised trauma score: 1–12

patient's palm to correspond to approximately 1% of the patient's BSA. The three common classifications of burn severity are:

- Minor: such as sunburn
- Moderate: an uncomplicated partial-thickness burn of less than 30% BSA of an adult or less than 15% BSA of a child
- Severe: requiring transport to a burn specialty center

Examples of severe burns include:

- Burns greater than 30% BSA of adults and greater than 15% BSA of children (Figure 5-3)
- Burns of the head, hands, feet, or perineum (Figure 5-4)
- Inhalation injuries
- Electrical burns (Figure 5-5)
- Burns associated with multiple trauma or serious medical problems

In most EMS systems that have a burn center, the severity of the burn is used to determine whether patients should be transported directly to the burn

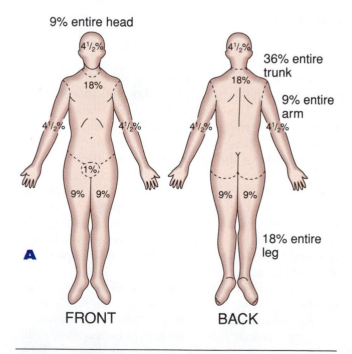

FIGURE 5-2 The rule of nines is used to determine the body surface area burned in an adult (**A**), child (**B**), and infant (**C**).

center or to a local hospital first. Review your local protocols and consult with your service medical director on this issue.

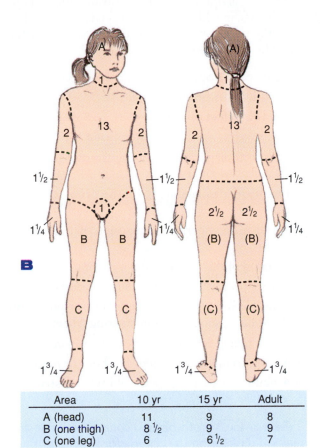

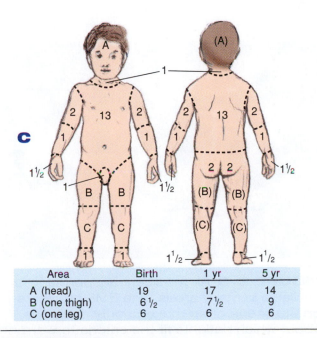

Area	10 yr	15 yr	Adult
A (head)	11	9	8
B (one thigh)	8 ½	9	9
C (one leg)	6	6 ½	7

Area	Birth	1 yr	5 yr
A (head)	19	17	14
B (one thigh)	6 ½	7 ½	9
C (one leg)	6	6	6

FIGURE 5-2 (continued)

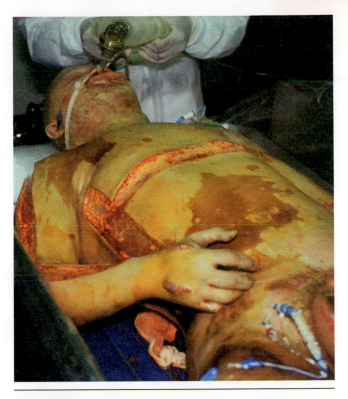

FIGURE 5-3 This severe burn required a complete **escharotomy** (surgical removal of necrotic tissue caused by a burn) of the chest and arms. (Courtesy of Ernest Grant, North Carolina Jaycee Burn Center, Chapel Hill, NC)

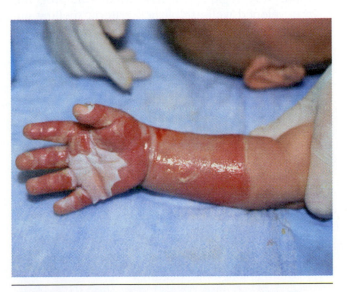

FIGURE 5-4 Intentional child abuse caused this burn. This is considered severe because it goes all the way around the arm and involves the hand. (Courtesy of Ernest Grant, North Carolina Jaycee Burn Center, Chapel Hill, NC)

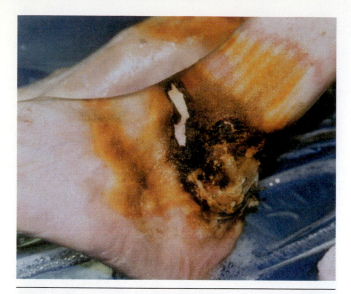

FIGURE 5-5 This is an electrical burn exit wound. (Courtesy of Ernest Grant, North Carolina Jaycee Burn Center, Chapel Hill, NC)

TRIAGE TO DETERMINE WHO RIDES THE HELICOPTER

The decision about which patients should be transported by a helicopter is another example of a medical priority decision. Most regions that have Med-Evac programs have developed well-established criteria spelling out which types of patients should be considered for helicopter transportation (Figure 5-6). The following medical criteria are often used to make this decision:

- Unconsciousness or decreased mental status
- A GCS score of less than 10
- A systolic blood pressure of less than 90 mm Hg with signs of shock
- A respiratory rate of less than 10 or greater than 30 breaths per minute
- A compromised airway
- A penetrating injury to the chest, abdomen, head, or neck
- Multiple long-bone fractures
- Flail chest
- Paralysis or suspected spinal cord injury
- Severe burns with or without trauma
- Chest pain or shortness of breath

- Active seizure
- Amputated extremities

Most helicopter programs also include circumstantial factors, in addition to medical criteria, as indications for the need for helicopter transport. Such factors might include the following:

- Distance to trauma center
- Lengthy extrications
- Falls of 15 feet or more
- Motor vehicle crash with significant MOI
- Rearward displacement of the front of the car by 20 inches or greater
- Rearward displacement of the front axle of a car
- Passenger compartment intrusion of 15 inches or more
- Ejection of the patient from a moving vehicle
- Car rollover with an unrestrained occupant
- Gross deformity at a patient's contact point with the vehicle, such as a bent steering wheel
- Death of any occupant in the same vehicle
- A pedestrian hit at 15 miles per hour or more
- A child less than 12 years old who is struck by a vehicle

Review local protocols and consult with the service medical director on the criteria for helicopter transport in your area.

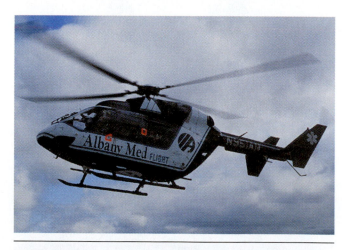

FIGURE 5-6 Air medical transportation is available in many areas. The EMS providers on the scene often make priority decisions about which patients fit the criteria to warrant this form of transportation.

TRIAGE IN MULTIPLE-CASUALTY INCIDENTS

At a multiple-casualty incident (MCI), triage is done on all patients to ensure that the most serious patients who can be saved are treated and transported first. In situations involving many high-priority patients and limited resources (ambulances, equipment, and personnel), the very critical patients who have a small chance of survival (e.g., cardiac arrest and mortal head wounds) are given the lowest priority.

The START System

START is an acronym for *simple triage and rapid treatment.* This is a method of triaging that was developed in Newport Beach, California, in the early 1980s. The START system separates patients into four categories: minor, delayed, immediate, and deceased. Step 1 of START is to clear an area and tell all of the walking wounded to walk to a specific location. After the scene has been cleared of the walking wounded, the remaining patients are assessed for respiratory status, hemodynamic status, and mental status (Figure 5-7). Each patient is triaged in less than 60 seconds.

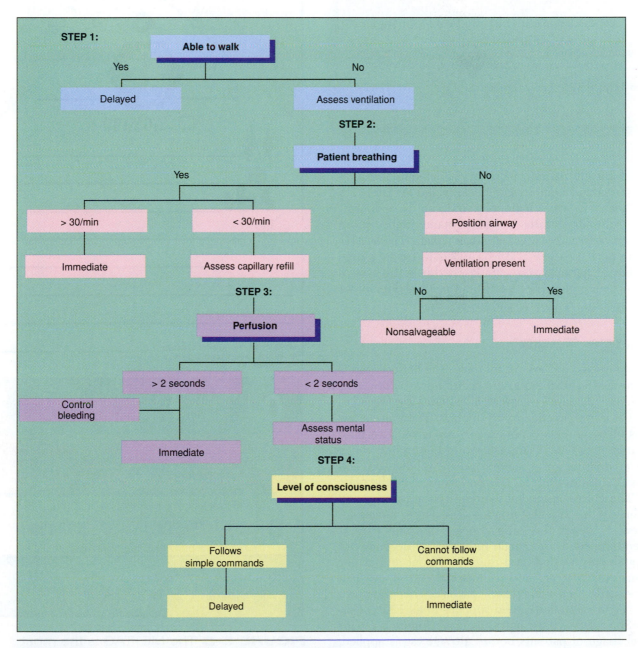

FIGURE 5-7 The algorithm used for START triage.

Exploring the Web

Explore the use and implementation of the START system. Are there similar systems that exist around the United States? Compare these systems with the START system. What are the advantages of each system? What are the disadvantages? What system is used in your area?

The following links may provide some assistance in your discussions:

- Take the sample quiz at http://www.citmt.org/education/Sample_Quiz.htm

- http://www.gc.maricopa.edu/emt-fsc/Start.htm

- http://www.start-triage.com

Basically, patients who have an adequate respiratory status and hemodynamic status and are alert are classified as delayed. Patients who do not have an adequate respiratory status or hemodynamic status or are not alert are usually classified as immediate. The START system permits a few EMS providers to triage a large number of patients very rapidly. If this is the system used in your region, check with your medical director for more specifics on how to use the system.

Triage Tags

Triage tags can be very useful tools. The hardest part is getting EMS providers to use them! Some EMS agencies have "tag days," on which all patients are tagged to give the crews practice using the tags. There are a few types of triage tags commercially available. The most common is the METTAG, shown in Figure 5-8, which uses a combination of colors (green, yellow, red, and black), priorities (0, I, II, III), and icons all on the same tag. The colors immediately identify the priority and urgency of the patient's situation. The dagger means the patient is dead; the rabbit means hospital care is urgently needed; the turtle indicates no urgency but hospital care needed; and the crossed-out ambulance means only first aid and no hospital care is needed. Some states, such as New York, have designed their own tags (Figure 5-9) and issued supplies to all EMS agencies. Some services use a priority label (Figure 5-10) for initial triage of patients before a triage tag is applied. These labels are similar to the priority packaging labels used by overnight services such as UPS, Airborne

Express, and Federal Express. Most tags and labels have four priorities: P-1 (immediate or red), P-2 (delayed or yellow), P-3 (hold or green, often referred to as the walking wounded), and P-0 (deceased or black). One useful aspect of triage tags is that they help prevent repeated assessments of the same patient. Once a patient has been tagged, it is clear that an EMS provider has seen the patient at least once. Examples of conditions that would fit into each of the triage categories are shown in Table 5-5.

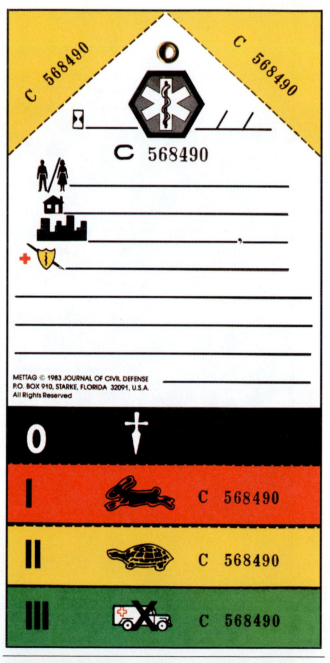

FIGURE 5-8 The METTAG is the most commonly used commercially available triage tag. (Courtesy of the American Civil Defense Association)

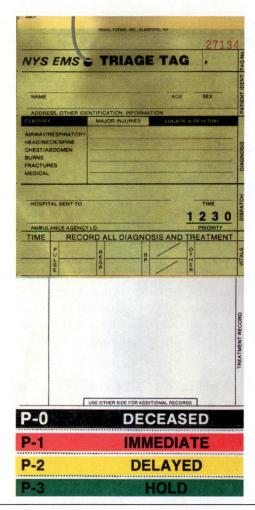

FIGURE 5-9 The New York State multiple-casualty incident tag.

TABLE 5-5
Examples of Triage Categories and Conditions

Category	Conditions
P-1, red, immediate	Airway or respiratory compromise, severe burns, cardiac problems, severe bleeding, open chest or abdominal wounds, severe head injuries, severe medical problems (e.g., heart attack, stroke)
P-2, yellow, delayed	Burns, multiple fractures, spinal injuries, uncomplicated head injury
P-3, green, hold	Minor fractures and wounds, burns on more than 10% of the BSA, psychological emergencies
P-0, black, deceased	Expired or cannot be saved

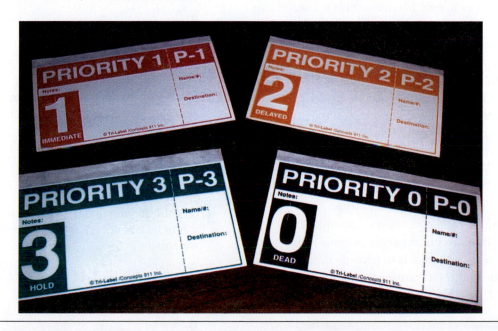

FIGURE 5-10 Priority label tags used for initial triage of patients at multiple-casualty incidents.

TRAUMA CENTERS

A **trauma center** is a hospital that has the capability of caring for the acutely injured patient. Hospitals must meet strict criteria to be designated as trauma centers. The criteria delineate the resources, personnel, equipment, and training necessary for an institution to provide quality trauma care. Every community has different needs and resources available, so trauma centers have been classified into four levels (see Table 5-6) based on the resources and programs available to each facility. In addition to being a trauma center, some hospitals specialize in burns, cardiac care (e.g., centers for heart transplantation), hyperbaric therapy, microsurgery, neurology, or pediatric trauma.

The needs of the patient and the capabilities of each trauma center are used to determine where to transport the patient. Criteria are based on the regional structure of the trauma care system and often can be found in local protocols. Criteria for transport to a level I trauma center include multiple-system trauma, severe burns, and trauma to a pediatric, geriatric, or pregnant patient.

 ## CONCLUSION

Making a priority decision is an important part of the EMS provider's assessment of the patient. Because care and transport decisions are based on the priority, the EMS provider must be well practiced and comfortable with making these decisions. Practice with the tools or systems of priority used in your region and consult your training officer or service medical director for advice. Above all, use the patient assessment algorithm (Figure 1-1) and remember to be flexible and to reevaluate regularly because patient conditions are dynamic and can change quickly, necessitating a change in patient priority.

 ## REVIEW QUESTIONS

TABLE 5-6
The Four Levels of Trauma Center

- **Level I.** Regional trauma centers serve as a leader in trauma care for a specific geographical area. Most level I trauma centers have a full range of resources, services, and programs 24 hours a day, 7 days a week.

- **Level II.** Area trauma centers can provide definitive patient care but may not have all of the resources of a level I trauma center. These centers stabilize specialty trauma cases and then transfer them to the regional center.

- **Level III.** Community trauma centers are designated in communities without level I or level II trauma centers. They can stabilize patients but, when necessary, will transfer patients to a level I or level II trauma center for further interventions and ongoing care.

- **Level IV.** These trauma centers were established for rural and remote communities. A level IV trauma center may be a clinic rather than a hospital. The goal is to provide initial stabilization and then transfer the patient to a level I, II, or III trauma center.

1. A French word that means "to sort" is:
   a. START.
   b. triage.
   c. priority.
   d. platinum 10.

2. If a trauma patient is deemed a high priority, the EMS provider should not spend more than _____ minutes on the scene of the call.
   a. 5
   b. 10
   c. 15
   d. 20

3. Setting the patient priority on the basis of the more serious of two potential conditions is known as:
   a. double triage.
   b. inverted prioritization.
   c. up triaging.
   d. pushing the platinum 10.

4. A patient who has cardiorespiratory instability might be considered any of the following priorities except:
   a. yellow.
   b. high.
   c. hot.
   d. severe.

5. A patient who has a psychological emergency could be considered any of the following priorities except:

   a. P.

   b. low.

   c. moderate.

   d. hot.

6. In the CUPS format, which of the following conditions would put an adult patient in the unstable category?

   a. impending cardiorespiratory arrest

   b. two or more long-bone fractures

   c. rising intracranial pressure

   d. general medical illness

7. Which of the following GCS scores would classify a patient as having a moderate head injury?

   a. 14

   b. 9

   c. 7

   d. 5

8. The trauma score takes into consideration the patient's:

   a. systolic blood pressure.

   b. respiratory expansion.

   c. GCS score.

   d. all of the above.

9. If an adult patient has a full-thickness burn involving the anterior torso and the complete anterior surface of both legs, this would be considered a _____ burn and a _____ priority.

   a. severe; high

   b. moderate; high

   c. moderate; low

   d. minor; low

10. Each of the following conditions qualifies a patient as a candidate for helicopter transport to the trauma center except:

    a. head injury with a GCS score of less than 11.

    b. multiple long-bone fractures.

    c. an amputated ring finger.

    d. a suspected spinal cord injury.

CRITICAL THINKING QUESTIONS

1. Prioritize the following patients using the CUPS system.

   a. A 4-year-old struck by a car backing out of a driveway

   b. A 15-year-old skateboarder who fell and has a leg fracture

   c. A woman who is giving birth to a premature infant

   d. A 35-year-old woman who fell 20 feet when rock climbing

   e. A 45-year-old man complaining of chest pain and shortness of breath

2. Are any of the above patients candidates for helicopter transport to the hospital? Why?

3. Explain why all services in a particular area should use the same triage system (START, for example). Should one system be used statewide? In light of the September 11, 2001, terrorist attacks, do you think there should be a national triage system? Why or why not?

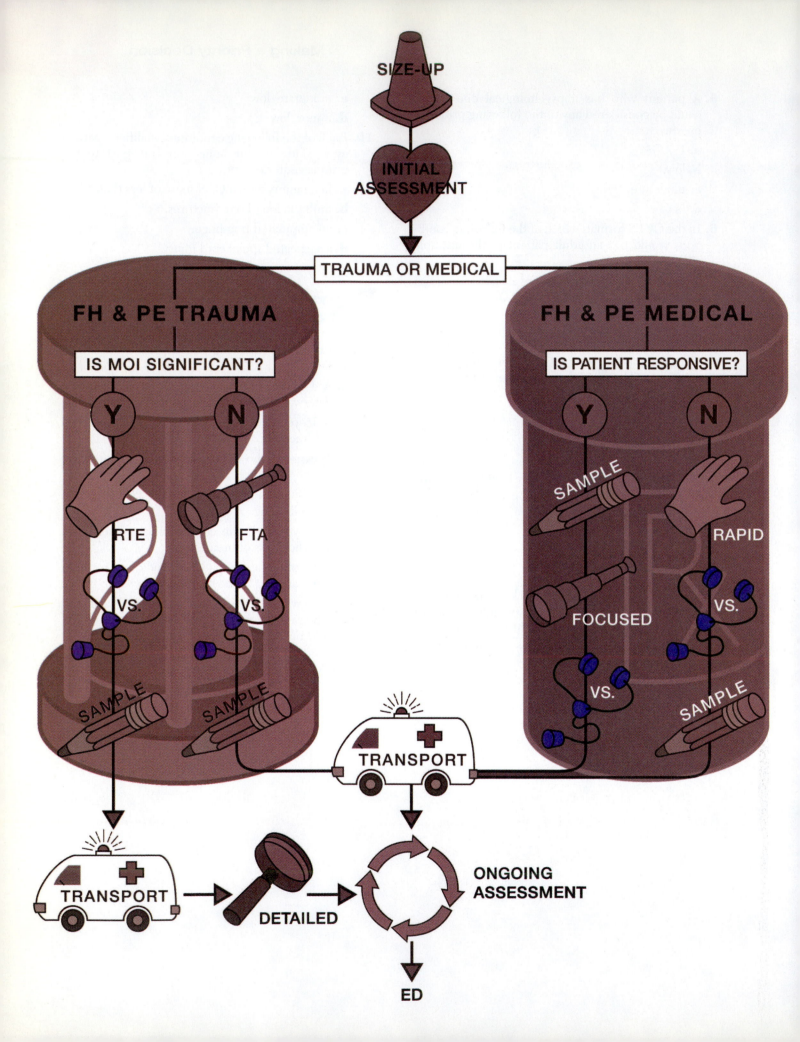

OBJECTIVES

Upon completion of this chapter, the reader should be able to:

- Describe the difference between a sign and a symptom and provide examples of each.
- List the devices EMS providers use to measure signs.
- Describe the method for assessing a patient's mental status using AVPU.
- Describe five abnormal breathing patterns and the typical causes of each.
- Specify why it is important to assess a distal pulse as well as a central pulse.
- Describe the difference between a blood pressure taken with a stethoscope and one taken without a stethoscope and when it is appropriate to use each technique.
- List examples of abnormal skin color, temperature, and condition and the possible indications or conditions for each.
- Define the mnemonic PERRLA and explain the consensual light reflex and normal accommodation of the eyes.
- Describe the principle of capillary refill in a pediatric patient.
- Describe the principle of pulse oximetry and provide examples of when a reading may be unreliable.
- Describe how capnography provides a true measurement of a patient's circulatory status.
- Explain how the Fick principle of oxygenation is relevant to the measurement of end-tidal carbon dioxide.
- Distinguish between a baseline set of vital signs and serial vital signs.
- Explain how the EMS provider develops trends by examining serial sets of vital signs.

KEY TERMS

accommodation

anisocoria

baseline

capnography

capnometer

conjugate gaze

consensual light reflex

converge

diastolic

diverge

end-tidal carbon dioxide (EtCO$_2$)

eupnea

Fick principle

hypercapnia

hypocapnia

minute volume

PERRLA

pulse oximetry

serial vital signs

sign

symptom

systolic

trends

vital signs

INTRODUCTION

Patient injuries and conditions are often described in terms of signs and symptoms. For example, as an EMS provider, you have already learned that the signs and symptoms of decompensated shock include tachycardia, anxiety, tachypnea, nausea, vomiting, thirst, pallor, diaphoresis (sweating), pupillary dilation, hypotension, and sometimes an altered mental status. Many illnesses and injuries require an EMS provider's understanding of their signs and symptoms. This chapter focuses on the importance of signs in the patient's overall assessment. Symptoms are covered throughout this book in discussions about the patient's description of the chief complaint and responses to questions about medical history. This chapter discusses the traditional vital signs of mental status, respirations, pulse, and blood pressure. Additional signs that are useful measurements in plotting a patient's condition—such as pupillary reaction, temperature, pulse oximetry readings, and end-tidal carbon dioxide—are also discussed.

SIGNS VERSUS SYMPTOMS

What exactly is the difference between a sign and a symptom? A **symptom** is a subjective finding that the patient tells the EMS provider. It is often difficult to accurately measure symptoms because they are subject to the individual interpretation of the patient. Examples of symptoms are pain, dyspnea, dizziness, and nausea. It would be difficult to measure exactly how nauseated a patient is. EMS providers can create a "yardstick" that works by comparison when used on the same patient. The best example is the evaluation of the quantity or severity of a patient's pain. With different patients having different pain thresholds, it would be difficult at best

to quantify pain. Repeatedly using the same yardstick (e.g., a 1 to 10 scale, with 1 being a minor pain and 10 being the worst ever) on each patient, however, enables the EMS provider to judge the severity of the patient's pain.

Signs can be measured accurately by hand or with a measuring device such as a sphygmomanometer (blood pressure cuff), oximeter, or thermometer. They can easily be compared with scales or charts as well as with what appears to be normal for the patient. These are referred to as objective findings and are more observable and measurable than the patient's descriptions. In a few instances, the findings may be both signs and symptoms, but such cases are rare. One such example would be the observable signs of respiratory distress (e.g., nasal flaring, tripod positioning, intercostal respirations, accessory muscle use, and pursed-lip exhalation) and the patient's description of the sensation of dyspnea, or difficulty breathing.

TRADITIONAL VITAL SIGNS

Because the triad of pulse, respiration, and blood pressure is often considered to be the starting point for assessment and a gauge of a patient's health status, they are called **vital signs**. Normal vital sign values are charted in ranges because values can vary and fluctuate for a variety of reasons. It is important to consider the particular patient when interpreting vital sign measurements and not take them out of context. Suppose a patient's radial pulse is noted as 42 to 48 and regular. On any vital sign chart, this would be considered bradycardia for adults. However, this might be the normal resting pulse rate of a trim, physically fit athlete. Before reacting to a single set of potentially abnormal vital signs and placing the pacing pads on the patient, the EMS provider should put the findings into the overall patient assessment picture. A good question to ask the patient is, "What's your normal pulse rate?"

Mental Status

A patient's mental status is by far the most important vital sign. A patient's mental status is first assessed in the initial assessment. Every patient's mental status should be evaluated along with pulse, blood pressure, and respirations. The easiest way for an EMS provider to evaluate the patient's mental status is to start by introducing herself and asking the patient his name. Follow up by asking, "How can I help you today?" After the patient answers, ask, "What day of the week is it?" and "Do you know where you are?" It is usually not necessary to ask the patient the date, or time; most people need to look at a watch for that information. A rough answer to where the patient is located will suffice (e.g., in the living room or at Joe's Diner).

The mental status is determined using the AVPU format: *a*lert, *v*erbally responsive, *p*ainful response, and *u*nresponsive. Later in the assessment of the patient who has a suspected head or spine injury, the Glasgow Coma Scale, related to eye opening, verbal, and motor responses, is used. Refer to Chapter 4, which includes comprehensive information pertaining to AVPU, and to Chapter 5 for information on the Glasgow Coma Scale.

Respirations

The respirations are evaluated in terms of rate, regularity, and quality or adequacy. Count the patient's rate of respirations by looking at his chest or abdomen (Figure 6-1). A patient who is conscious of an EMS provider's counting can easily change the respiratory rate, so attempt to count without the patient's knowledge. One way to do so is to take the patient's wrist and hold his radial pulse against his belly. For the first 30 seconds, count the respirations, and for the next 30 seconds count the pulse. The normal adult and pediatric respiratory rates are listed in Table 6-1.

The respirations are also assessed in terms of their regularity and their quality. Two terms that are commonly used to describe quality of respirations are *labored* (requiring observable work of breathing and the use of accessory muscles) and *shallow* (very little movement of the chest). Another abnormal pattern is paradoxical respirations, as might be observed in a patient who has a flail segment. Normally, the chest rises on inspiration, however, the chest of a flail segment patient would fall on inspiration and rise on exhalation.

Adequacy is determined by the amount of gas inspired in a minute, called the **minute volume**. An

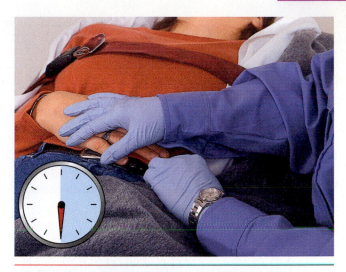

FIGURE 6-1 Count the number of complete breaths taken (one inhalation and one exhalation count as one breath) over a 30-second period.

TABLE 6-1
Normal Respiratory Rates

Patient Age (yr)	Breaths/Minute
Infant (birth–1)	Initially 40–60; rate drops to 30–40 after a few minutes; slows to 20–30 by 1 year
Toddler (1–3)	20–30
Preschooler (3–5)	20–30
School-ager (6–10)	15–30
Adolescent (11–14)	12–20
Young or middle-aged adult (15–64)	12–20
Older adult (65+)	Depends on patient's health

inadequate minute volume occurs if the respirations are shallow and the rate is too slow, as in hypoventilation. Normal breathing is referred to as **eupnea**. Respiratory

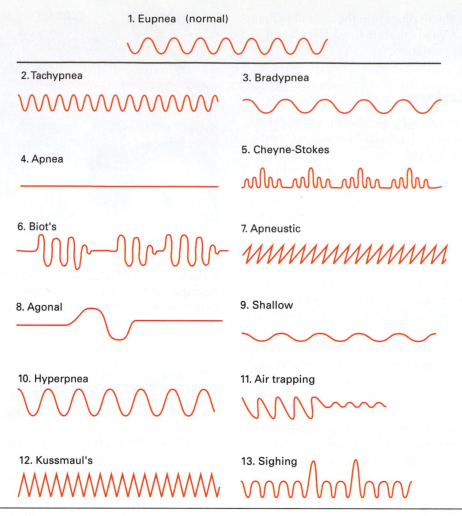

FIGURE 6-2 Respiratory patterns.

patterns are illustrated in Figure 6-2. Some common respiratory patterns and their causes are described in Table 6-2. Examples of descriptions of respiration are "16 and regular," "24 shallow and irregular," and "28 and labored."

Pulse

The pulse is evaluated in terms of rate, regularity, and quality. When counting the pulse, if the rhythm is regular, count for 30 seconds and then multiply by 2 or count for 15 seconds and multiply by 4 (as shown in Figure 6-3). If the pulse rhythm is not regular, count it out for a full minute. During the initial assessment of an unconscious patient, the pulse is taken at the carotid artery for a quick check to determine whether the patient has a pulse. For infants, this quick check is done at the brachial artery in the upper arm. Once it has been determined that the patient actually has a pulse or signs of circulation, the radial pulse is usually measured. The radial

pulse is more useful than a carotid pulse because it gives information about the effectiveness of the distal circulation. In some shock states, the patient may have a palpable carotid pulse, but the distal circulation might be so poor (hypoperfusion) that the radial pulse cannot be palpated. Palpating the radial pulse helps the EMS provider to initially estimate the systolic blood pressure without applying a blood pressure cuff. In an adult, it takes approximately 80 mm Hg of pressure for a radial pulse to be palpable. A femoral pulse takes about 70 mm Hg, and a carotid takes approximately 60 mm Hg.

Rate

In general, adult pulse rates below 60 are called bradycardia and above 100 are called tachycardia. Pulses are often evaluated as a comparison between the central (femoral and carotid) and the peripheral or distal (radial or pedal) pulse. A difference in the rate may be an indication of poor peripheral perfusion. The normal adult and pediatric pulse rates are shown in Table 6-3.

TABLE 6-2
Selected Respiratory Patterns and Their Description and Cause

Pattern	Description and Cause
Cheyne-Stokes	Gradually increasing rate and tidal volume, which increases to a maximum, then gradually decreases; occurs in brain stem injuries
Biot's	Irregular pattern and volume, with intermittent periods of apnea; found in patients with increased intracranial pressure
Agonal	Slow, shallow, irregular respiration; results from brain anoxia
Kussmaul's	Deep gasping respirations, representing hyperventilation, "blowing off" of excess carbon dioxide and compensation for an abnormal accumulation of metabolic acids in the blood; though possible in any patient with metabolic acidosis, best known with diabetic ketoacidosis
Central neurogenic hyperventilation	Deep, rapid, regular respiration; found in patients with increased intracranial pressure

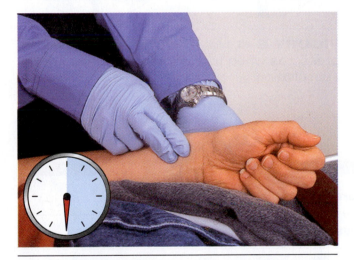

FIGURE 6-3 Taking the radial pulse of an adult patient.

Regularity

When feeling a pulse, try to determine whether it has a regular rhythm or an irregular rhythm. Some EMS providers have become proficient at noting the pulse rhythm and can actually feel the compensatory pause after a premature ventricular contraction (PVC). Any patient who has an irregular heart rhythm or an exceptionally fast or slow heart rate should be placed on an electrocardiogram (ECG) monitor. Some of the procedures that EMS providers perform on patients can slow

TABLE 6-3
Normal Pulse Rates

Patient Age	Beats/Minute
Newborn	120–160
Infant (0–5 months)	90–140
Infant (6–12 months)	80–140
Toddler (1–3 years)	80–130
Preschooler (3–5 years)	80–120
School-ager (6–10 years)	70–110
Adolescent (11–14 years)	60–105
Young or middle-aged adult (15–64 years)	60–100
Older adult (65+ years)	Depends on patient's health

down their pulse rate. Children are especially sensitive to vagal nerve stimulation. The vagus is the tenth cranial nerve, and one of its responsibilities is to slow down the heart rate. (For more on the vagus and other cranial nerves, see Chapter 14.) The vagus can be stimulated by any pressure on the eyes, stimulation of the back of the throat, as might occur during suctioning, and carotid sinus massage (which is no longer routinely used in the field owing to the potential of causing an embolism). The patient can stimulate the vagus nerve without actually planning to do so. For example, bearing down and then quickly relaxing, as when pushing hard to move one's bowels, causes a sudden change in the intrathoracic pressure and causes the vagus nerve to be stimulated. The reason that many cardiac arrest patients are found in the bathroom is probably related to this maneuver. Another example of a patient who may be found to have had a syncopal episode in the bathroom would be a man with a sensitive carotid sinus who stimulates his vagus when shaving his neck and then has a syncope spell. Yet another example would be a person having difficulty putting in contact lenses and passing out from the vagal stimulation.

Quality

The pulse quality is usually described as weak, thready, bounding, or strong. Examples of pulse descriptions are "88 and regular," "110 thready and irregular," "68 and bounding." A weak or thready pulse is difficult to feel and may accompany hypoperfusion. A bounding pulse feels as if it will throw your finger off the artery and is usually an indication of hypertension or heat stroke.

Blood Pressure

The blood pressure (BP) is taken either by auscultation using a stethoscope or by palpation without a stethoscope. Palpation is sometimes a more practical method to use in noisy environments. When taken by auscultation, the BP is reported as a fraction, with the systolic reading over the diastolic reading. The **systolic** is the peak pressure in the arterial system as the left ventricle

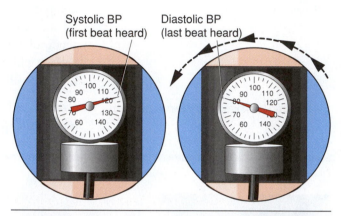

FIGURE 6-4 Note the systolic and diastolic pressures when taking the blood pressure by auscultation.

TABLE 6-4
Normal Blood Pressures

Patient Age (Years)	Blood Pressure (mm Hg)	
	Systolic	Diastolic
Infant and toddler (0–3)	80 + (2 times age in years)	Two-thirds systolic
Preschooler (3–5)	78–116	average 55
School-ager (6–10)	80–122	average 57
Adolescent (11–14)	88–140	average 59
Young and middle-aged adult (15–64)	90–150	60–90
Older adult (65+)	Depends on patient's health	Depends on patient's health

contracts, and the **diastolic** is the residual pressure left in the system as the left ventricle relaxes (Figure 6-4).

Patients who have a history of high blood pressure are said to have hypertension, which is a systolic over 150 mm Hg or a diastolic over 90 mm Hg in an adult patient. Patients who have a history of low blood pressure are said to have hypotension, a systolic under 90 mm Hg and a diastolic under 60 mm Hg. The normal adult and pediatric blood pressures are given in Table 6-4. In documentation of the BP that is taken by palpation, the convention is to write 120/palp or 120/p.

ADDITIONAL VITAL SIGNS OF SIGNIFICANCE

To complete the overall patient assessment picture, the EMS provider considers additional vitals signs such as skin color, temperature, and condition; core body temperature; eye movements; capillary refill; oxygen saturation; and end-tidal carbon dioxide.

Skin Signs

Skin signs are indications of the patient's perfusion. They are assessed with three things in mind: color, temperature, and condition (CTC). The skin color is assessed by looking at the nail beds, lips, and eyes. Abnormal skin color indications are shown in Table 6-5. The skin temperature is routinely taken by the triage nurse on every patient entering an emergency department. In the field, temperature is often estimated by placing the back of the hand on the patient's forehead (Figure 6-5).

Exploring the Web

- Explain why vital signs are key indicators of a patient's health status. Search for information on pulse, respirations, and blood pressure and the effects alterations in these vital signs have on a person's health. Create index cards that list the health factors to consider if you identify alterations in a patient's pulse, respirations, and blood pressure during your assessment. For example:

Blood Pressure

Rate	Indication
High <150 systolic	Hypertension, at risk of stroke or heart attack

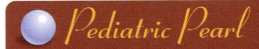

Pediatric Pearl

- Temperature is an important vital sign in the young. Immature thermoregulatory systems make body temperature regulation more critical. Be sure to closely assess the temperature of the pediatric patient.

TABLE 6-5
Abnormal Skin Colors, and Their Indications

Color	Indications
Pale	Constricted blood vessels, blood loss, shock, hypotension, hypothermia, emotional distress
Blue (cyanotic)	Lack of oxygen from inadequate breathing or heart function
Red (flushed)	Heat exposure, hypertension, emotional excitement
Yellow (jaundiced)	Abnormalities of the liver (e.g., hepatitis, liver failure)

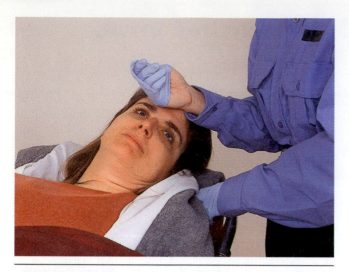

FIGURE 6-5 The EMS provider should use the back of her hand on the patient's forehead to assess the skin temperature.

Normally, the skin should be warm and dry, although the temperature may vary a bit with the ambient air temperature and weather conditions. Abnormal skin temperature and conditions are listed in Table 6-6.

Core Body Temperature

The core body temperature is measured most accurately by using a rectal thermometer. Other devices for temperature measurement, such as oral, axillary, and tym-

panic thermometers, are less accurate. The palpated skin temperature of cool, warm, or hot does not always correspond to a measured core body temperature.

The normal body temperature is 37°C (98.6°F). Critically high temperatures are above 40.6°C (105°F), and critically low body temperatures are below 30°C (86°F). Any patient suspected of having an elevated or decreased temperature should have the core temperature taken with a rectal thermometer. Cases of suspected hypothermia will require a thermometer that reads below 32°C (90°F).

Eye Movements

The pupils should be equally round and 3–5 mm in diameter (Figure 6-6). A difference of more than 1 mm is considered abnormal. The term **anisocoria** means unequal pupils and may indicate a central nervous system disease; however, a small percentage of the popula-

TABLE 6-6
Abnormal Skin Temperature, Conditions, and Potential Causes

Temperature and Condition	Potential Cause
Cool or cold and moist (clammy)	Shock or the body may be losing heat
Cold and dry	Exposure to cold, hypothermia, poor peripheral circulation
Hot and dry or moist	High fever or heat exposure
Piloerection and shivering, chattering teeth, blue lips, and pale skin	Chills, exposure to cold, communicable disease, pain, or fever
Tenting	Dehydration

is shone into one eye, both pupils should constrict as a normal response; this is the **consensual light reflex**.

Accommodation is the ability of the lenses of the eyes to adjust to focus on objects at different distances. The normal position of the eyes as they focus on a distant object is called the **conjugate gaze**. Normally the eyes move apart (**diverge**) as they focus on a distant object. As the object comes closer to the face, the eyes should move toward each other (**converge**) and the pupils should constrict. The patient should first focus on a distant object, then focus on the EMS provider's finger as it is held in front of the face; watch for accommodation and constriction. For recording purposes, the letters **PERRLA** are commonly used to document normal findings with the eyes: *p*upils *e*qually *r*ound, *r*eactive to *l*ight and *a*ccommodation.

Capillary Refill

For years, the capillary refill time has been used as an indicator of distal perfusion. Recently, the efficacy of this test on adults has come into question because many factors, such as a history of heavy smoking, can interfere; thus, it is now recommended that it be used only for infants and children. To obtain the capillary refill time, simply squeeze with the thumb and index finger on the child's finger or toe and then let go (Figure 6-8). It should take less than 2 seconds, or the amount of time it takes to say "capillary refill," for the color to return. A refill time of longer than 2 seconds is considered a positive finding of delayed capillary refill. To check the capillary refill on an infant, press on the bottom of the foot.

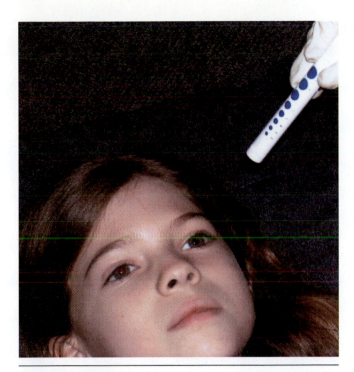

FIGURE 6-6 A pupil gauge, such as the one on this penlight, can be used to note changes in the pupil size.

tion normally has anisocoria (Figure 6-7). The pupils should constrict as a normal reaction to a light source. When the ambient light is bright, the EMS provider uses the hand to shield the patient's eyes, blocking out the light source, and observes for dilation. When a light

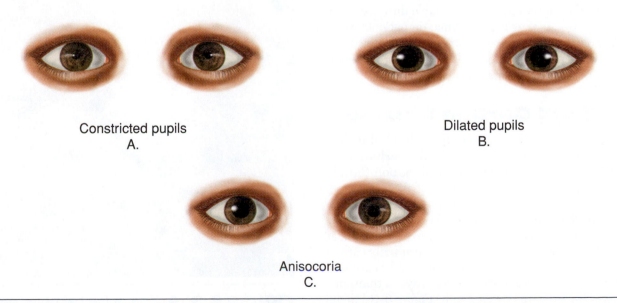

Constricted pupils
A.

Dilated pupils
B.

Anisocoria
C.

FIGURE 6-7 Abnormal pupils may be (**A**) constricted, (**B**) dilated, or (**C**) unequal (anisocoria).

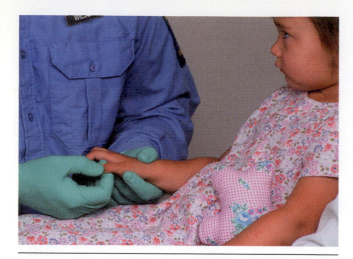

FIGURE 6-8 Capillary refill is an indication of the perfusion in a pediatric patient.

Oxygen Saturation

Pulse oximetry is a noninvasive technique in which an electrode is placed on the patient's fingertip and an infrared light beam measures the oxygen saturation of the blood. The normal reading is 95% or greater. Patients whose saturation values are below 90% usually need supplemental oxygen. Pulse oximeters are small, portable, and easy to apply to the patient's finger, ear, or nose, as shown in Figure 6-9.

The principle of pulse oximetry assumes normal capillary blood flow, normal hemoglobin concentration, and a normal hemoglobin molecule. Any abnormality or alteration of these conditions may lead to false values. Thus, pulse oximetry may not be reliable during cardiac arrest, hypovolemia, or hypothermia; on patients wearing nail polish; or in cases of carbon monoxide poisoning (or any other condition with an altered hemoglobin molecule), shock, or severe anemia.

End-Tidal Carbon Dioxide

Capnography is an assessment of the level of carbon dioxide exhaled by the patient. **End-tidal carbon dioxide (EtCO$_2$)** is the concentration of carbon dioxide (CO$_2$) in the exhaled gas at the end of the exhalation. Some experts say that this is a true measurement of the circulatory status of the organism because adequately functioning cells must not only take in oxygen and sugar but must also excrete waste products, primarily carbon dioxide and water. Therefore, an abnormal level of carbon dioxide indicates a dysfunction in oxygen transport. Although the use of the capnograph (Figure 6-10) in the field has been focused on the monitoring of an endotracheal tube, it can be helpful in many other situations in which circulatory status is in question. There is also a

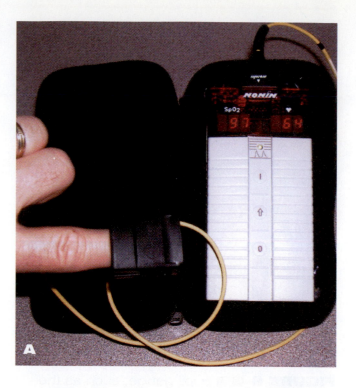

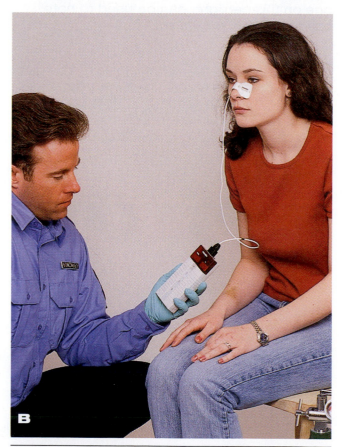

FIGURE 6-9 (A) The pulse oximeter probe is placed on the patient's fingertip. **(B)** If circulation is diminished, a disposable nose probe can be used.

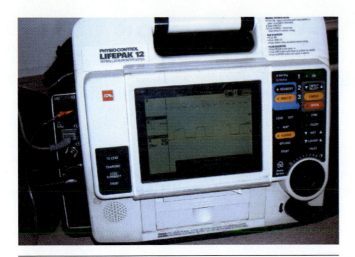

FIGURE 6-10 Capnography is becoming a standard for prehospital care.

device called a **capnometer**, which has a digital readout, but the capnograph usually contains both the digital readout and a waveform, which can be studied and analyzed for various conditions.

The normal capnograph waveform has four phases, as shown in Figure 6-11. The **Fick principle** of oxygen transport states that in order for there to be adequate cellular perfusion four components must be present and working: (1) There must be an adequate amount of oxygen. (2) The patient must have an adequate number of red blood cells because the RBCs carry hemoglobin, which carries the oxygen molecules. (3) The red blood cells must be able to bind and release oxygen. Conditions such as carbon monoxide poisoning and cyanide poisoning inhibit their ability to bind and release oxygen molecules. (4) There needs to be an adequate BP to move the blood to the cells. Shock states affect one or more of the four components of the Fick principle.

A patient can be ventilating but not adequately perfusing. The $EtCO_2$ tells us whether the patient is perfusing. If the cells are releasing carbon dioxide, they are being perfused. The normal reading for the $EtCO_2$ is 35–45 mm Hg, with higher readings defined as **hypercapnia** and lower readings as **hypocapnia**. A very low or nonexistent reading would indicate that the endotracheal tube had been placed into the esophagus instead of the trachea, provided the patient had not just ingested a carbonated beverage. A sudden loss of the waveform (Figure 6-12) could indicate endotracheal tube obstruction, a dislodged endotracheal tube, and respiratory arrest in a nonintubated patient or malfunction of the capnograph. A waveform that shows fast complexes consistently below 30 mm Hg (Figure 6-13) indicates hyperventilation syndrome, a pulmonary embolism, or an overzealous bagging of the patient.

A "shark fin" pattern (Figure 6-14) indicates obstructed exhalation and the loss of the alveolar

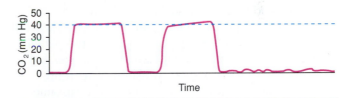

FIGURE 6-12 A sudden loss of the capnograph waveform indicates an absence of carbon dioxide.

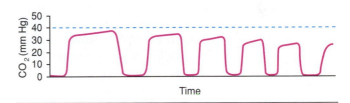

FIGURE 6-13 A fast, narrow capnograph waveform with a low $EtCO_2$ may be due to hyperventilation, pulmonary embolism, or aggressive bagging.

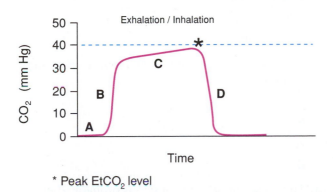

* Peak $EtCO_2$ level

FIGURE 6-11 The four phases of the normal capnography waveform are (**A**) respiratory baseline, (**B**) expiratory upstroke, (**C**) expiratory plateau, and (**D**) inspiratory downstroke.

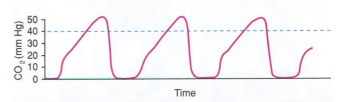

FIGURE 6-14 The "shark fin" pattern in the capnograph waveform indicates a loss of the alveolar plateau, found in conditions involving bronchoconstriction.

plateau. It may be an indication of chronic obstructive pulmonary disease (COPD), asthma, partial upper airway obstruction, or bronchoconstriction.

BASELINE VERSUS SERIAL VITAL SIGNS

The emphasis in obtaining all measurements, such as vital signs, should be on the trends that develop from examining serial sets, as opposed to reacting to a single set of measurements. The first set of a patient's signs that are measured is referred to as the **baseline**. All additional measurements, or **serial vital signs**, are comparisons against the initial, or baseline, measurements. The frequency with which additional sets of vital signs are obtained is determined by the patient's priority. For patients who are considered stable, it is routine to obtain vital signs every 15 minutes in the emergency setting (Figure 6-15). For patients who are considered unstable, the vital signs should be evaluated every 5 minutes, provided there is ample help to do so.

The concept of obtaining serial vital signs is used to establish **trends** (changes over time) in the patient's condition. Two sets of vital signs are a comparison, but at least three sets are needed to establish a trend. For example, the mental status of a patient who sustained a blow to the head might change from alert to verbally responsive to painful response during treatment and transport. Another example would be a continual increase in the pulse rate and decrease in BP of a patient who has sustained considerable blood loss. For both of these patients, it might be hard to establish their priority solely on the basis of one baseline set of vital signs. However, the trends in both examples depict patients who are in serious trouble and need to be considered a high treatment and transportation priority.

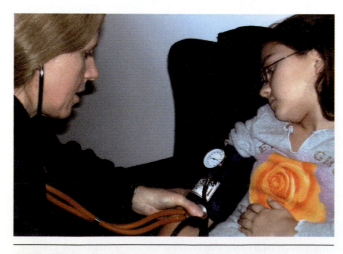

FIGURE 6-15 Obtain multiple sets of vital signs from every patient treated.

CONCLUSION

Assessment of the baseline vital signs and comparisons with the serial vital signs for analysis of trends can provide essential information about the status of the patient's condition. Before reacting to a single set of potentially abnormal vital signs, consider the findings in the overall patient assessment picture. For unstable patients, reassess vital signs every 5 minutes, and for stable patients every 15 minutes. Be sure to document the findings to determine trends. When documenting, note the time the signs were taken.

REVIEW QUESTIONS

1. A subjective finding described by the patient is called a:

   a. sign.

   b. symptom.

   c. presenting problem.

   d. diagnosis.

2. To determine a sign, the EMS provider may have to use a:

   a. penlight.

   b. thermometer.

   c. BP cuff.

   d. all of the above.

3. A sign is considered _____ finding.

   a. a subjective

   b. a terminal

   c. an objective

   d. a disputable

4. It takes _____ sets of vital signs to determine a trend.

   a. 1

   b. 2

   c. 3

   d. 0

5. The most important vital sign is probably the:

   a. glucose level.

   b. pupil reactions.

   c. mental status.

   d. pulse oximeter reading.

6. An adult patient who is alert is oriented to:

   a. person.

   b. place.

   c. day.

   d. all of the above.

7. It usually takes a systolic BP of at least _____ mm Hg for the radial pulse to be felt.

   a. 60

   b. 70

   c. 80

   d. 90

8. Stimulation of the _____ cranial nerve will _____ the heart rate.

   a. fourth; increase

   b. tenth; increase

   c. tenth; slow

   d. fourth; slow

9. The residual pressure left in the cardiovascular system as the left ventricle relaxes is called the:

   a. minute volume.

   b. diastolic.

   c. stroke volume.

   d. systolic.

10. As an object comes closer to the face, the eyes normally:

   a. accommodate.

   b. conjugate.

   c. dilate.

   d. converge.

CRITICAL THINKING QUESTIONS

1. You are caring for a patient with head trauma due to a fall on an ice-covered sidewalk. Your initial assessment finds the patient alert and verbally responsive. Vital signs are good. How often should you reassess vital signs on this patient? Why?

2. Which is more accurate, auscultating blood pressure or palpating blood pressure? Why? What factors may determine which method to use in the field?

3. If an EMS provider fails to acquire a trend in vital signs while managing the care of a patient, is she at legal risk?

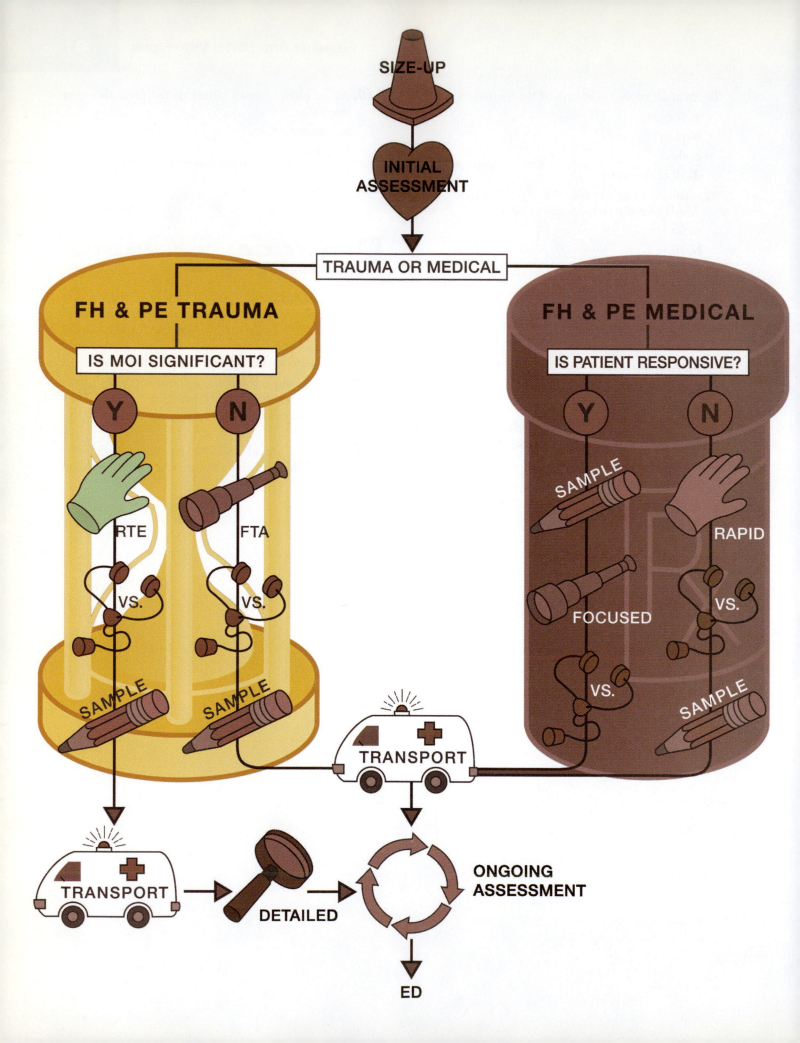

7

The Focused History and Physical Examination of the Trauma Patient

OBJECTIVES

Upon completion of this chapter, the reader should be able to:

- State how the EMS provider's assessment of the mechanism of injury is critical to the management of the trauma patient.
- Discuss how the EMS provider's index of suspicion is related to the mechanism of injury.
- Describe the two major factors affecting injuries to the body.
- Describe how the golden hour and the platinum 10 minutes pertain to the critical trauma patient.
- Explain why the SAMPLE history is important to the management of the critical trauma patient.
- Explain why the EMS provider should complete a full assessment on the minor trauma patient who appears to be intoxicated or to have an altered mental status.

KEY TERMS

altered mental status (AMS)
index of suspicion
rapid trauma examination (RTE)

INTRODUCTION

In the United States, trauma is the leading cause of death for people 1 to 44 years of age, with nearly 150,000 unexpected deaths occurring each year (according to National Safety Council statistics). Motor vehicle crashes, falls, poisonings, burns, and drownings are the top five causes of trauma death. After the EMS provider has conducted a scene size-up to ensure personal safety and an initial assessment of the patient's airway, breathing, and circulation (ABCs), the MOI must be evaluated for all trauma patients. The MOI is important because many MOIs have predictable injury patterns, and getting a complete and accurate history of the incident can help identify as many as 95% of the injuries present. This chapter discusses the importance of the MOI and how the EMS provider can determine whether the MOI is significant or minor.

RECONSIDER THE MECHANISM OF INJURY

Early evaluation of the MOI is the foundation of assessment for the trauma patient. When an EMS provider assesses the MOI at the scene of a trauma, he should suspect that certain injury patterns will be found. From these injury patterns, one can look for specific injuries and anticipate the potential for shock or other problems. This process is referred to as the **index of suspicion**. An example would be to suspect spinal injury in a motor vehicle accident that resulted in a cracked windshield, bent steering wheel, dented dashboard, or side-door intrusion.

The two major factors for injuries are the amount of energy exchanged with the body and the anatomical structures that are involved. (Review the discussion of physics in Chapter 3: Mechanism of Injury or Nature of Illness.) When energy is exchanged with the body, tissue damage occurs. The energy that is absorbed by the body during an impact produces damage to the body. The extent of the damage caused by this energy depends on the specific organs that have been affected. Examples of significant MOIs are:

- Penetrating trauma to the head, neck, chest (Figure 7-1), abdomen, or pelvis
- Major burn injury (Figure 7-2)
- Head trauma with altered mental status
- Car rollover with unrestrained occupants
- Death of an occupant in the same vehicle
- Fall of greater than three times the patient's height
- Evidence of increased intracranial pressure (Figure 7-3)

Decisions made regarding the MOI will determine the course of action in taking a focused history and performing the physical examination, so the finding of a significant MOI is a key decision point in the assessment algorithm. This decision can save the life of a critical trauma patient by minimizing time on the scene and ensuring performance of a rapid trauma assessment, life-saving procedures, and transport of the patient to a

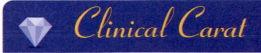

Clinical Carat

- Inappropriate identification of the MOI and incorrect treatment may result in high mortality rates among trauma patients.

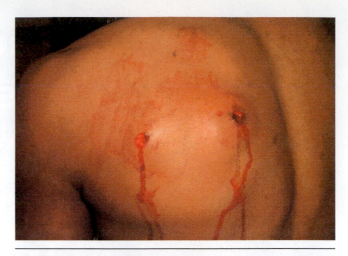

FIGURE 7-1 A gunshot wound in the chest is a potentially life-threatening injury. (Courtesy of Deborah Funk, MD, Albany Medical Center, Albany, NY)

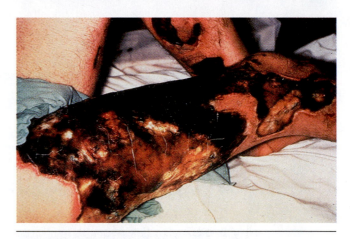

FIGURE 7-2 Full-thickness burns are potentially life threatening. (Courtesy of the Phoenix Society for Burn Survivors, Inc., Phoenix, AZ)

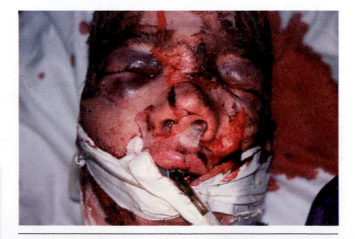

FIGURE 7-3 Significant facial and head injuries are potentially life threatening. (Courtesy of Kevin Reilly, MD, Albany Medical Center, Albany, NY)

Clinical Carat

- The finding of a significant MOI is a key decision point in the assessment algorithm.

facility appropriate for the patient's needs. The EMS provider should ask himself the following questions about the MOI:

- How long ago did this happen?
- What velocity was involved?
- How hard was the surface hit?
- From what height did the patient fall?
- How far did the patient travel before stopping?

SIGNIFICANT TRAUMA

Managing a trauma patient takes practice and discipline by the EMS provider, who must be able to construct a detailed observation of the MOI and assess and manage both the patient and the scene. Distracting injuries such as serious bleeding and obvious fractures can keep more serious injuries (e.g., internal hemorrhage or head injury) from being discovered quickly. The patient, multiple patients, relatives, bystanders, and even other rescuers can distract the EMS provider with yelling, crying, or physical disruptions. Often, minor trauma appears to be significant. To accurately make the distinction between major and minor trauma, the EMS provider follows a systematic approach using the patient assessment algorithm.

For example, EMS providers are called to the local hockey rink for a fall. Upon arrival, they are met by excited fans and security personnel, who lead them onto the ice to a hockey player who was body checked, slammed into the sideboards at a high rate of speed, fell,

Exploring the Web

- Search the Web for additional information on various mechanisms of injury. Create index cards that specify the injury patterns likely to be seen with each mechanism. Include notes on what assessments are needed for each mechanism.

and struck his head. The EMS providers see a bleeding wound from the forehead and an unconscious patient on the ice. This patient has a significant MOI. Now suppose that, on a different day, EMS providers respond to a call to the same hockey rink and are met by one security officer, who leads them to a corner of the sidelines where a hockey player has taken off her right skate and is icing the ankle she twisted when she fell. She did not strike her head or injure any other body part, and she has good pulse, motor, and sensory function distal to the injury site. This patient has an isolated extremity injury without a significant MOI.

For the patient with a significant MOI, time is a critical factor. Barring any need for extrication, the rules of the golden hour and the platinum 10 minutes will apply. The **golden hour** begins at the time of injury, and the goal is to get the patient to the operating room within 1 hour for the best chance of survival (Figure 7-4). The **platinum 10 minutes**, originally from both Montana's and New York State's Critical Trauma Care courses in the mid-1980s, is the goal of a maximum of 10 minutes spent at the scene for a critical trauma patient. The EMS provider needs to conduct the **rapid trauma examination (RTE)**, a systematic, quick examination of the major body sections (head, neck, chest, abdomen, pelvis, back, buttocks, and extremities) for injuries. The RTE is described in detail in Chapter 8.

The EMS provider next needs to obtain baseline vital signs and a SAMPLE history. The SAMPLE history is especially important because the trauma patient with significant MOI may become unconscious or, owing to medication or intubation, may no longer be able to speak for herself. Many critical trauma patients ultimately go to surgery, so the importance of the time of

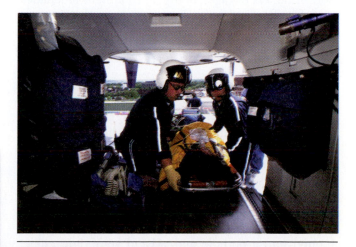

FIGURE 7-4 Helicopter transportation may be needed to get the critical trauma patient into surgery to control internal bleeding within the golden hour.

their last food intake cannot be understated. When a patient is unresponsive throughout assessment and management, the EMS provider can try to quickly obtain information from relatives or bystanders if any are present. Transport should not be delayed, however. Police, fire personnel, or other rescuers can stay and attempt to obtain patient information and then relay that information to the EMS provider during transport or at the emergency department.

The EMS provider should now begin to transport the patient and prepare to do the detailed physical examination as described in Chapter 11. The decision of where to transport the patient depends on the needs of the patient and the capabilities of a trauma center. The criteria for transportation (transport protocols) to a specific level of trauma center are based on the regional structure of the trauma care system and can be found in local protocols. (Review the discussion of trauma centers in Chapter 5.) A short scene time, management of the ABCs, a rapid trauma exam, baseline vitals signs, and a SAMPLE history may all be for naught when a severe trauma patient is transported to an inappropriate facility. Criteria for transport to a level I trauma center include multiple-system trauma, severe burns, and trauma to a pregnant, pediatric, or geriatric patient.

In a critical trauma case, the ongoing assessment is repeated every 5 minutes en route to the hospital until the ambulance arrives at the emergency department. The ongoing assessment includes repeating the initial assessment and reassessing the vital signs and interventions. Personnel, treatment, and transport time will often affect both the detailed physical examination and the ongoing assessment. It would not be unusual for an EMS provider not to have completed the detailed physical examination, for example when transport time is short or he was engaged in urgent treatment modalities or had inadequate help. In these cases, the ongoing assessment of life-threatening injuries takes priority over the detailed physical examination.

MINOR TRAUMA

For the patient in the second hockey rink scenario, the minor trauma case, the examination will be focused on, or aimed at, the injured body part, which in this case is her ankle. It is not necessary to perform a detailed physical examination or to spend time doing a head-to-toe examination on this patient. Think of it this way: if you limped into your doctor's office and said you had stepped into a pothole and twisted your right ankle, would he start palpating your head, neck, chest, pelvis, or arms? Absolutely not! The physician might compare the injured leg with the uninjured leg, but it would not

Clinical Carat

● Any patient who appears to be intoxicated or to have an altered mental status with a potential nonsignificant MOI needs to be evaluated completely.

be necessary to do a detailed examination of the uninjured left leg. The examination would focus on the injured body part. Examples of minor traumatic injuries are isolated extremity injury, minor burns, and small lacerations or abrasions.

The exception to that rule is the patient who appears to be intoxicated or to have an **altered mental status (AMS)** with a potential nonsignificant MOI. Just to be on the safe side, it is strongly recommended that the EMS provider examine this patient fully because the intoxicant or cause of AMS may mask pain elsewhere or the patient may not fully recall what happened to her.

In the focused physical examination of a minor trauma patient, the emphasis is on examination of the injured part for deformity, contusions, abrasions, penetrations or punctures, burns, tenderness, lacerations, and swelling (abbreviated DCAP-BTLS). Range of motion (ROM); neurological status and distal pulse, motor, and sensory (PMS) function; and skin color, temperature, and condition (CTC) are also assessed. Then a treatment plan is developed, which, in the case of our second hockey player, would include splinting the foot in the position of function, with the splint extending above the knee, reassessing distal PMS, and applying cold while transporting the patient to the emergency department. It is also necessary to obtain baseline vital signs and a SAMPLE history from this patient. En route, the EMS provider performs an ongoing assessment every 15 minutes. The ongoing assessment is discussed in detail in Chapter 20.

 ## CONCLUSION

The EMS provider can save the life of a critical trauma patient by minimizing scene time, performing a rapid assessment, performing lifesaving interventions, and transporting the patient to a facility that is appropriate for her needs, such as a trauma center. The decision of whether the MOI is significant will determine the extent of the examination, the speed or priority of transport, and the destination for the patient.

REVIEW QUESTIONS

1. The leading cause of death for people 1 to 44 years of age is:

    a. choking.

    b. heart disease.

    c. trauma.

    d. drowning.

2. Many MOIs have:

    a. little to no value in patient care.

    b. predictable injury patterns.

    c. value in identifying significant illness.

    d. none of the above.

3. Examples of an index of suspicion of significant injury would include:

    a. a bent steering wheel.

    b. a cracked windshield.

    c. side-door intrusion into the vehicle.

    d. all of the above.

4. Of the following, which is not considered an example of a significant MOI?

    a. penetrating injury to the head

    b. car rollover with a restrained occupant

    c. head trauma with altered mental status

    d. death of another occupant in the same vehicle

5. A patient who twisted her ankle but did not strike her head probably has a:

    a. significant MOI.

    b. significant health assessment.

    c. nonsignificant MOI.

    d. nonsignificant illness.

6. The period of time from the time of the injury to surgical intervention should not exceed the:

    a. patient's age in minutes.

    b. golden hour.

    c. platinum 10 minutes.

    d. silver 30 minutes.

7. Why is it important for the EMS provider to obtain the "L" in the SAMPLE history of a trauma patient?

    a. all lacerations must be controlled

    b. the fluid loss can be considerable

    c. many trauma patients will need to go to surgery

    d. none of the above

8. Criteria for transport to a level I trauma center include all of the following except:

    a. a fracture of the humerus.

    b. trauma to a pregnant patient.

    c. multiple-system trauma.

    d. severe burns.

9. Each of the following is a criterion for transport to a level I trauma center except:

    a. multiple-system trauma.

    b. child with a fracture.

    c. severe burns.

    d. geriatric trauma patient.

10. Examples of minor traumatic injury include:

    a. an isolated extremity injury.

    b. minor burns.

    c. small lacerations or abrasions.

    d. all of the above.

CRITICAL THINKING QUESTIONS

1. You arrive on the scene of a motor vehicle accident. The police are directing traffic. A car traveling south on a divided highway crossed the median and struck a car headed north. You have been instructed to care for the two occupants of the northbound car. The car has significant front-end and passenger-side damage. Upon your initial assessment, you determine that the passenger has died. The driver is unconscious and bleeding profusely. What injuries might you expect this patient to have? Is this a significant MOI? What transport decisions should be made about this patient?

2. You are dispatched to the high school soccer field, where a player has been injured. Upon arrival, you see the player sitting on the ground holding his knee and in obvious pain. The player tells you he was kicked behind the knee by another player going for the ball. He said he felt something pop, and the knee is swelling. Is this a significant MOI? What transport decision should be made regarding this patient?

3. Why is the time period between ongoing assessments shorter for a patient with a significant MOI than for a patient without a significant MOI?

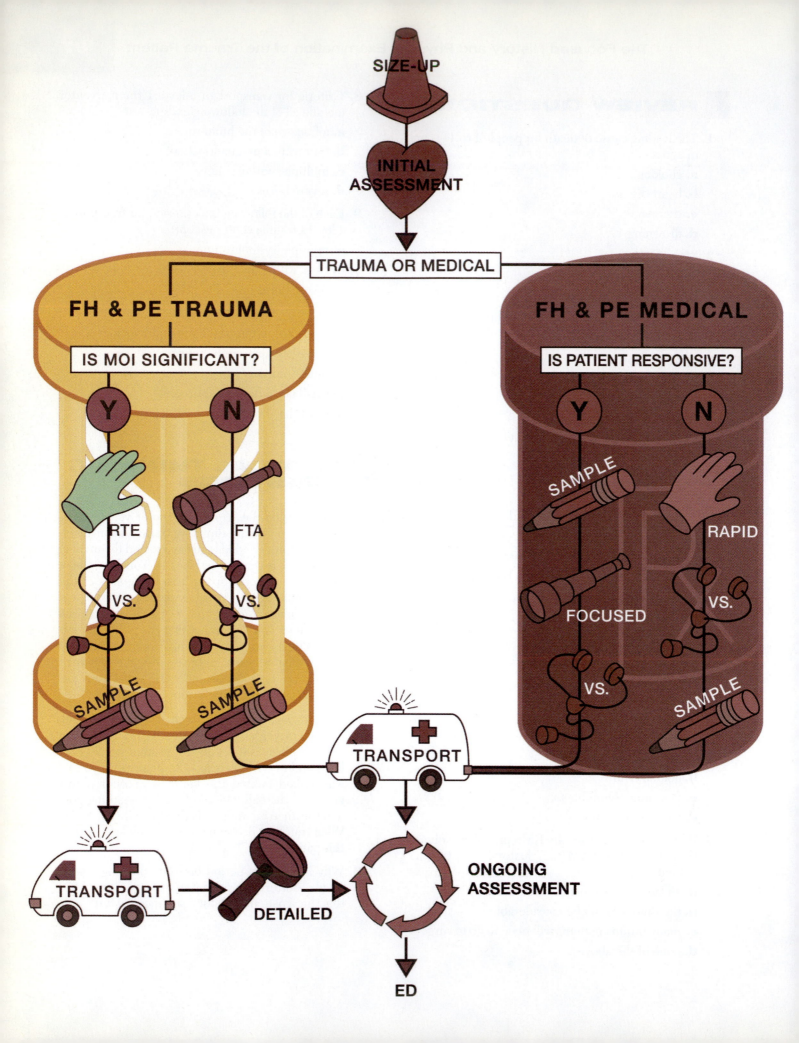

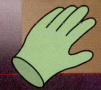

Chapter 8

The Rapid Trauma Examination

OBJECTIVES

- Upon completion of this chapter, the reader should be able to:
- Describe when it is appropriate for the EMS provider to perform the rapid trauma examination.
- Explain the objectives of the rapid trauma examination.
- Describe how DCAP-BTLS is used during the rapid trauma examination.
- Explain the steps of the rapid trauma examination.
- Explain why it is necessary to remove various articles of the patient's clothing during the rapid trauma examination and what considerations should be taken in removing any clothing.
- List several examples of significant mechanisms of injury.

KEY TERMS

crepitation
DCAP-BTLS

rapid trauma examination (RTE)
subcutaneous emphysema

INTRODUCTION

Once the initial assessment has been completed and it has been determined that the patient is a trauma victim who has suffered a significant mechanism of injury (MOI), the rapid trauma examination (RTE) will need to be completed. The RTE needs to be completed quickly—in no more than a few minutes—and, in most instances, performed on the scene before moving the trauma patient. In some rare situations, the patient may have already been moved because of hazards uncovered in the scene size-up or emergency resuscitation if a life threat (e.g., a crushed airway, a tension pneumothorax, flail chest, or uncontrolled external arterial bleeding) was uncovered during the initial assessment. In these circumstances, the patient may have already been moved to the ambulance on a stretcher or long backboard.

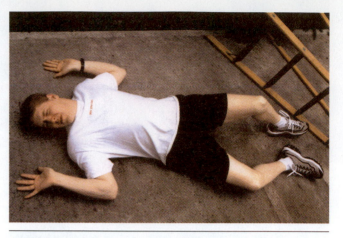

FIGURE 8-1 This patient might have a head, neck, or back injury from a fall.

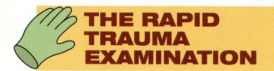

THE RAPID TRAUMA EXAMINATION

The objective of the **rapid trauma examination (RTE)** is to quickly examine the patient's head, neck, chest, abdomen, pelvis, extremities, back, and buttocks. Because of the potential for head, neck, and back injuries in many circumstances (Figure 8-1), two rescuers will be needed. Manual head and neck immobilization in a neutral position should have been started during the initial assessment and will need to be maintained throughout the examination. Stabilization can be accomplished by standing behind the seated patient (Figure 8-2) or kneeling at the head of the supine patient (Figure 8-3) and holding the head still with both hands in the area of the ears. If the airway also needs to be maintained in an open position, a jaw thrust maneuver can be done.

If the patient is responsive, the EMS provider can continue to gather information as the RTE is conducted. If at any time an initial assessment problem (mental status–airway, breathing, circulation; MS-ABC) is uncovered that was overlooked or has resulted from the deterioration of the patient's condition, it is appropriate to manage any life threats and readjust the patient's priority and transportation decision.

During inspection and palpation of the patient during the RTE, the EMS provider will be looking and feeling for injuries and signs of injuries the patient may have sustained. One abbreviation commonly used to remind the EMS provider what to assess in soft tissue is **DCAP-BTLS**. The letters stand for *d*eformities, *c*ontusions, *a*brasions, *p*enetrations or *p*unctures, *b*urns, *t*enderness, *l*acerations, and *s*welling. The EMS provider should also listen or feel for **crepitation** (the sound or sensation of broken bone ends grating on each other) when palpating bones.

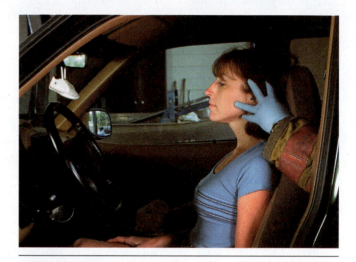

FIGURE 8-2 A patient found in the seated position will need manual stabilization of the head.

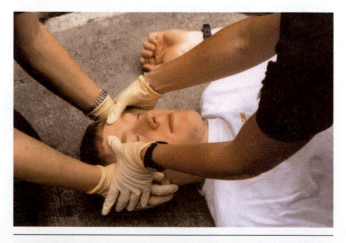

FIGURE 8-3 The head should be manually stabilized throughout the assessment of the head.

STEPS IN THE RAPID TRAUMA EXAMINATION

The rapid trauma examination is performed from head to toe. DCAP-BTLS is assessed in each region. The steps to follow in performance of the RTE are outlined next.

Body Substance Isolation Precautions

Before beginning the RTE, the EMS provider must first take body substance isolation (BSI) precautions. Minimally, the EMS provider should don disposable gloves. A mask and eye shield should be worn if there is any possibility of spurting blood, vomiting, or exposure to oral secretions. If the patient is covered in foreign material or is bleeding profusely, the EMS provider may also choose to don a disposable gown to protect the uniform from getting soiled. If the patient is lying in or seated in glass from a broken window or automobile windshield, lightweight leather gloves may be helpful to prevent cutting the hands on the glass. If the EMS provider suspects there may be drug paraphernalia or weapons hidden on the patient, care should be taken in removing clothing.

Clothing

In conducting the RTE, the EMS provider will have to remove some of the patient's clothing to look at his skin. The environmental conditions should be taken into consideration. If it is pouring rain or snowing, it is most appropriate to carefully move the patient on a long backboard out of the weather into the ambulance.

Be considerate of the patient's privacy and modesty and obtain permission from conscious patients before taking any action. In some situations, especially when a patient needs to be exposed in a very public location, the EMS provider may want to consider using first responders to hold up a blanket to shield the patient from the eyes of curious bystanders.

The Mechanism of Injury

Next, reconsider the mechanism of injury (MOI). Recall from Chapter 4 that the MOI should have been considered during the initial assessment, so life threats have already been identified; there may be a little more time at this point to identify other injuries. If the MOI is significant, proceed with the RTE. Continue manual stabilization of the head and neck; consider requesting advanced life support (ALS) personnel, and reconsider the transportation decision. (Ask, "Do we need to transport the patient now, or can we wait a few more moments?") Reassess the patient's mental status and ABCs and perform the RTE. Examples of common significant MOIs appear in Table 8-1.

Head and Neck

Beginning with the head (Figure 8-2) assess for DCAP-BTLS and crepitation that may be felt when there is a fracture to the skull (frontal, parietal, temporal, or occipital bone), jaw, or facial bones. When palpating the skull, the EMS provider should carefully use the pads of her gloved fingers and should not poke her fingertips into the bones. If there is an open fracture or bone fragment below the skin, poking could drive the fragment into the brain tissue. Take note whether there is any fluid exiting the nose or ears.

Next, while maintaining stabilization of the head, assess the patient's neck (Figure 8-4) for DCAP-BTLS and jugular venous distension (JVD). If the patient is found in the supine position, one would expect there to be blood in the neck veins. Flattened veins may indicate significant blood loss or hypoperfusion. Engorged veins may indicate an obstruction to the blood flow into the heart as might be seen with a tension pneumothorax or a cardiac tamponade. Feel for crepitation in the front and back of the neck. Is the trachea crushed or out of the midline? Is there muscular guarding in the cervical spine? Guarding might indicate an injury to the bones, muscles, or supporting ligaments in the neck. Once assessment of the neck has been completed, one EMS provider places a rigid collar on the patient's neck while the other rescuer continues to manually stabilize the head and neck. The only time it is appropriate to let go of the manual immobilization is after the torso and then the head and neck have been properly affixed to a long backboard, or to the Kendrick Extrication Device (KED) for the seated patient.

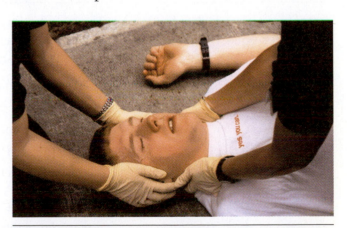

FIGURE 8-4 One EMS provider continues to maintain manual stabilization of the head while the other EMS provider examines the neck. A collar will be placed on the neck after it has been assessed.

TABLE 8-1
Common Significant Mechanisms of Injury

Feet-first impact	The initial injuries are to the heel, with fractures of ankles, legs, and hips. If the patient fell from more than three times his own height or there is an open ankle fracture, also suspect spine fracture (Fx).
Head-first impact	Injuries will be to the cranium and cervical spine. Also consider thoracic aortic disruption if rapid deceleration was involved.
Fall on outstretched arm	Wrist, elbow, and Colles' fracture (dinner fork deformity) are common.
Fall on or twisting of the knee	These injuries are from physical activities that involve planting the foot as the body is still twisting (e.g., basketball, skiing, racquetball). These often injure the supporting structures of the knee.
Up and over the steering column or dashboard	These injuries occur to unrestrained passengers in the front seat of a vehicle. Suspect facial lacerations and head and cervical spine injuries. The secondary injuries are to the chest and abdomen.
Down and under the steering column or dashboard	These injuries occur to unrestrained passengers in the front seat of a vehicle. Suspect knee, femur, hip, pelvis, and spine injuries.
Lateral impact (broadside)	The injury on side of impact is more serious if there is 12 inches or more of vehicular intrusion. This type of impact usually causes fractures of the humerus, ribs, pelvis, and femur on the same side as the impact and may involve a head injury.
Coup-contrecoup head injury	Striking one side of the head often causes blunt trauma to the brain in the area that was struck (coup) as well as the opposite area of the brain (contrecoup).
Penetration by a high-velocity (>200 ft/second) projectile (usually a bullet)	The severity of the injury is determined by what was hit (e.g., the heart, the lung, soft tissue) and by the tumble, fragmentation, and profile of the projectile. Cavitation may also occur. • Tumble. The bullet tumbles or rolls through space, so the side of the bullet, rather than the point, may enter the patient's skin. • Fragmentation. The projectile bursts into many smaller pieces, and each causes its own injury path. • Profile. This is the shape of the bullet. Does it have a solid or a soft hollow nose? Solid-nosed bullets penetrate farther. Soft-nosed bullets mushroom out, causing very large temporary spaces (20 times the diameter of the bullet) and a large permanent injury tract.

(continues)

TABLE 8-1 *(continued)*

	• Cavitation. This is the momentary acceleration of tissue laterally away from the projectile tract, similar to the ripple effect of a rock dropped into a pond. These waves of tissue can cause damage and explain why a bullet near the spine can injure the spine. It also explains why the exit wound is usually larger than the entrance wound.
Injury that suggests other underlying injuries	Examples include a contusion over the left side of the ribs with a possible underlying liver or spleen injury and a steering wheel imprint on the chest with underlying lung contusion.
Physical signs on the vehicle that suggest underlying injuries	Examples include a starred or cracked windshield, a broken steering wheel, a broken dashboard, and intrusion into the side of the passenger compartment.
Physical abuse	These are injuries in areas that are not usually injured (e.g., upper arms, upper back) or that have unusual patterns (e.g., dipping burn lines, cigarette burns, or rope burns from being restrained).
Waddell's triad	This is an injury pattern in children struck by a vehicle. The legs are injured from a direct blow; the chest, from being thrown onto the car hood; and the head, from being thrown clear of the vehicle when the vehicle came to a stop.
Blow to the side of the head	Striking the temples of the cranium with a blunt object causes the middle meningeal artery to bleed and an epidural hematoma to develop.
Ejection from a vehicle	It is estimated that the chances of a spinal injury are up to 1,300 times greater for a person who is thrown clear of the vehicle than for a person who is not.
Partial ejection	Often, the patient's arms and legs are severely crushed when the vehicle rolls and extremities flop outside the vehicle.
Motorcycle accident	Injuries include road rash (serious abrasions) from laying the bike down, two fractured femurs from being propelled over the handlebars, crushing injuries to the leg from sideswiping a vehicle.

Chest

Next examine the chest. It is necessary to expose the chest during this part of the exam, but it is not necessary to remove a female patient's bra. Examine the chest for DCAP-BTLS and feel for crepitation (Figure 8-5).

Sometimes the EMS provider may palpate **subcutaneous emphysema**, air bubbles under the skin from a pneumothorax. Do the two sides of the chest move the same amount in a coordinated manner? Listen to the patient's breath sounds to see whether they are present

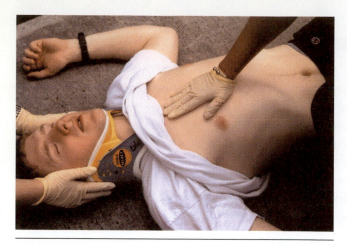

FIGURE 8-5 Assess the ribs and sternum for crepitation while manual stabilization is being maintained.

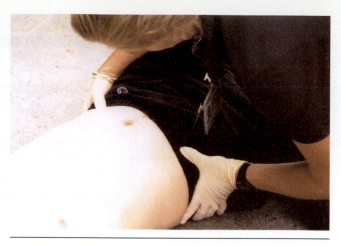

FIGURE 8-7 Examine the pelvis by pressing inward.

on both sides and equal. At this point in the examination of the trauma patient, the EMS provider is listening to a minimum of four locations (in the midclavicular second rib area and then where the anterior axillary line and the nipple level intersect, as shown in Figure 8-5). Be sure to compare the corresponding locations on the right and left sides of the chest. If any life threats are identified, manage them right away. These would include holes in the chest wall, impaled objects, and flail segments.

Abdomen

Examine the patient's abdomen next. The abdomen can be examined without removing underwear. Check for

DCAP-BTLS and note whether the four quadrants of the abdomen are firm, soft, or distended (Figure 8-6). If the patient's abdomen is large and bloated in appearance, it is appropriate to ask, "Is this normal for you?" Now examine the pelvis for DCAP-BTLS and use gentle compression inward (Figure 8-7), then downward (Figure 8-8); place some pressure over the symphysis pubis. Remember, the pelvic structure consists of three bones (the ilium, the ischium, and the symphysis pubis) and the lower spine (sacral and coccygeal) all fused together, so the patient may not complain of any pain until pressure is applied directly to the bones. This part of the examination is important because an unrecognized pelvic injury may be masking some 1,500 ml of blood loss into the pelvic cavity.

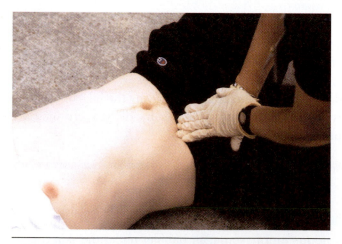

FIGURE 8-6 After listening to lung sounds in at least four locations, examine and palpate all four abdominal quadrants.

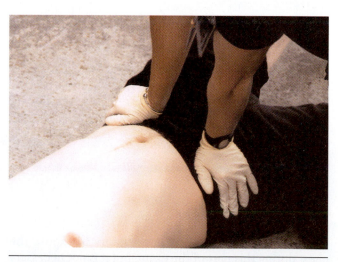

FIGURE 8-8 Examine the pelvis by pressing downward.

Extremities

The four extremities are checked for DCAP-BTLS and the presence of distal pulse, motor, and sensory (PMS) function (Figure 8-9). Sometimes it is hard to find the pulse in the foot; once the EMS provider finds it, it is helpful to make a small mark with a pen on the area it was found. This mark will make reassessment much easier at a later time. When assessing for motor activity, always try to check both hands and both feet at the same time. Simultaneous checking will help determine whether there is a weaker extremity or a weaker side of the body. Test the patient's hands for their grip strength. To determine the motor strength of the legs, have the patient pull his toes up toward his nose and then press down his feet "on the pedals."

Posterior

At this point, the patient's entire front, or anterior, has been assessed. To avoid unnecessary steps, before assessing the posterior have a crew member get the long backboard and place it alongside the patient. Next, at the direction of the rescuer maintaining manual stabilization of the head and neck, carefully logroll the patient toward the rescuer who is performing the RTE (Figure 8-10) and check the back and buttocks for DCAP-BTLS. Consideration of which way to roll the patient must involve the size of the room the patient is in (e.g., tight bathroom), the presence of injuries to one side of the body (e.g., do not roll the patient onto a fractured hip or humerus), the available number of rescuers, and the size of the patient. Once examination of the posterior has been completed, carefully roll the patient back onto the long backboard for immobilization of the torso and then the head and neck. Once the patient is on the board, it is a good idea to cover him with a blanket to help maintain body heat.

After examining the patient, the EMS provider will need to get some serial vital signs, ask the SAMPLE history questions, perform the appropriate interventions (e.g., splinting, bandaging, dealing with pain), and package and transport the patient to the most appropriate facility. Be prepared to document assessment findings and interventions once the patient is delivered to the emergency department.

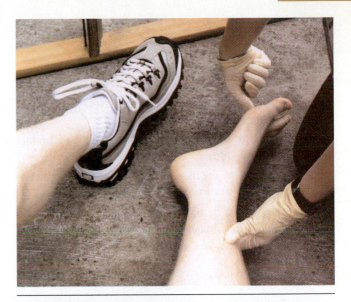

FIGURE 8-9 Remove each shoe, and check the foot for distal pulse, motor, and sensory function.

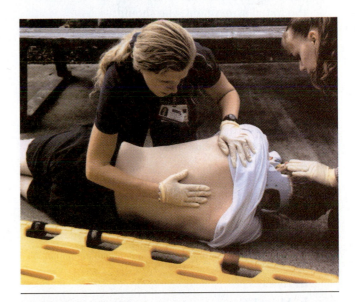

FIGURE 8-10 Roll the patient and examine his back and buttocks while manual stabilization is maintained.

rapid trauma examination (RTE). Because time is often of the essence for the trauma patient with a significant MOI, the EMS provider's ability to conduct the RTE quickly and accurately will be very important in the prehospital care of the patient. It is best to practice this examination often in teams using a mock patient found in various positions (e.g., supine, prone, seated in a car, at the base of a stairwell). Practice helps keep EMS providers prepared for the time patients need them!

▮ CONCLUSION

After performing the patient's initial assessment and determining that the patient has a significant mechanism of injury (MOI), the EMS provider will need to do the

REVIEW QUESTIONS

1. The rapid trauma examination is completed:

   a. before the initial assessment.

   b. immediately after the initial assessment of all trauma patients.

   c. after the initial assessment of a patient who has a significant mechanism of injury.

   d. during the focused history of the responsive medical patient.

2. If the patient sustained a _____ , it may be necessary to complete the rapid trauma examination en route to the hospital.

   a. crushed trachea

   b. tension pneumothorax

   c. flail chest

   d. all of the above

3. If, while conducting the rapid trauma examination, the EMS provider uncovers a life threat missed in the initial assessment, she should:

   a. make a note of it.

   b. immediately manage the lift threat.

   c. continue with the detailed physical examination.

   d. locate the EMS provider who did the initial assessment.

4. The objective of the rapid trauma examination is to quickly examine each of the following except the:

   a. ears.

   b. chest.

   c. posterior.

   d. pelvis.

5. The letters used to remember what to observe when examining soft tissue are:

   a. AVPU.

   b. MS-ABC.

   c. DCAP-BTLS.

   d. OPQRST.

6. In addition to the usual body substance isolation precautions, the EMS provider should consider wearing _____ when assessing a patient in a car crash.

   a. a gown

   b. lightweight leather gloves

   c. a mask

   d. a Tyvek suit

7. If the patient is lying in the snow and apparently very cold, the rapid trauma examination should be:

   a. eliminated.

   b. done at the hospital.

   c. done in the back of the ambulance.

   d. replaced with the detailed physical examination.

8. Guarding of the neck muscles could indicate a:

   a. fracture.

   b. strain.

   c. torn or stretched ligament.

   d. all of the above.

9. The sensation of bubbles under the skin of the chest wall is called:

   a. pulsus paradoxus.

   b. a flail segment.

   c. subcutaneous emphysema

   d. a hematoma.

10. Examination of the four extremities during the rapid trauma examination should always include evaluation of:

    a. the range of motion.

    b. cold sensation.

    c. distal pulse, motor, and sensory function.

    d. all of the above.

CRITICAL THINKING QUESTIONS

1. For which of the following patients would a rapid trauma examination be indicated? Explain why.

   a. 7-year-old with a head injury caused by falling while rollerblading

   b. 65-year-old male patient with chest pain and shortness of breath

   c. 20-year-old with a knee injury due to a fall when skiing

   d. unconscious patient involved in a car crash who was not wearing a seat belt

2. Explain the rationale for always assessing from head to toe during the rapid trauma examination. How long should this assessment take? Explain your answer.

3. You are called to respond to a snowmobile crash in which one rider struck a tree and was thrown from the vehicle. The rider lost consciousness but had regained consciousness before your arrival. Should you conduct a rapid trauma examination on this patient? Why or why not? What are the potential injuries this patient could have suffered? What things other than the patient's injuries do you need to consider?

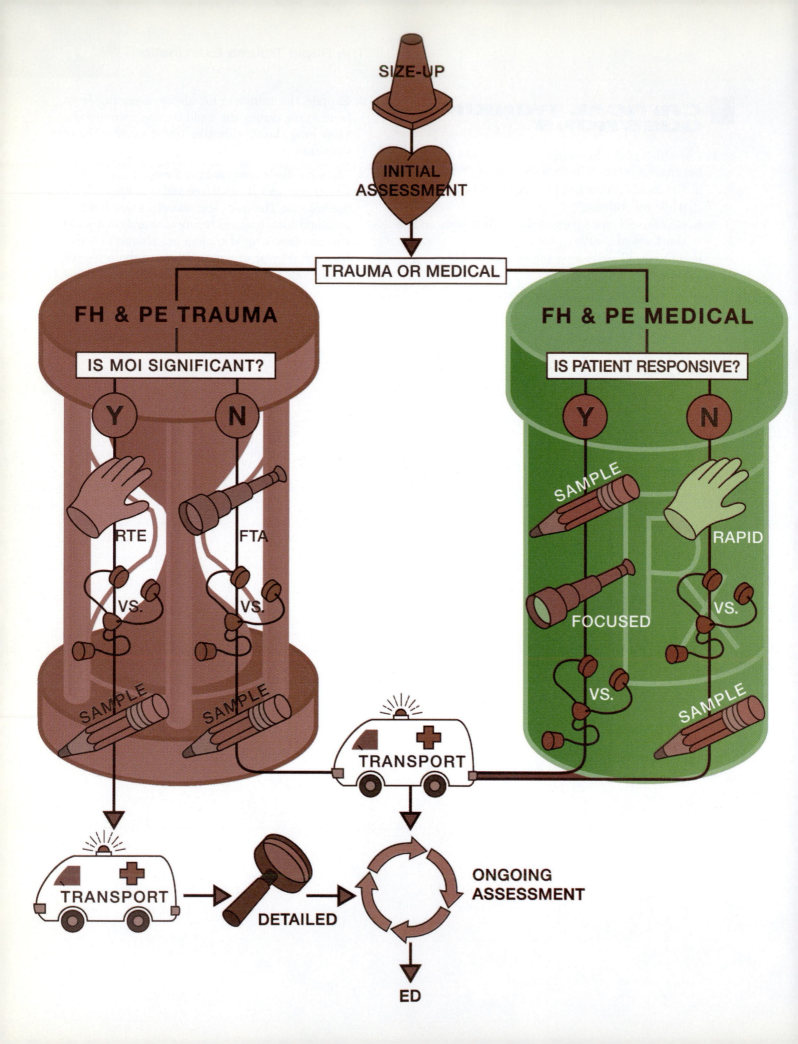

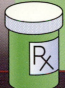

Chapter 9

The Focused History and Physical Examination of the Medical Patient

OBJECTIVES

Upon completion of this chapter, the reader should be able to:

- Describe the approach for obtaining a focused history from a responsive medical patient.
- Explain how the EMS provider might obtain a focused history from an unresponsive patient.
- Provide examples of positive findings and pertinent negatives for a medical patient.
- Describe how the abbreviations OPQRST and SAMPLE are used to obtain essential medical history information.
- List the components of the focused physical examination for the medical patient.
- Describe how the approach to the physical examination of a responsive medical patient differs from the approach for the unresponsive medical patient.

KEY TERMS

chief complaint (CC)
Global Med-Net
history of the present illness (HPI)
Medic Alert Foundation
pertinent negatives

positive findings
post-ictal
rapid physical examination (RPE)
Vial of Life

INTRODUCTION

Following the patient assessment algorithm, note that after the scene size-up and initial assessment have been completed, the next step in the assessment for a medical patient is to focus on the patient's **chief complaint (CC)**. The chief complaint is the reason EMS was called; it is best described in the patient's own words. Examples of a CC include: "I can't breath," "My chest hurts," and " I feel like I am going to pass out." In the absence of trauma and a mechanism of injury (MOI), the patient most often will have a medical complaint. This chapter discusses the focused history and physical examination of the medical patient who is either responsive or unresponsive. A key decision point in the patient assessment algorithm is the determination of the medical patient's responsiveness.

DETERMINING RESPONSIVENESS

In general, if the patient is responsive, the EMS provider is able to talk to the patient and ask questions before beginning a hands-on physical examination. In most cases, it is necessary to establish a rapport and get consent for treatment before touching a patient. Talking to a medical patient before touching builds trust and cooperation and is necessary to demonstrate professionalism and show respect. If the patient is not responsive, the physical examination comes first; the questions for relevant historical information are secondary because most information will probably be obtained from relatives, caretakers, or any bystanders present.

A responsive patient is one who responds to the EMS provider in a manner that is reasonable for the current situation. It does not always have to be a patient who is alert to her name (person), the day of the week (day), and physical location (place). An awake patient who is slightly confused or intoxicated may not be an A on the AVPU (alert, verbally responsive, painful response, unresponsive) scale, but she would be considered responsive. Confusion about the date or her surroundings may be a completely normal finding for a patient with Alzheimer's disease, so she would be considered responsive.

THE FOCUSED HISTORY

Upon determining that the patient's complaint is medical in origin and that the patient is responsive, the EMS provider should begin to obtain the focused history while simultaneously performing the physical examination. Gather a SAMPLE history and the **history of the present illness (HPI)**. Collect the **positive findings**, or the information that is clearly relevant to the chief complaint, as well as the **pertinent negatives**, symptoms the patient does not have that may be relevant to the case. Examples of positive findings and pertinent negatives are listed in Table 9-1.

The Responsive Patient

Two mnemonics, OPQRST and SAMPLE, can help the EMS provider remember what medical history information is essential. The chapters in this book that discuss specific medical complaints (such as respiratory, cardiac, neurological, behavioral, or altered mental status problems) have modified questions tailored within the OPQRST and SAMPLE history to address that particular complaint. Sample pocket cards, with these mnemonics, are helpful to use while interviewing a patient; they appear in Appendix A. Tables 9-2 and 9-3 provide a list of the general questions that are asked of

---

TABLE 9-1
Examples of Positive Findings and Pertinent Negatives

Positive Findings

- Shortness of breath in a patient with chest pain
- Pain on inspiration in a patient with chest pain
- Distension in a patient with abdominal pain
- Constipation in a patient with abdominal pain
- Pain with urination in a patient with flank pain

Pertinent Negatives

- Absence of chest pain in a patient with shortness of breath
- Lack of sputum (nonproductive cough) in a patient with an upper respiratory infection
- Normal bowel movement in a patient with abdominal pain
- No loss of consciousness
- No prolonged bed rest or immobilization in a patient with shortness of breath

TABLE 9-2
OPQRST Questions for the Medical Patient

Information	Questions
Onset	When did (the symptom/chief complaint) begin?
Provocation	What seems to provoke it (e.g., exercise, fever)?
Quality	How would you describe the sensation (e.g., crushing, stabbing, pressure)?
Region, **r**adiation, **r**elief, **r**ecurrence	Where is the pain, and where does it go (e.g., chest pain that reaches into the neck, jaw, or left arm)? Have you tried anything to get relief, such as take medication or rest? Has this type of event ever happened before? If it has, when and what was done at that time?
Severity	How would you rate this experience on a scale of 1 to 10 (with 1 being a minor pain and 10 the worst pain ever experienced)?
Time	How long has the symptom been present (e.g., since last night, a half hour ago)?

Note: If the patient is not responsive, a bystander or family member may have answers to some of these questions.

TABLE 9-3
SAMPLE Questions for the Medical Patient

Information	Questions
Symptoms	Describe what you are feeling (e.g., nausea, vomiting, blurred vision, or dizziness).
Allergies	Are you allergic to anything (e.g., drugs, insects, plants, foods)?
Medications	Are you currently taking any medications (e.g., Lasix, potassium, digoxin, insulin, penicillin)? Have you used any home remedies (e.g., herbal, over-the-counter, or homeopathic medications)?
Pertinent past medical history	Has anything like this ever happened before? Do you have any medical problems you are currently being seen for?
Last oral intake	When did you last have anything to eat or drink (i.e., meal, drinks, or medications)?
Events	What led up to this episode (e.g., emotional or physical stress)?

Note: If the patient is not responsive, a bystander or family member may have answers to some of these questions.

TABLE 9-4:
Relevant Past Medical History

Recent surgery

Recent illness

Recent trauma

Recent period of immobilization (e.g., long-bone cast, confined to bed)

Any hospitalization

Change in mental status

Change in physical ability

Change in medications

Change in daily routine or activities

Family history (similar to the current event, epilepsy, diabetes)

Disabilities or handicaps

Blood transfusions

Medical devices (e.g., pacemaker)

the responsive medical patient for the OPQRST and SAMPLE history. Table 9-4 lists the type of medical history information that is relevant.

The Unresponsive Patient

When a medical patient is not responsive, the EMS provider begins the focused history and physical examination by touching then talking. That is to say, the physical examination is done before questions are asked of family or bystanders. Remember, this point in the assessment algorithm is reached only after the life threats have already been managed. Although the patient is not responsive, she does have an open airway, is not in respiratory distress, and has adequate circulation.

Consider the patient experiencing a seizure on a carpeted floor. Bystanders moved furniture away while waiting for EMS to arrive. EMS providers moved the patient into the recovery position during the initial

assessment to allow fluid to drain, and now the patient is **post-ictal** (the third phase of a seizure, during which the patient is extremely exhausted and confused while slowly regaining consciousness). The patient remains unresponsive, so the EMS provider will perform a **rapid physical examination (RPE)** to ensure that there are no injuries and to listen to the appropriate body regions. The RPE involves examining the head, neck, chest, abdomen, pelvis, back, buttocks, and extremities; this procedure is described in detail in Chapter 10.

The RPE is similar to the rapid trauma examination (RTE) but is conducted on medical patients for whom trauma is not suspected or has not been identified during the initial assessment. Once the RPE has been completed, obtain a set of baseline vital signs (respiration, pulse, blood pressure, skin signs [CTC]) and reevaluate the mental status. If there is sufficient assistance from other EMS providers, the RPE, baseline vital sign measurements, and reevaluation of mental status can be done simultaneously. Consider the need for other means of evaluating the patient's condition if necessary, such as pulse oximetry, capnography, temperature reading, electrocardiography, and blood sugar testing.

Speaking with Family and Bystanders

For the unresponsive patient or the patient who is unable to communicate, the SAMPLE history is obtained by interviewing the family, caretakers, or bystanders and by incorporating clues that may help tell the story for the patient. Ask the relatives or caretakers about the patient's general health status and any major conditions for which she is under a doctor's care. Ask whether they can provide a list of the patient's medications or the actual medication containers. Ask about any advance directives or patient wishes when appropriate (e.g., if the patient has a preexisting terminal condition or a life-threatening injury). Take a moment to explain to the relatives what is happening, and consider taking one family member on the transport to provide any additional information.

Looking for Clues

A number of information sources may be found on patients in the field. Some wear necklaces or bracelets; others use smart cards or computer chips, carry wallet cards, or keep a Vial of Life in the refrigerator. These devices are usually found during the initial assessment or the RPE. Take a quick look at the medical identification device to see whether it offers any information pertinent to today's problem.

Of all the devices available, the most common ones are the necklaces and bracelets available from the **Medic Alert Foundation** (http://www.medicalert.org), which maintains a 24-hour emergency response center (Figure 9-1). The toll-free Medic Alert phone number (1-800-629-3780) specifically for EMS providers is answered by a trained representative. The representative can fax copies of the patient's medical data and can assist with language translation services, via AT&T's translation service. Conditions noted on these devices include allergies, diabetes, hypertension, blood-clotting disorders, seizure disorders, Alzheimer's disease, and implanted devices (e.g., automatic internal cardiac defibrillator, pacemakers).

Another service is the **Global Med-Net**, to which patients may subscribe. The patient wears a symbol that is supplied as a sticker (Figure 9-2) to put on a key chain or wallet. On calling the toll-free phone number (1-800-650-0409) with the patient's membership identification number, EMS providers can receive the patient's complete medical profile.

Look for medication containers because they can tell a lot about a patient. For example, the EMS provider can learn whether patients have a cardiac or respiratory history, hypertension, or diabetes. The EMS provider can also determine whether the patient is compliant with medications by checking the date and amount of prescription fill and counting the remaining amount. Many EMS providers carry a pocket medication reference so they can check medications found in the field.

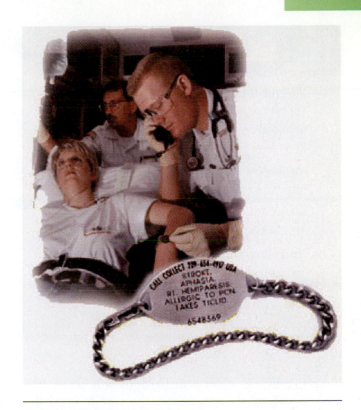

FIGURE 9-1 Always check for a Medic Alert bracelet or necklace on the patient. (Courtesy of Medic Alert Foundation, Turlock, CA)

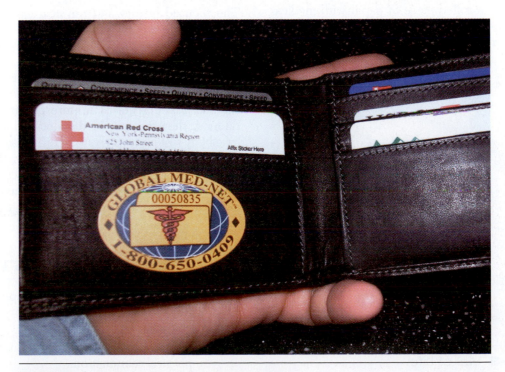

FIGURE 9-2 Global Med-Net sticker.

If such a reference is not available or there is not enough time to look up the medications, be sure to bring the medications or a list of all medications and doses to the hospital. If the medication is not in plain view, have a crew member look in the medicine cabinet, bedroom, or kitchen. Be sure to look in the refrigerator. There you may find insulin for the diabetic patient, other medications requiring refrigeration, or a Vial of Life. The **Vial of Life** is a small plastic container similar to a medicine bottle. It contains a rolled piece of paper with medical information about the patient (Figure 9-3). Patients are told to keep their Vial of Life in the refrigerator.

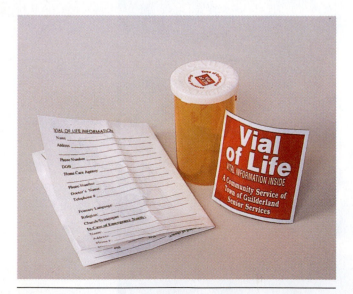

FIGURE 9-3 Vial of Life.

THE FOCUSED PHYSICAL EXAMINATION

The focused physical examination does just what its name implies; it focuses on the specific body system that needs to be examined on the basis of the patient's chief complaint and the findings of the initial assessment. Skill sheets are provided in Appendix D for exams based on specific medical complaints. The various focused physical examinations used by EMS providers include the respiratory, cardiac, neurological, behavioral, abdominal, geriatric, and pediatric exams. The components of the focused physical examination are guided by the chief complaint, the findings of the initial assessment, and the findings discovered during the exam. For example, when a patient has a chief complaint of chest pain, after the initial assessment has been conducted, the examination will focus on the cardiac system. If, while listening to breath sounds, the EMS provider detects wheezing in the bases of the lungs, he will modify the focused physical examination to also include the respiratory system. Thus, the focused physical examination is a dynamic process that will often cover multiple body systems. For example, in the assessment of a patient with abdominal pain, the exam includes evaluation of the skin and of the musculoskeletal, circulatory, and gastrointestinal systems.

CONCLUSION

The focused history and physical examination of the medical patient follows one of two paths, depending on decisions made in the patient assessment algorithm. The determination of whether the patient is responsive or unresponsive will dictate the order of assessment steps. The examination may be general and rapid, owing to the potential urgency of an unresponsive patient's condition or the exam may be detailed and focused on specific body systems, which are determined on the basis of the interview or focused history with the responsive patient. During transport, all medical patients are reevaluated as part of their ongoing assessment. The ongoing assessment is covered in Chapter 20.

REVIEW QUESTIONS

1. When the medical patient is responsive, in what order should the focused history and physical examination be done?

   a. First get the baseline vital signs, and then do a physical examination.

b. Interview the patient, and then get the vital signs and do a physical examination.

c. Do a physical examination, and then ask the SAMPLE history questions.

d. none of the above

2. If the patient is unresponsive, the SAMPLE history may be obtained from:

a. relatives.

b. bystanders.

c. caretakers.

d. all of the above.

3. A patient who just struck his head is asked by the EMS provider, "Did you pass out?" The EMS provider is looking for:

a. a pertinent negative.

b. an obvious neurological deficit.

c. an irregularity in the cranial nerves.

d. a positive finding.

4. What does the *P* in OPQRST stand for?

a. prior to treatment

b. provocation

c. previous intervention

d. pertinent negative

5. What does the *R* in OPQRST stand for?

a. radiation

b. referral

c. relief

d. all of the above

6. When determining the severity of pain, the EMS provider should:

a. develop the pain scale and fit the patient into it.

b. ask the patient to describe the pain as high or low priority.

c. ask the patient to rate the pain on a scale of 1 to 10.

d. assign a 5 to all patients who do not look as if their pain is severe.

7. Why does the EMS provider ask the patient about allergies?

a. Treatment may include medication administration.

b. The patient may be experiencing an allergic reaction.

c. An allergy may be relevant to the patient's symptoms.

d. all of the above

8. After completing the initial assessment on an unresponsive medical patient, the EMS provider should:

a. do the physical examination.

b. interview the family.

c. take a full set of vital signs.

d. do the rapid trauma examination and transport immediately.

9. If a patient is not responsive, the EMS provider should search for a bracelet, anklet, or necklace known as a:

a. Global Med-Net.

b. Vial of Life.

c. Medic Alert.

d. advance directive.

10. If an EMS provider is searching in a patient's refrigerator, he is most likely looking for a:

a. Global Med-Net.

b. Vial of Life.

c. Medic Alert.

d. supply of cardiac medication.

CRITICAL THINKING QUESTIONS

1. You are one of two EMS providers from your service area who are scheduled to speak at a senior citizens center on medical emergencies. What information can you discuss with this group that will enable you to better serve them in the event they have a medical emergency and need to call EMS? Explain the importance of your having access to medical information from your point of view and how it will help them in an emergency. Distribute handouts that have contact information for the various organizations that store medical information mentioned in this chapter.

2. You are called to a residence for a patient who appears to be having a severe allergic reaction. She does not live at the residence but was visiting. She started breaking out in hives and experienced facial swelling after eating a seafood dinner. What questions should you ask this patient and the bystanders? If the patient is unable to provide information on her medical history, how might you be able to get that information?

3. Consider the patient having chest pain. What positive findings might you expect? What pertinent negatives should you be alert to? What questions are relevant to this patient?

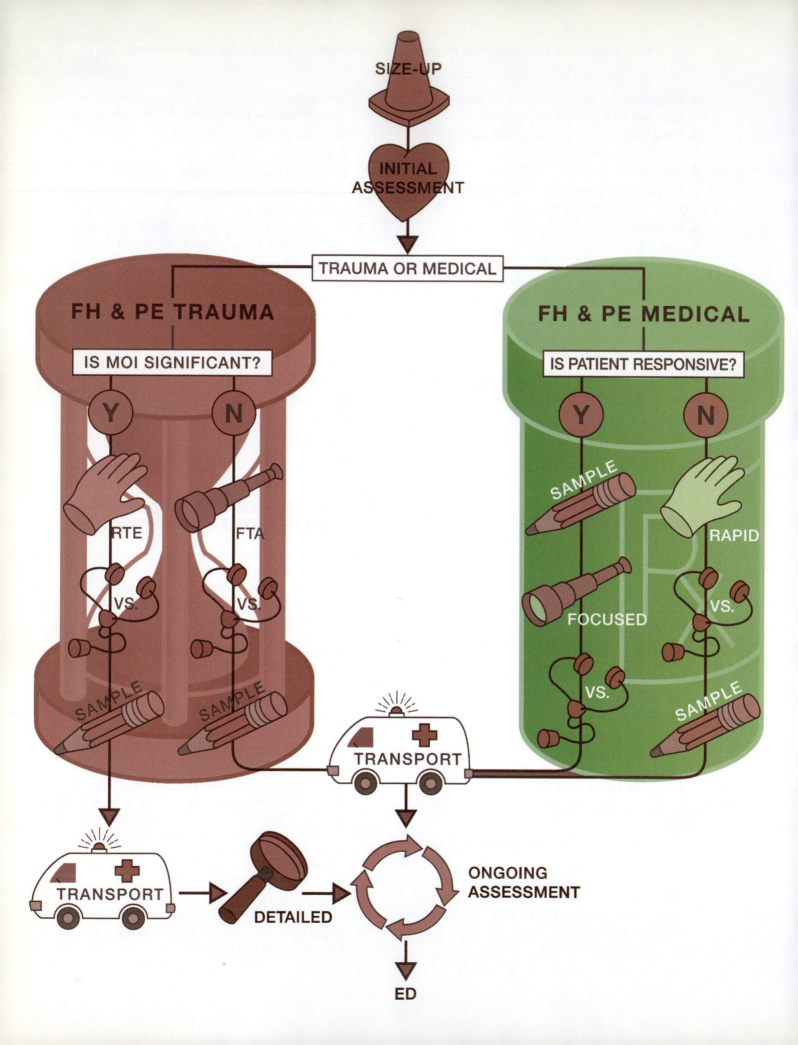

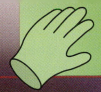

Chapter 10

The Rapid Physical Examination

OBJECTIVES

Upon completion of this chapter, the reader should be able to:

- Describe when the EMS provider would perform the rapid physical examination.
- List factors to consider when removing patient clothing as part of the rapid physical examination.
- Describe the sequence for evaluation of body parts or regions as part of the rapid physical examination.
- Identify people from whom the EMS provider can gather pertinent information when a patient is unable to provide it.
- Describe how the EMS provider can best gain proficiency in conducting the rapid physical examination quickly and accurately.

KEY TERMS

guarding

rapid physical examination (RPE)

symphysis pubis

syncopal episode

INTRODUCTION

Once the initial assessment has been completed and it has been determined that the patient has a medical problem and is not responsive, a rapid physical examination will need to be completed. The **rapid physical examination (RPE)** needs to be completed quickly and, in most instances, performed on the scene before moving the medical patient. In some rare situations, the patient may have already been moved to the ambulance owing to hazards uncovered in the scene size-up or emergency treatment of life threats uncovered during the initial assessment (e.g., crushing chest pain combined with hypotension, flagrant pulmonary edema, or a compromised airway).

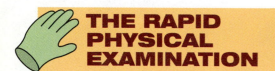

THE RAPID PHYSICAL EXAMINATION

The objective of the RPE is to quickly and systematically examine the patient's head, neck, chest, abdomen, pelvis, extremities, back, and buttocks. It is similar to the rapid trauma examination (RTE) that is conducted on a trauma patient with a significant mechanism of injury (MOI) but is called a physical examination when the chief complaint is medical in nature. Both trauma and nonresponsive medical patients need to be quickly examined for injuries. One difference between the two assessments is that all trauma patients with a significant MOI are given an RTE, and medical patients who are not responsive are given an RPE.

One example of a medical patient who needs to be examined for injuries would be a patient who had a stroke and was found on the floor. This patient may have been injured while falling to the floor. Another example would be the diabetic patient who has bruises that he is unaware of owing to his neuropathy. Yet another example would be the child who sustains a lacerated tongue or bloody nose during a seizure (Figure 10-1). The rapid physical examination would be conducted also for a patient who, during a **syncopal episode**, fell from the couch onto the carpeted floor. Another example would be the office worker who had a seizure and whose coworkers helped the patient to the floor. In some of these examples, there might be no obvious injury, but in all of them there could be a hidden injury. For example, the patient who had a syncopal episode and fell onto a carpeted floor might not have hit his head on the nearby coffee table but might have sustained an extremity injury.

If the EMS provider has any reason to suspect there is an injury to the neck or back, spinal immobilization will need to be manually maintained throughout the

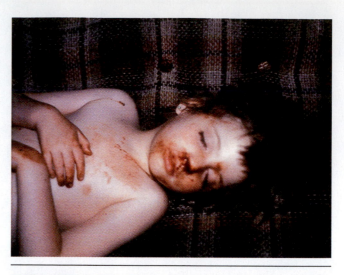

FIGURE 10-1 This child hit her face during seizure activity, sustaining a laceration and a bloody nose.

examination by assigning one rescuer to manually stabilize the head and neck in a neutral position. Manual stabilization can be accomplished by kneeling at the head of the supine patient or behind the seated patient and holding the head still with both hands in the area of the ears. If the airway needs to be maintained in an open position because the patient cannot do this himself, a jaw thrust maneuver can be used.

If at any time during the RPE an initial assessment problem (MS-ABC) is uncovered that resulted from deterioration of the patient's condition, it is appropriate to manage any life threats and readjust the patient's priority and transportation decision.

During the RPE, the EMS provider inspects and palpates the patient from head to toe (from toe to head with small children), looking and feeling for abnormal findings and signs of injury. The mnemonic that is used to remember what the EMS provider is assessing as the RPE is conducted is DCAP-BTLS. Recall from Chapter 8 that this stands for deformity, contusions, abrasions, penetrations or punctures, burns, tenderness, lacerations, and swelling. There are also some body regions in which it is appropriate to listen or feel for crepitation, which is the sound or sensation of broken bone ends grating on each other. Some conditions that are traditionally thought of as a traumatic injury can also be found on the patient presenting with a medical complaint. An example would be the patient who complains of dyspnea and sharp pleuritic chest pain that came on suddenly. When examined, this patient could have subcutaneous emphysema and absent lung sounds on one side from a spontaneous pneumothorax.

STEPS IN THE RAPID PHYSICAL EXAMINATION

To begin the RPE, first take body substance isolation (BSI) precautions. Don disposable gloves; a mask and eye shield should be worn if there is any possibility of spurting blood, a productive cough, vomiting, or exposure to any body secretions. If the patient is covered in foreign material, has lost control of his bladder or bowels, or is bleeding profusely, consider wearing a disposable gown to protect the uniform from getting soiled. Seizure patients often bite their tongue and may have some blood mixed with oral secretions. Sometimes patients who have just had a seizure or medical incident lose control of their bladder or bowels, so be prepared, not surprised, upon reaching underneath the patient. If you suspect there may be drug paraphernalia or weapons hidden on the patient, be careful when removing clothing to avoid being cut by or stuck with an infected sharp.

In conducting the RPE, the EMS provider will have to remove some of the patient's clothing to look at the skin. The environmental conditions (e.g., ski slope, rain, direct baking sunlight) should be taken into consideration. If it is pouring rain or snowing, it is most appropriate to carefully move the patient on a long backboard out of the weather into the back of the ambulance to conduct the RPE.

Be considerate of the patient's privacy and modesty; the patient may regain consciousness and become scared, confused, or embarrassed. In some situations, especially when a patient needs to be exposed in a public location (e.g., church, restaurant, sports arena), consider using first responders to hold up a blanket to shield the patient from the eyes of curious bystanders and the media's cameras.

Nature of the Illness

Next reconsider the nature of the illness (NOI) and the potential for a mechanism of injury (MOI). There may be a little more time at this point because the life threats were attended to in the initial assessment. Ask yourself, "Could this have been a combination of a medical problem and trauma?" For example, a seizing patient might have hit his head while convulsing or an elderly woman who fainted might have lacerations and bleeding from falling and striking an object.

Head and Neck

The RPE involves sequentially evaluating each of the following body parts or regions: head, neck, chest, abdomen, pelvis, extremities, and posterior. First assess the head for DCAP-BTLS and crepitation, which may be felt when there is a fracture to the skull, jaw, or facial bones. When palpating the skull, carefully use the pads of your gloved fingers and do not poke your fingertips into the bones. If there is an open fracture or if there are bone fragments below the skin, poking with your fingertips could drive them into the brain tissue. Pay attention to the color of the patient's face; it may give an indication of high blood pressure or inadequate perfusion.

Next, examine the patient's neck by assessing for DCAP-BTLS and jugular venous distension. When the patient is found in the supine position, one would expect there to be blood in the neck veins. Flattened veins may indicate blood loss or hypoperfusion. Engorged veins (Figure 10-2) may indicate an obstruction to the blood flow into the heart, as might be seen with a tension pneumothorax, cardiac tamponade, or right-sided heart failure. Feel for crepitation in the front and back of the neck. Is the trachea crushed or out of midline? Is there muscular **guarding** (a particular position to protect a body part from pain) in the cervical spine, possibly indicating an injury to the bones, muscles, or supporting ligaments in the neck? Upon completion of the assessment of the neck, apply a rigid collar and make sure that one rescuer continues to manually stabilize the head and neck if there is any indication of a neck injury. The only time it is appropriate to discontinue the manual immobilization is after the torso, head, and neck have been properly affixed to a long backboard. If bystanders' descriptions of how the patient ended up on the floor leave no doubt that there was no injury to the patient's

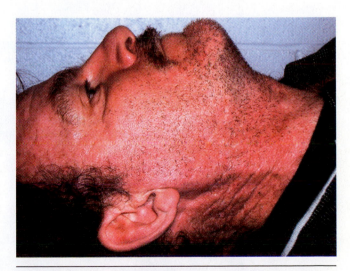

FIGURE 10-2 Engorged or distended neck veins can indicate obstruction to the flow of blood into the right side of the heart.

neck or back, then it may be appropriate to discontinue the neck immobilization and use the stretcher rather than the long backboard. For the medical patient who was found in bed, note whether there is swelling of the neck as could be found in a patient who is having an allergic reaction.

Chest

Next, expose the chest to assess it. (It is not necessary to remove a woman's bra.) Examine the chest for DCAP-BTLS and feel for crepitation. Do the two sides of the chest move the same amount in a coordinated manner? Take a quick listen to the patient's breath sounds to see whether they are present on both sides and equal. At this point in the examination of the medical patient, the EMS provider is listening in the second intercostal space in the midclavicular area (Figure 10-3) and where the anterior axillary line and the nipple level intersect. Be sure to compare the location on the right side of the chest with the corresponding location on the left side of the chest. If any previously undetected life threats are found, deal with them right away. These would include holes in the chest wall, impaled objects, and unstable or flail segments. Note any obvious rash possible from an allergic reaction as well as evidence of swelling or puffiness under the skin, such as subcutaneous emphysema. Take note of any obvious scars, which may be helpful clues to the patient's past medical history (e.g., a CABG scar indicates a significant cardiac history).

Abdomen

Examine the patient's abdomen next. This examination can be done without removing underwear. Check for DCAP-BTLS and note if the four quadrants of the abdomen are firm, soft, or distended. If the patient's abdomen is large and bloated in appearance, consider asking the family or caretaker whether this is the patient's normal belly size. Also look for a pulsing mass, which could indicate the patient has dissecting abdominal aortic aneurysm. Take note of any scars that could be helpful clues to the cause of pain in the abdomen, such as those from prior surgery.

Pelvis

Now examine the pelvis for DCAP-BTLS, using gentle compression inward and downward, and place some pressure over the **symphysis pubis** (the area where the two pubic bones grow together). Remember, the pelvic structure consists of three bones (the ilium, the ischium, and the pubis) and the lower spine (sacrum and coccyx) all fused together, so the patient may not display any sensation of pain until pressure is applied to the bone structure. This part of the examination is important because an unrecognized pelvic injury may result in 1,500 ml of blood loss into the pelvic cavity.

Extremities

Next, examine the four extremities, checking for DCAP-BTLS and the presence of distal pulse, motor, and sen-

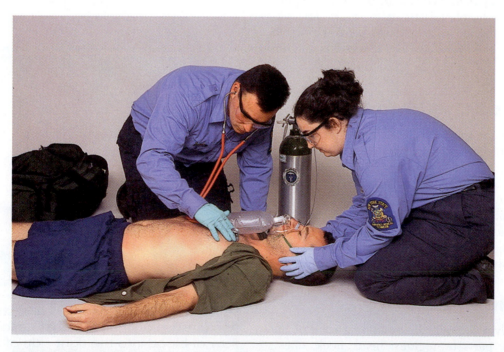

FIGURE 10-3 Breath sounds should be assessed bilaterally.

sory (PMS) function. Sometimes it is hard to find the pulse in the foot, so once it has been found make a small mark with a pen at the point it was found. This mark will make reassessment much easier at a later time. Assess reflexes to evaluate nervous control; test for Babinski's response in each foot, and test for a response to pain in the upper extremities.

If the patient begins to regain consciousness, test for equal grip strength. When assessing for motor activity, always try to check both hands at the same time. Do the same with both feet. Simultaneous checking will help determine whether there is a weaker extremity or a weaker side of the body. To determine the motor strength of the legs, ask the patient to pull up his toes toward his nose and then to press his feet down "on the pedals."

Posterior

At this point, the patient's entire front, or anterior, has been assessed. To avoid unnecessary steps when a neck or back injury is suspected, before assessing the posterior have a crew member get the long backboard and place it alongside the patient. Next, at the direction of the rescuer maintaining manual stabilization of the head and neck, carefully logroll the patient toward you and check the back and buttocks for DCAP-BTLS. Consideration for which way to roll the patient must involve the size of the room (e.g., tight bathroom), the presence of injuries to one side of the body (e.g., do not roll the patient onto a fractured hip or humerus), the available number of rescuers, and the size of the patient.

Once the posterior examination has been completed, carefully roll the patient onto the long backboard for immobilization of the torso and then the head and neck. If there is no potential for neck or spine injury, the patient can be lifted onto the stretcher and placed in the recovery position so that fluids can drain from the mouth. Once the patient is on the board or stretcher, it is a good idea to cover him with a blanket to help maintain body heat.

After examining the patient, obtain serial vital signs. If the patient has not yet regained consciousness, ask the family, caretaker, or bystanders (Figure 10-4) the SAMPLE history questions appropriate to the patient's chief complaint (discussed in detail in Chapters 12 through 19). Next, perform the necessary interventions (e.g., airway positioning, oxygen administration, continuation of suction, ECG monitoring, pain management) and package and transport the patient to the most appropriate facility. Be prepared to provide an oral report to the emergency department personnel and to document assessment findings and interventions once the patient has been transferred to the hospital emergency department.

GAINING PROFICIENCY

Because time is often of the essence in the case of an unstable medical patient who is not responsive, the ability to conduct the RPE quickly and accurately is very important in prehospital patient management. To

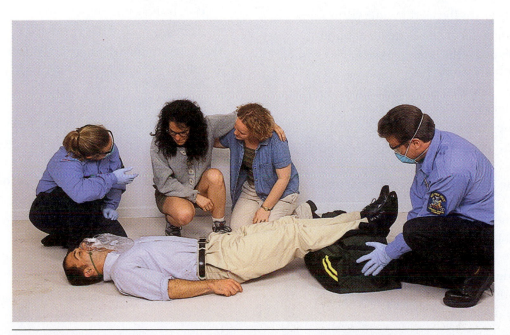

FIGURE 10-4 The family or bystanders should be asked the SAMPLE history questions if the patient is not yet alert.

become proficient, practice the RPE in teams using mock patients found in various positions (e.g., supine or prone on the floor or bed, seated in a wheelchair). If you practice before an actual emergency, then when your patients need you most, you will be prepared to help them.

 ## CONCLUSION

After performing the patient's initial assessment and determining that the patient has a medical emergency and is not responsive, complete the rapid physical examination (RPE). The purpose of the RPE is to uncover injuries that the patient cannot tell you about or that might not be readily apparent. The RPE is a systematic sequential examination of the head, neck, chest, abdomen, pelvis, extremities, back, and buttocks.

REVIEW QUESTIONS

1. When or for whom should the rapid physical examination be used?
   a. in preparation for the initial assessment
   b. in place of the detailed physical examination
   c. for the medical patient who is not responsive
   d. for all medical patients

2. The objective of the rapid physical examination is to:
   a. locate and manage all life threats.
   b. quickly assess the alert trauma victim.
   c. determine the patient's treatment priority.
   d. quickly assess the unresponsive medical patient's major body parts.

3. If you are sure that the patient did not injure his neck, you can:
   a. continue to immobilize the neck with a collar.
   b. roll the patient onto his side to allow fluid to drain.
   c. ask the patient to get up and walk to the ambulance.
   d. skip the assessment of the neck area.

4. If you believe the patient who just had a seizure may have injured his head or neck, you should:
   a. provide in-line manual stabilization.
   b. open the airway with the jaw thrust maneuver.
   c. apply a cervical collar.
   d. all of the above.

5. If the patient has a productive cough, during the RPE the EMS providers should wear all of the following except:
   a. self-contained breathing apparatus.
   b. disposable gloves.
   c. eye shield.
   d. disposable mask.

6. When would it be sensible to wear a gown in the RPE of a seizure patient?
   a. when it is very cold outside
   b. when it is raining
   c. if the patient lost control of his bladder or bowels
   d. all of the above

7. Why is it necessary to consider the MOI if the patient is a medical patient?
   a. In addition to the medical condition, the patient may have been injured.
   b. Most medical patients have hidden injuries.
   c. The patient who has an injury will not get the RPE.
   d. all of the above

8. What is another name for crepitation felt under the skin of the chest wall?
   a. a flail chest
   b. compartment syndrome
   c. subcutaneous emphysema
   d. a dissecting aortic aneurysm

9. To determine whether the patient has equal lung sounds during the RPE, the EMS provider should listen in the:
   a. right lower rib area.
   b. midaxillary line at the fourth rib.
   c. anterior axillary line at the second intercostal space.
   d. midclavicular line at the second intercostal space.

10. The best way to practice the RPE is to:
    a. conduct one on all patients.
    b. practice in teams using mock patients.
    c. ask the patient to assist you.
    d. examine every detail as meticulously as you can.

CRITICAL THINKING QUESTIONS

1. For which of the patients listed below should you conduct a rapid physical examination?

   a. a patient who fainted at work

   b. an unconscious victim of a head-on car collision

   c. an 85-year-old man found unconscious in bed

   d. a 6-year-old who fell and broke his arm

2. Explain the differences between the rapid physical examination and the rapid trauma examination. How are the two assessments similar?

3. Explain why a medical patient may also have traumatic injuries. Provide an example.

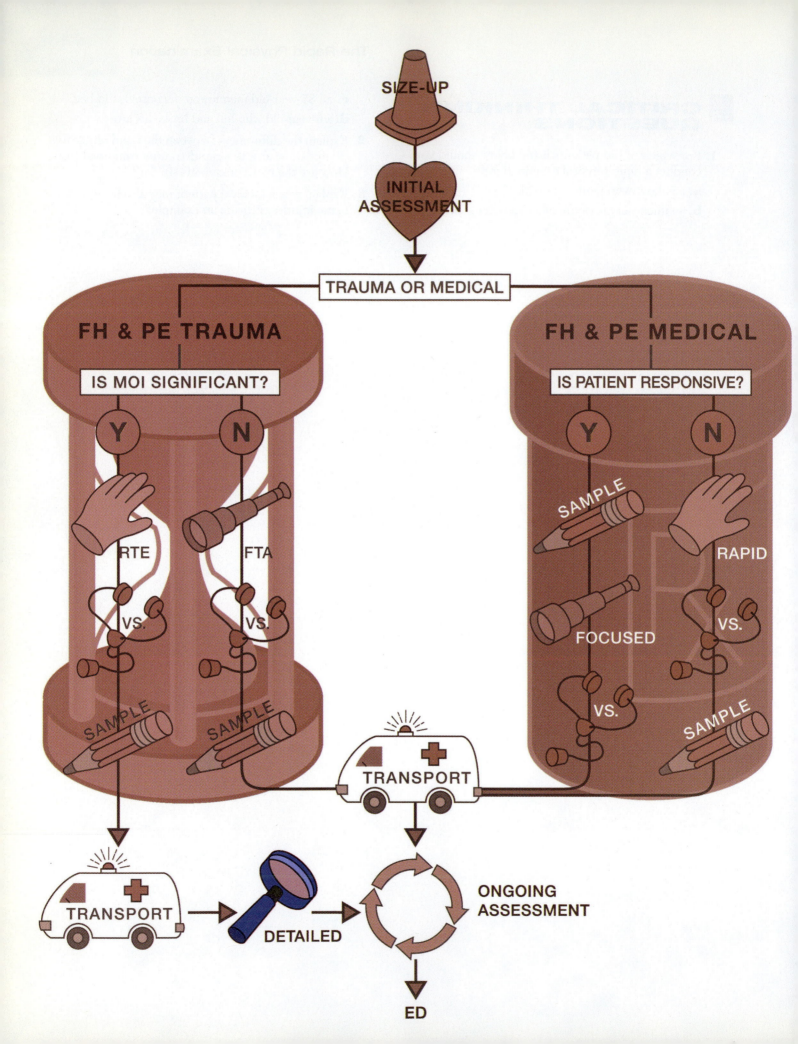

Chapter 11

The Detailed Physical Examination

OBJECTIVES

Upon completion of this chapter, the reader should be able to:

- Describe patients on whom the EMS provider should perform a detailed physical examination.

- Explain when in the assessment process the EMS provider would perform a detailed physical examination.

- Describe how and why the approach to the detailed physical examination is modified for children.

- List the three general types of closed soft-tissue injury the EMS provider might discover during an examination.

- Describe the various types of open soft-tissue injury the EMS provider might discover during an examination.

- List the body areas and specific assessment points for each area.

- Explain how the mnemonic DCAP-BTLS is used during the detailed physical examination.

- Provide an example of when the detailed physical examination would not be performed by the EMS provider.

KEY TERMS

abrasion
amputation
ascites
atelectasis
avulsion
cerebrospinal fluid (CSF)
contusion

crushing injury
degloving
detailed physical examination (DPE)
extravasate
hemotoma
hyphema
impaled object

(continues)

INTRODUCTION

The **detailed physical examination (DPE)** is a complete head-to-toe examination for injuries that have been determined to be neither life threatening nor limb threatening. The EMS provider should complete a DPE on the trauma patient who has a significant mechanism of injury (MOI). Following the patient assessment algorithm, note that the DPE is listed as a step to be completed during transport time. If transport is delayed for any reason, however, the DPE should be performed on the scene. This chapter discusses the components of the DPE.

THE DETAILED PHYSICAL EXAMINATION

Because the patient's injuries and the situation are consistent with a significant MOI, the patient will most likely be packaged on a spine board, with full immobilization of the neck and spine. In addition, most patients with a significant MOI will already be receiving oxygen by a non-rebreather mask. The EMS provider begins the DPE by taking body substance isolation (BSI) precautions and donning a fresh pair of gloves if needed. The EMS provider will begin the examination at the head for most patients and will work downward toward the feet. The toe-to-head approach, with a parent present, may be used for young children because it often decreases the young patient's fear and anxiety.

Soft-tissue injuries that might be discovered during the examination are classified as closed or open. The three general categories of closed soft-tissue injuries are **contusions**, **hematomas**, and **crushing injuries** (Table 11-1). The various types of open soft-tissue injuries include **abrasions**, **avulsions**, **deglovings**, **incisions**, **lacerations**, **punctures** and **penetrations**, **amputations**, **impaled objects**, crushing injuries, and major artery lacerations. These injuries are described in

TABLE 11-1
Three General Categories of Closed Soft-Tissue Injury

- **Contusion.** The skin is intact, the cells are damaged, and the blood vessels in the dermis are usually torn, causing ecchymosis (an accumulation of blood under the skin). The resulting swelling and pain can be delayed for up to 24 to 48 hours after the injury.

- **Hematoma.** This is a collection of blood beneath the skin caused, generally, by a larger amount of tissue damage than in a contusion. The vessels that are damaged are usually larger, and the patient could lose one or more liters of blood.

- **Crushing injury.** The pressure from a crushing force applied to the body can cause internal organ rupture and is often associated with severe fractures. Although the overlying skin appears intact, there often is internal bleeding that can be severe and can involve shock.

Table 11-2. The following areas of the body are examined for deformities, contusions, abrasions, penetrations or punctures, burns, tenderness, lacerations, and swelling. The mnemonic DCAP-BTLS is used to help one remember the points of assessment.

Pediatric Pearl

- The DPE will be easier to do with a parent present and in a toe-to-head order on an infant, toddler, or preschooler.

Clinical Carat

- Two areas of soft tissue that can mask or hide a potentially critical injury are the thigh and underneath the scalp. A person can bleed to death by **extravasating** (escaping) blood within either area, and the clinical findings (except for shock) may be minimal.

TABLE 11-2
Types of Open Soft-Tissue Injury

- **Abrasion.** The epidermis (outermost layer of the skin) is damaged by shearing forces. This is a painful injury that is usually superficial and involves only minor bleeding. Contamination is the major problem.

- **Avulsion.** This is a flap of loose, torn tissue that may not be viable for reimplantation.

- **Degloving.** This is the removal of the epidermis of the skin in a manner similar to removing tight gloves—inside-out.

- **Incision.** This is a clean break in the skin, usually caused by a very sharp object such as a knife, sharp metal, or scalpel. The incision can be deep or superficial.

- **Laceration.** This is a break in the skin of varying depth that may be regular or irregular. The jagged wound is caused by forceful impact with a sharp object, causing the ends to bleed freely.

- **Punctures and penetrations.** These are caused by a foreign object entering the body. External bleeding is usually minimal or absent if the injury occurs in an extremity. Bleeding can be severe if there is an object impaled in the thorax or abdomen. The underlying thoracic injuries can be extensive (e.g., simple, open, or tension pneumothorax; hemothorax; pericardial tamponade; penetrating heart wound; rupture of the esophagus, aorta, diaphragm, or mainstem bronchus). Underlying abdominal injuries can involve either hollow or solid organs. The potential for infection is great.

- **Amputation.** This involves loss of an extremity or other body part. Jagged skin or bone edges are typically present at the site of amputation. The patient may have massive bleeding, or the bleeding may be controlled (e.g., patient run over by a subway train has a leg amputated, but there is little bleeding because the heat of the train cauterized the wound).

- **Impaled object.** An object that punctures the skin and remains in the wound.

- **Crushing injuries.** These are caused by a compressive force sufficient to interfere with the normal metabolic function of the involved tissue. Crushing injuries can be caused by the collapse of heavy materials, industrial accidents, and any prolonged compression in a chronic situation (e.g., prolonged application of MAST/PASG, improperly applied cast, or an unconscious patient lying on an extremity).

- **Major artery laceration.** When a major artery is lacerated, the bleeding is severe, spurting, and bright red. The artery may spasm, decreasing the blood flow, but most of the patient's blood volume can be spurted out. The result may be shock or death when a major artery is lacerated with a gaping cut.

Head

Assess for DCAP-BTLS and crepitation of the head and scalp. Crepitation is the grating of broken bones. Common traumatic injuries associated with the head include contusions and lacerations, which can bleed profusely owing to the high vascularity of the scalp. Pay particular attention to injuries to the temporal area of the skull. The cranium is very thin, and a skull fracture can easily cause damage to the middle meningeal artery, with subsequent development of epidural hematoma.

Face

Assess for DCAP-BTLS, crepitation, and symmetry of the face. Is one side of the face swollen or disfigured?

The facial bones should be palpated for stability. Unstable facial bones can cause airway problems due to bleeding and obstruction. Vision problems can result from a loss of facial structure.

Eyes

Assess for DCAP-BTLS; check the response of the pupils with a penlight; observe eye movement; and note any discoloration. Can the patient follow your fingers with her eyes in all four directions (up, down, right, and left) without moving her head? (At this point in the examination, the head and neck should be immobilized with a collar and full spine board if there was any reason to suspect neck injury.) Examine the eyes for discoloration; **hyphema** (bleeding into the anterior chamber of the eye, as shown in Figure 11-1); and ecchymosis, such as raccoon's eyes, or periorbital (around the eyes) ecchymosis (Figure 11-2), which may be indicative of a basilar skull fracture.

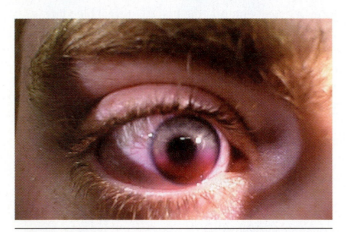

FIGURE 11-1 Blood in the front of the eye is called a hyphema. (Courtesy of Kevin Reilly, MD, Albany Medical Center, Albany, NY)

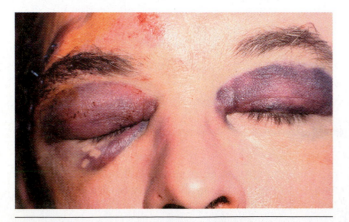

FIGURE 11-2 Raccoon's eyes are indicative of a basilar skull fracture. (Courtesy of Wayne Triner, DO, Albany Medical Center, Albany, NY)

Nose

Assess for DCAP-BTLS and any drainage, such as blood or **cerebrospinal fluid (CSF)**. (Cerebrospinal fluid is a clear fluid, manufactured in the brain, that bathes the brain and spinal cord.) When a patient is supine on a backboard, the EMS provider must be alert so that drainage from the nose does not become an airway problem. The EMS provider should suction the patient as often as needed.

Ears

Assess for DCAP-BTLS and any drainage such as blood or CSF. Cerebrospinal fluid is a clear fluid that separates out from blood because the two fluids do not mix well (like oil and water), so when bleeding is collected on a gauze pad the CSF forms a halo around the bloodstain. Drainage from the ears should be allowed to flow and should never be occluded because dangerous pressures in the head may result from occlusion.

Mouth

Assess for DCAP-BTLS, crepitation of the mouth and jaw, loose or broken teeth, swelling or laceration of the tongue or throat, unusual odors, discoloration, and drainage. A patient with a skull fracture that leaks CSF might complain of a salty taste in the back of her throat because CSF is about as salty as seawater. Pay particular attention to airway control and the need for suctioning and drainage of the patient with a possible jaw fracture. Often the patient cannot spit or clear the blood effectively from the airway because of the pain and deformity.

Neck

Assess for DCAP-BTLS, crepitation, and jugular venous distension (JVD). It is not possible to properly assess JVD if the patient is immobilized supine on a long backboard because the presence of JVD in a supine patient is a normal finding. To properly assess for JVD, the EMS provider must put the patient in a 45-degree position. If there is the possibility of neck or spine injury, do not sit the patient up to assess for JVD. If the patient has to be repositioned, another EMS provider must hold manual stabilization so as not to compromise the spine. To properly assess the neck, the EMS provider may have to open the patient's collar.

Chest

Assess for DCAP-BTLS; crepitation; symmetry; and **paradoxical motion** (one section of the rib cage moves in the opposite direction of the rest of the rib cage dur-

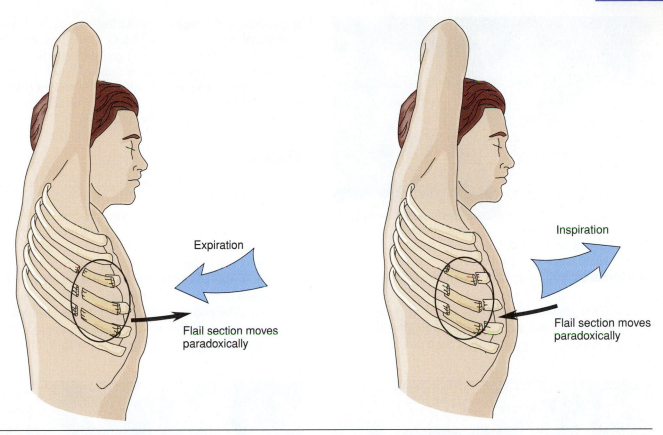

Expiration

Flail section moves
paradoxically

Inspiration

Flail section moves
paradoxically

FIGURE 11-3 A flail segment impairs breathing because its paradoxical motion decreases the tidal volume.

ing respirations), as found with a flail segment (Figure 11-3) and listen for the presence of breath sounds. Although the EMS provider will have assessed the breath sounds during the initial assessment, this assessment should be more thorough and will alert the EMS provider to any changes occurring. Observe the chest for old scars, which may be clues to the patient's medical history (e.g., heart surgery, CABG, pneumonectomy). Gentle chest compression will reveal rib fractures (Figure 11-4). Carefully evaluate the respiratory excursion (one complete movement of expansion and contraction in a single breath) of the chest because the fracture of even a single rib can seriously decrease the tidal volume and result in **atelectasis** (collapse of lung tissue).

Abdomen

Assess for DCAP-BTLS, guarding, rigidity, masses (pulsing or firm), and distension. Before palpating the abdomen, listen for the absence of bowel sounds, if feasible. Often, it is hard to hear bowel sounds because of the noises in a traveling ambulance. Next, palpate the abdomen (Figure 11-5). If the patient indicates there is pain in one of the four quadrants, palpate that area last. Ask the overweight or obese patient whether her

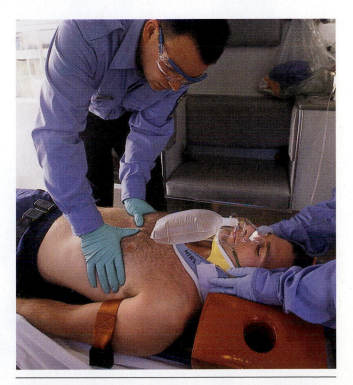

FIGURE 11-4 Palpate the ribs to locate tenderness and possible rib fractures.

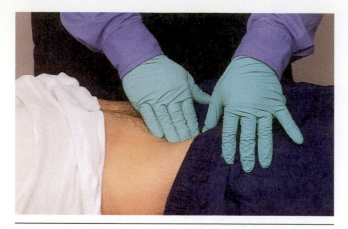

FIGURE 11-5 Careful examination of each of the four abdominal quadrants can reveal tenderness.

stomach is normal or bloated. Assess for the presence of **ascites** (an abnormal accumulation of fluid in the peritoneal cavity). A firm mass may be a tumor or fecal impaction. If the mass is pulsating, it may be from an abdominal aortic aneurysm (AAA). Look for scars, which may indicate prior surgery and give clues to the patient's history (e.g., an appendectomy scar rules out appendicitis as a cause of abdominal pain). If the patient is female and of childbearing age, consider that she could be pregnant or may have an ectopic pregnancy.

Pelvis

Assess for DCAP-BTLS, crepitation, and stability. Apply downward pressure (compress the two hips posteriorly) on the pelvic ring of the supine patient. Then apply inward pressure (compress the two hips medially), and then apply pressure on the symphysis pubis. This sequence should elicit some tenderness or instability if a fracture of the pelvis is present (Figure 11-6). If the mechanism of injury (MOI) is suggestive of pelvic instability (e.g., the patient was crushed under a vehicle), do not put pressure on the pelvis because doing so will only cause unnecessary pain and possible further injury.

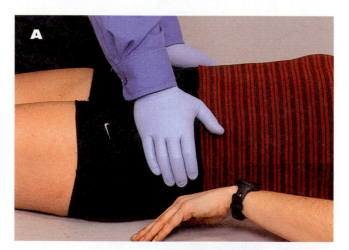

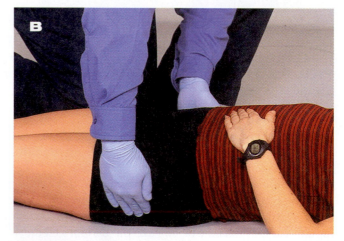

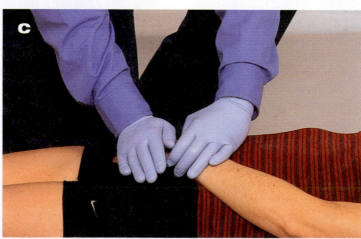

FIGURE 11-6 When palpating the pelvis, press down (**A**), press in (**B**), and press on the symphysis pubis (**C**).

Posterior

Assess the back and buttocks for DCAP-BTLS and crepitation. A trauma patient who has a significant MOI might already have been placed on a long spine board, so the ability to assess the back and buttocks will be limited. In most cases, the back is checked before the patient is rolled onto the board. For the patient on a spine board, the EMS provider can reach around beneath the patient to palpate with his fingertips (Figure 11-7). Of course, a patient who does not have spinal involvement can easily be rolled onto her side for assessment of the back and buttocks.

Extremities

Assess for DCAP-BTLS; crepitation; and distal pulse, motor, and sensory (PMS) function. Determine whether the patient has equal strength by comparing the two sides simultaneously, and examine for range of motion. If the patient has a major injury, such as a degloving injury (Figure 11-8) or an amputation of an extremity, make sure that the bleeding has been controlled and that the hand or stump has been properly dressed and

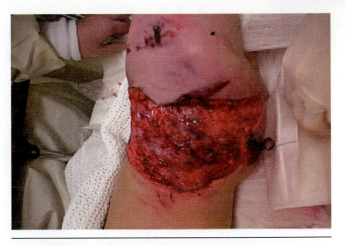

FIGURE 11-8 A degloving injury is commonly seen around machinery. (Courtesy of Kevin Reilly, MD, Albany Medical Center, Albany, NY)

bandaged. If the extremities have been crushed for a lengthy time, the EMS provider should be prepared for the possibility of potentially dangerous substances (e.g., acids and electrolytes) rushing back into the patient's system when the crushing weight is removed. If the crush period was lengthy, the patient's condition may deteriorate rapidly, progressing from acute shock to cardiac arrest.

PRIORITY DETERMINES CARE

The DPE is conducted only if time permits and usually en route to the hospital. When a patient is critical, the necessary interventions, serial assessments, trending of vital signs, and transport time sometimes do not allow enough time to perform the DPE. Those components of the management process take priority over the DPE. Consider the patient found in traumatic cardiac arrest. The interventions required to support this patient probably will not permit enough time to complete a DPE. As the patient is transferred to the emergency department, the multiple personnel working the resuscitation are likely to find additional injuries (e.g., fractured arm, swollen ankle, multiple lacerations, blunt trauma). These are lower priorities that will be attended to after the higher priorities have been stabilized. However, only about 10% of trauma patients are so critical that the DPE is omitted.

Now consider the small pediatric patient who was struck by a vehicle. Small children, such as preschoolers, often have an injury pattern known as **Waddell's triad**, which involves the legs, chest, and head. In this case, the legs sustained direct injury from the bumper of the car; the chest was injured from being thrown up onto the

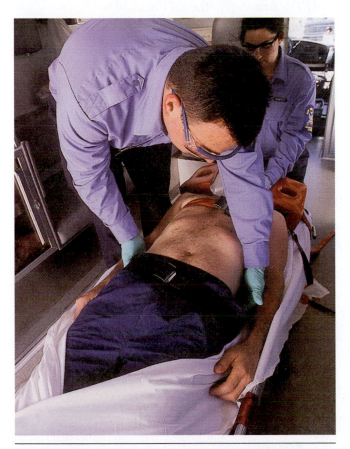

FIGURE 11-7 Reach beneath the immobilized patient and palpate with your fingertips to assess the posterior.

Exploring the Web

● Search the Web for traumatic injuries to each of the body regions assessed in the detailed physical examination. What types of injuries in each area can pose a life threat? For each region, create an index card listing the types of injuries you might find and the significance of the finding to the overall assessment and well-being of the patient.

car hood; and the head was injured when the child was thrown clear of the vehicle when it came to a stop. Because children have a proportionately large head, they fly head first—like a javelin. This patient will most likely need immediate field resuscitation and rapid transport to a trauma center. The EMS provider will ensure scene safety, perform an initial assessment and the rapid trauma examination (RTE), and obtain baseline vital signs and a quick SAMPLE history from a bystander or family member. The DPE of this patient should be done en route to the hospital. If personnel are limited or involved in higher-priority management (e.g., resuscitation of the ABCs), the DPE can be delayed until arrival at the emergency department or trauma center, where the DPE will be done once the highest-priority life threats have been stabilized.

CONCLUSION

The DPE is a thorough head-to-toe examination of the trauma patient who has a significant MOI. It is usually accomplished en route to the hospital after higher priorities have been addressed. The approach of the DPE on the small child differs in that the order of assessment is from toe to head. This approach helps reduce fear and anxiety for the patient and is usually more effective for the EMS provider. Upon arrival at the emergency department, all findings are reported to the next caregiver and are accurately documented on the prehospital care report. It is important to emphasize that conducting the DPE is not a high priority on a patient who has life-threatening problems requiring resuscitation. If the DPE cannot be done en route, do not worry; the staff in the emergency department will do it.

REVIEW QUESTIONS

1. A head-to-toe examination for non-life- or non-limb-threatening injuries is called the:
   a. initial assessment.
   b. rapid physical examination.
   c. detailed physical examination.
   d. rapid trauma examination.

2. Generally, the DPE is conducted:
   a. at the scene of a medical emergency.
   b. en route to the hospital for trauma patients.
   c. at the scene of a minor injury.
   d. en route to the hospital for medical patients.

3. When conducting the DPE on a toddler, the EMS provider should:
   a. examine from head to toe.
   b. hold the patient absolutely still.
   c. examine the patient from toe to head.
   d. keep the child as quiet as possible.

4. The first step in the DPE should be:
   a. examining the neck.
   b. examining the head.
   c. examining the feet.
   d. ensuring that BSI precautions are taken.

5. Types of closed soft-tissue injuries include all of the following except:
   a. contusions.
   b. punctures.
   c. crushing injuries.
   d. hematomas.

6. Types of open soft-tissue injuries include all of the following except:
   a. bruises.
   b. penetrations.
   c. lacerations.
   d. incisions.

7. Bleeding into the anterior chamber of the eye is called a:
   a. glaucoma.
   b. cataract.
   c. perfusion.
   d. hyphema.

8. If a patient complains of a salty taste in her throat immediately after being involved in a car crash in which she struck the windshield, this taste could be due to:

    a. a hyphema.

    b. hallucination caused by head trauma.

    c. CSF leakage caused by a skull fracture.

    d. none of the above.

9. If your patient complains of abdominal pain, what is the significance of examining for surgical scars?

    a. They will predict medical problems.

    b. They may help rule out certain causes of pain.

    c. Patients with scars usually have an automated implanted cardiac defibrillator.

    d. none of the above

10. When examining the extremities, always compare strength from side to side and assess:

    a. distal PMS function.

    b. the ability to walk.

    c. the length of the extremity.

    d. the ability to bend a broken joint.

CRITICAL THINKING QUESTIONS

1. What is the importance of conducting the detailed physical examination while en route to the hospital? What could the detailed physical examination uncover? Might you change a patient's priority on the basis of findings in the DPE? When and why?

2. Explain why it is necessary to start the detailed physical examination at the patient's head. What could happen if you started the exam on any other body region?

3. For which of the following patients would a detailed physical examination be appropriate?

    a. a 19-year-old male who drove into a telephone pole head-on and appears to be intoxicated

    b. a 5-year-old who fell off a swing and is having pain in her arm

    c. a 60-year-old male complaining of chest pain after shoveling snow

    d. a 90-year-old woman who slipped and fell at bingo

    e. a 23-year-old skier who fell and aggravated a knee injury

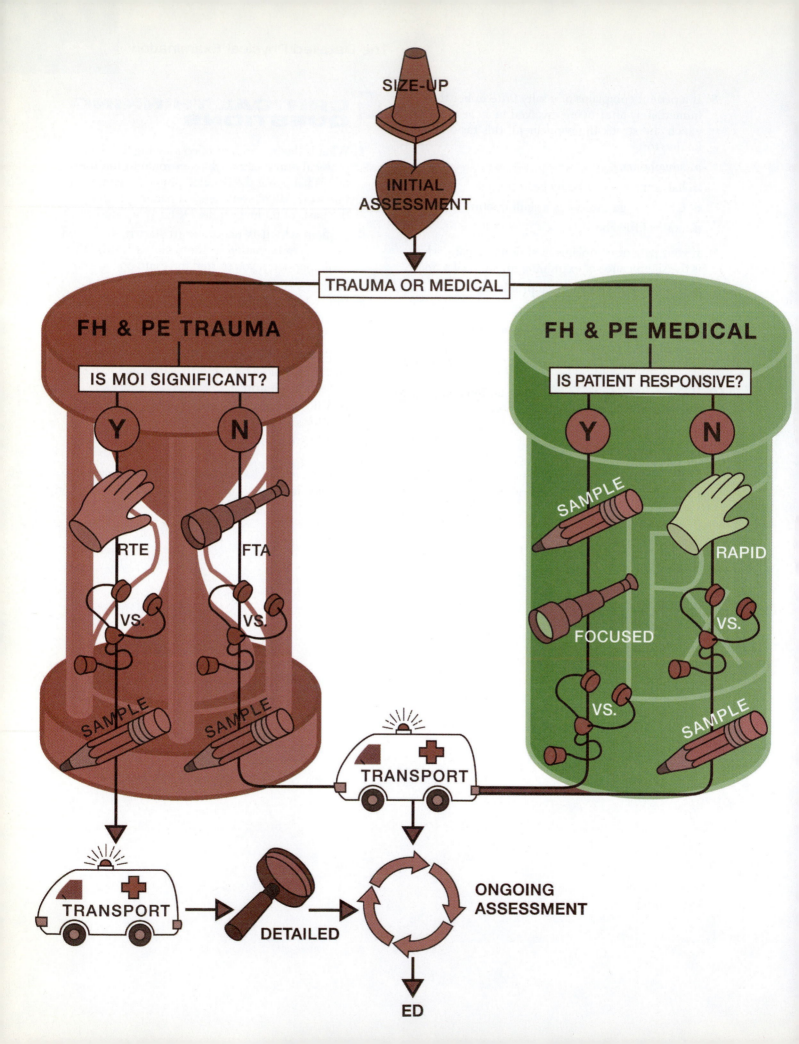

Chapter 12

The Focused History and Physical Examination of the Respiratory Patient

OBJECTIVES

Upon completion of this chapter, the reader should be able to:

- Describe how and when the focused history and physical examination of a patient with a respiratory complaint are integrated into the patient assessment algorithm.
- List some of the common respiratory chief complaints.
- Discuss the importance of quickly obtaining pertinent medical information about the patient with respiratory distress.
- List examples of relevant information the EMS provider needs to obtain in the focused history of the patient with respiratory distress.
- Describe physical findings about the patient's ability to speak that would indicate signs of mild, moderate, and severe respiratory distress.
- Describe findings that indicate an immediate life threat for a patient with respiratory distress, including the patient's mental status; breathing effort; position of comfort; and skin color, temperature, and condition.
- Describe the technique for listening to lung sounds.
- Describe the physical examination of the chest using visualization, auscultation, palpation, and percussion.
- List additional diagnostic tools that may be used and describe how these tools may or may not be helpful in the assessment of a patient with respiratory distress.
- List and describe both normal and abnormal lung sounds.
- List and describe both normal and abnormal breathing patterns.
- List abnormal physical findings associated with the patient diagnosed with a pulmonary disorder and describe the significance of each.
- List some of the most common acute respiratory conditions.
- Describe the signs and symptoms associated with the most common acute respiratory conditions.

KEY TERMS

acute pulmonary edema (APE)

adventitious

agonal respirations

allergy

anaphylaxis

angioedema

apnea

asthma

Biot's respirations

bradypnea

carpopedal spasms

Cheyne-Stokes respirations

chronic obstructive pulmonary disease (COPD)

crackles

dyspnea

eupnea

exacerbation

foreign body airway obstruction (FBAO)

grunting

hemoptysis

hypercarbia

hyperventilation

hypocapnia

hypoventilation

hypoxia

Kussmaul's breathing

nasal flaring

orthopnea

paroxysmal nocturnal dyspnea (PND)

peak flow

pleural friction rub

pleurisy

pneumonia

pneumothorax

pulmonary embolism (PE)

pursed-lip breathing

rales

retraction

rhonchi

stridor

tachypnea

tactile fremitus

tension pneumothorax

tripod position

wheezing

INTRODUCTION

The EMS provider has completed a scene size-up, determined that the scene is safe to enter, and called for any additional resources necessary. The EMS provider has taken the appropriate body substance isolation (BSI) precautions and is wearing gloves, eye protection, and a mask. The initial assessment is complete, and life threats have been addressed and managed. The priority for the patient has been established, and a transportation plan is in place. The EMS provider is now ready to begin the focused history and physical examination based upon the patient's chief complaint.

This chapter discusses specific clinical signs, symptoms, and history taking unique to the patient with an acute respiratory problem. A Skill Sheet for Respiratory Assessment is included in Appendix C.

Respiratory problems are either acute—such as an obstruction, bronchospasm, or acute pulmonary edema (APE)—or chronic—such as chronic obstructive pulmonary disease (COPD) or congestive heart failure (CHF). Specific signs and symptoms of these conditions will be addressed later in this chapter. Chronic respiratory conditions often present with an acute **exacerbation** (increased seriousness) of the con-

dition. Thus, most of the EMS provider's patients with respiratory problems will have an acute condition. Some of the most common respiratory chief complaints found in the prehospital setting appear in Table 12-1.

TABLE 12-1
Common Prehospital Respiratory Chief Complaints

- **Dyspnea.** "My breathing is worse today." "I can't breathe." "I can't get my breath."

- **Chest pain.** "My chest feels tight." "It hurts to take a deep breath."

- **Cough.** "I've been coughing a lot the last few days, and now my chest hurts."

- **Wheezing.** "My wheezing is back again."

- **Signs of infection.** "I recently had pneumonia." "I have the chills." "I feel hot."

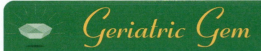

Geriatric Gem

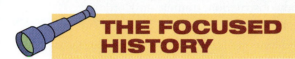

- A chief complaint of shortness of breath may be the only clue that an elderly patient is having a cardiac problem.

must ask for the most pertinent information right away in the event the patient becomes unable to answer questions because of a rapidly deteriorating condition. When family or caretakers are present, obtain as much information as possible from them. When the patient is severely distressed, ask questions that require a yes or no answer and have the patient respond by nodding his head. Speaking requires a great deal of effort for the patient with difficulty breathing.

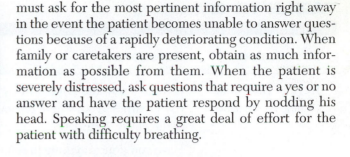

THE FOCUSED HISTORY

The EMS provider obtains the history of the present illness by using the mnemonic OPQRST and the acronym SAMPLE. When obtaining a focused history from a patient with a respiratory problem, the EMS provider

The OPQRST History

The relevant information that is most crucial pertains to the *o*nset; *p*rovocation; *q*uality; *r*egion, *r*adiation, *r*elief, *r*ecurrence; *s*everity; and *t*ime of the current episode: OPQRST. Table 12-2 lists some examples of questions to ask the patient with a respiratory complaint and provides some information on their significance.

TABLE 12-2
OPQRST for the Respiratory Patient

Information	Questions	Remarks
Onset	How did the difficulty breathing begin? Did it develop rapidly or over a period of time?	The classic presentation of cardiogenic hydrostatic pulmonary edema is a rapid onset (over minutes) of severe shortness of breath (SOB). Exacerbations of asthma or chronic obstructive pulmonary disease (COPD) typically develop over hours or days.
Provocation	What were you doing when the breathing problem began? Are you short of breath all the time or only when you exert yourself?	Some have exercise induced bronchoconstriction.
Quality	What does the shortness of breath feel like? Is it worse on inhalation or exhalation? Is it hard to take a breath in or a breath out? Can you take a deep breath? Is there any chest pain or pressure when you take a deep breath? Is this event similar to any previous events?	If they are asthmatic, find out if they ever had to be tubed.

(continues)

TABLE 12-2 *(continued)*

Information	Questions	Remarks
Region, **R**adiation, **R**elief, **R**ecurrence	Is there a sensation of tightness when you breathe? If so, where do you feel it: in the chest or throat? Have you done anything to relieve the current episode (e.g., use an inhaler or nebulizer or move to a more comfortable position)? Did it work? If so, for how long? Has this happened before?	Generally, dyspnea does not radiate. The EMS provider should determine whether the difficulty breathing is due to an upper airway problem (e.g., foreign body obstruction, trauma, epiglottis dysfunction, or tonsillitis), lower airway problem (e.g., trauma, obstructive lung disease, bronchospasm), impairment of chest wall movement (e.g., trauma, multiple sclerosis, muscular dystrophy), or neurological problem (e.g., stroke, central nervous system depressant drugs, spinal nerve dysfunction).
Severity	How does this compare with any previous similar events?	Obtain a baseline assessment followed by serial assessments to determine whether the condition is improving.
Time	For how long have you been short of breath?	Even if the onset was acute, the patient may have waited a long time before calling for help because he thought the problem would get better.

 ## The SAMPLE History

Use the acronym SAMPLE (Table 12-3) to obtain additional information that is relevant and recent about the patient's past medical history. A patient who tells the EMS provider he had his tonsils removed 20 years ago is not providing information that is relevant to the EMS provider. Be careful not to cut off the patient but rather focus his history on what is most relevant to today's chief complaint. Examples of relevant information include recent surgery, illness, immobilization, or trauma; a change in mental status, physical ability, medications, or daily activities; and a family history similar to the current event.

TABLE 12-3
SAMPLE for the Respiratory Patient

Information	Questions	Remarks
Signs and **S**ymptoms	Do you have a cough? Does the cough produce sputum?	Dyspnea is often accompanied by chest pain, fever, weakness, dizziness, nausea, fatigue, sleep disturbance, anxiety.

(continues)

TABLE 12-3 *(continued)*

Information	Questions	Remarks
Signs and Symptoms *(continued)*	What color is the sputum?	The sputum color and amounts are significant pieces of information. Clear or white is normal; yellow or green indicates infection; and pink or red usually indicates blood (**hemoptysis**).
Allergies	Do you have any allergies to medication? Have you been exposed to anything you're allergic to? Have you been bitten or stung by a spider or an insect?	Medications that might be used to treat a respiratory problem (e.g., inhalers, steroids, epinephrine, Benadryl) or cardiac medications may have caused the current incident.
Medications	What medications are you taking?	Check especially for respiratory, cardiac, and antihypertensive medications. Ask about all medications taken. Look for recent or sudden changes in dosages and for discontinued medications. Include prescribed, over-the-counter (OTC), herbal, and homeopathic medications; home oxygen; and the use of someone else's medication.
Pertinent past medical history	Do you have or have you ever had a lung disease (e.g., asthma, emphysema, bronchitis, pneumonia, tuberculosis, cancer) or cardiac disease?	How many packs/years of smoking?
Last oral intake	When did you last eat, drink, or take medication or a home remedy?	Is dehydration a factor?
Events leading up to this incident	Do you have any associated conditions that may have precipitated this condition such as limited mobility, fluid volume excess, ineffective ability to clear the airway, or other preexisting risks for infection? What were you doing when symptoms began (resting, sleeping, physical work)?	Did the symptoms come on suddenly in the middle of the night (paroxysmal nocturnal dyspnea [PND])?

THE PHYSICAL EXAMINATION

In most cases, the EMS provider will conduct the physical examination while simultaneously interviewing the patient and continuing to assess the patient's mental status and level of distress. When more hands are available, oxygen saturation (SpO_2), temperature, serial vital signs (blood pressure, heart and respiratory rates), end-tidal carbon dioxide ($EtCO_2$), and ECG findings can be obtained simultaneously.

Determining Life Threats

If a patient looks as if he is working to breathe, he usually is! A patient in moderate to severe respiratory distress will have difficulty with lengthy sentences. During the interview with the patient, the EMS provider may find that the patient can say only a few words between breaths. This finding is described as one- or two- or three-word dyspnea depending on how many words the patient can say between breaths. The inability to speak in full sentences because of respiratory distress indicates an immediate life threat and should be managed in the initial assessment.

Other findings that indicate an immediate life threat in a patient with respiratory distress are changes in mental status, such as anxiety or confusion indicative of **hypoxia** (inadequate oxygen in the blood cells); **hypercarbia** (carbon dioxide retention); signs of poor perfusion, such as cyanosis, pallor, or diaphoresis; absent or **adventitious** (abnormal) breath sounds; use of accessory muscles or the presence of **retractions** (skin pulls inward during inhalation), tachycardia, bradycardia, or hypotension. These findings should be found and managed during the initial assessment.

General Impression

Throughout the assessment, note the patient's facial expression and position or posture. These findings can help determine the patient's level of distress. Levels of respiratory distress are commonly described as mild, moderate, or severe. Patients with dyspnea will almost always be sitting upright. The more distressed the patient is, the more he will resist lying back; the inability to breathe in a recumbent position is referred to as **orthopnea**. A patient in severe respiratory distress may be sitting in a **tripod position** (see Figure 4-6); the patient sits with his elbows outward, his body leaning forward, and his hands on his knees. A patient in respiratory distress should not be forced out of a position of comfort because doing so will increase anxiety and the effort to breathe. Ask the patient about orthopnea at night; chronic conditions often worsen during the night.

Ask the patient how many pillows he uses to prop himself up; the more pillows the patient uses, the worse the condition is.

Inspection

Further examination of the patient should now include noting the presence and degree of any peripheral edema, ascites, use of transdermal patches, surgical scars (Figure 12-1), implanted devices such as an automated implanted cardiac defibrillator (AICD), intracatheters, Medic Alert tags, and general hygiene. Inspect the skin color, temperature, and condition (CTC) for signs of poor perfusion. If not already done, loosen and open any clothing covering the neck and upper torso. Visually inspect the neck and chest for symmetry, deformity, and excessive use of accessory muscles. Specifically look for retractions in the suprasternal, supraclavicular, and intercostal areas.

During the inspection of the neck and upper chest, evaluate for the presence of jugular venous distension

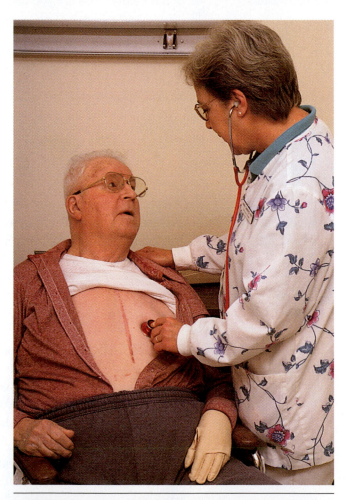

FIGURE 12-1 Always inspect the patient's chest for scars from previous surgery, such as coronary artery bypass graft (CABG).

(JVD). This is a quick measure of central venous pressure, and distension indicates backpressure from the right ventricle. Jugular venous distension is commonly seen with left ventricular failure, primary right heart failure, COPD, massive pulmonary embolism, and cardiogenic shock. It is measured as mild (showing just above the clavicle), moderate (halfway up the neck), or severe (all the way up to the angle of the jaw).

Auscultation

Next, evaluate the respiratory rate, pattern, and depth. Auscultate the lung sounds beginning at the apices. Always compare side to side for equality or deficit. Auscultate for the presence of normal and adventitious breath sounds and the absence of breath sounds. Observe the type of breathing pattern. Proceed to listen bilaterally from apex to base on both the anterior and posterior chest. Posterior chest sounds are louder and clearer than anterior sounds because of the absence of breasts and adipose tissue, and the wedge shape of the lower lobes of the lungs makes auscultation best on the posterior side. (For a detailed description of lung sound assessment, see Chapter 21.)

Palpation and Percussion

The physical exam of the chest should include palpating the thorax for tenderness, **tactile fremitus** (a vibration of the chest wall during breathing), masses or lumps, and symmetrical expansion. Percussion is another assessment technique that may be of value if time permits. The EMS provider taps the patient's skin with short, sharp strokes to assess the underlying structures. This technique enables the EMS provider to depict the size, location, and density or consolidation of underlying organs. Percussion is done over the same areas that are auscultated, from apex to base at 5-centimeter intervals, comparing side to side and estimating diaphragmatic excursion. (For a detailed description of this procedure, see Chapter 21.)

Diagnostic Tools

Performing the physical examination often includes the use of diagnostic tools such as pulse oximetry and electrocardiography. Whether taking vital signs, assessing for lung sounds with a stethoscope, or using more advanced tools, the EMS provider should remember that if the patient looks sick he probably is, and trending is more important than isolated readings.

Pulse oximetry is a noninvasive technique for measuring oxygen saturation (SpO_2). An electrode is placed on the patient's fingertip, and an infrared light beam measures the oxygen saturation of the blood. Pulse oximetry may be of value, but it is not consistently reliable, especially in the patient with respiratory distress. Visual inspection for perfusion should never be deemphasized or disregarded for a meter reading. The normal reading is 95% or greater. Patients whose saturation values are below 90% usually need supplemental oxygen.

An electrocardiogram (ECG) reading can alert the EMS provider to the presence of cardiac dysrhythmias.

Core body temperature is an important sign, especially in children and the elderly. Even modestly elevated or subnormal temperatures are indications for concern, especially when combined with other symptoms.

Capnography measures the level of carbon dioxide exhaled by the patient. End-tidal carbon dioxide ($EtCO_2$) is the concentration of carbon dioxide (CO_2) expelled at the end of exhalation; it can be measured intermittently or continuously depending on the device. The reading obtained can help determine whether a patient is breathing effectively or whether an airway adjunct is properly inserted. The normal reading is 36–44 mm Hg.

Peak flow is a measurement of how rapidly a patient can exhale. Peak flow meters are routinely used for patients with bronchoconstriction due to an obstructive lung disease such as asthma or COPD. The measurement is made by asking the patient to inhale deeply and then exhale as quickly as possible through the peak flow meter. A reading of less than 150 liters per minute in an adult indicates the need for immediate treatment. Peak flow meters are inexpensive and easy to use and provide a baseline assessment to follow during therapy.

ABNORMAL FINDINGS

During the assessment of a patient in respiratory distress, the EMS provider will observe abnormal findings. Adventitious, or abnormal, breath sounds have been described in numerous terms and definitions. The use of simple terms to describe sounds usually works best.

When listening to the chest, place the stethoscope on the skin to minimize external noises. Begin by listening to the apices of the lungs at the top of the chest; listen and compare one side of the chest with the other while moving down the chest to the bases of the lungs. Listen to the front and the back and describe any differences from one side to the other; for example, the left lower lobe produces fainter sounds than the right lower lobe.

Wheezing

Wheezing is a continuous whistling sound caused by narrowing of the lower airways that is usually heard at the end of exhalation. Severe wheezing often can be heard without a stethoscope. Wheezing is associated with many conditions (e.g., asthma, croup, airway obstruction, pulmonary edema, COPD), or it can be brought on with exercise by causing airway muscle spasm. Wheezing alone is not a significant sign. The key questions to ask about the wheezing are "Do you have chronic wheezing?" and "Is the wheezing today worse than or different from normal?" Wheezing heard on inspiration may be caused by a foreign body or edema, whereas wheezing heard on expiration is more often related to asthma.

Stridor

Stridor is a high-pitched sound associated with upper airway obstruction. Stridor is usually heard on inspiration and may be heard even without a stethoscope. This is a significant finding and should alert the EMS provider to the possibility of an upper airway obstruction (e.g., foreign body obstruction, croup, epiglottitis).

Grunting

Grunting is a sound that occurs primarily in infants and small toddlers when the child breathes out against a partially closed epiglottis; grunting is usually a sign of respiratory distress.

> ### Pediatric Pearl
>
> - Grunting is a sound that occurs primarily in infants and small toddlers when the child breathes out against a partially closed epiglottis. It is often a sign of respiratory distress.

Wet or Dry Lungs

When the EMS provider places a stethoscope on the patient's chest, one of the first signs noticed is the presence or absence of fluid in the airways, interstitial tissue, or both. *Wet lungs* and *dry lungs* are simple but effective words to describe this finding. Fluid in the airways directly obstructs diffusion of oxygen and carbon dioxide, resulting in states of hypoxemia and hypoxia.

Crackles

Crackles sound similar to the sound made by the crumpling up of a candy wrapper; they can be heard on expiration. Crackles are not continuous and can be heard only with a stethoscope. Crackles are produced by air passing over retained airway secretions. These sounds are described as fine (short and soft, high-pitched) or coarse (longer and louder, low-pitched). Crackles are wet sounds! Some clinicians use the term **rales** to describe this sound.

Rhonchi

Rhonchi are rattling noises in the upper airways caused by mucus or other secretions. A rhonchus is a wet sound and often can be cleared by coughing.

Absent Sounds

The absence of sounds in the lungs may be due to consolidation of edema or pneumonia, complete **foreign body airway obstruction (FBAO)**, or a severe state of asthma when the patient has become too tired to effectively move air in or out. Absent sounds unilaterally may be due to a pneumothorax, and absent sounds in the apices may result from increased consolidation, decompensated COPD, or FBAO.

Pleural Friction Rub

A **pleural friction rub** is not a lung sound but is heard in the chest as a grating sound over the area that is painful for the patient. This condition is caused by inflamed pleural surfaces and associated with the early stage of **pleurisy**.

Dyspnea

One- or two-word dyspnea indicates severe respiratory distress. A more detailed discussion of dyspnea follows.

Pursed-Lip Breathing

Pursed-lip breathing creates resistance to exhalation and helps to build up airway pressure (positive end-expiratory pressure, or PEEP) in the lungs. It helps to open airways by keeping alveoli from collapsing and thus improves oxygenation. This finding is associated with asthma and acute exacerbation of COPD (Figure 12-2).

The Use of Accessory Muscles and Retractions

The use of accessory muscles to breathe and retractions occur with increased breathing effort. When the chest is exposed, the EMS provider can see retractions during inspiration by the way the skin is pulled in between the ribs, above the clavicles, and at the sternum.

Nasal Flaring

Nasal flaring is a widening of the nostrils during inspiration. It is a sign of increased respiratory effort

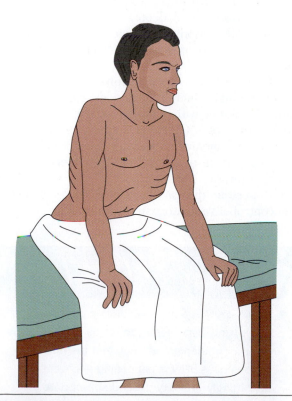

FIGURE 12-2 This patient is exhibiting pursed-lip breathing.

indicating a partial airway obstruction. This finding is more common in children than in adults.

Carpopedal Spasms

Carpopedal spasms are spasmodic contractions of the hands, wrists, feet, and ankles associated with alkalosis and hypocapnia that can result from prolonged hyperventilation (whatever the cause) or any condition that leads to respiratory alkalosis. The safest approach is to assume that the patient has something seriously wrong (e.g., pulmonary embolism, diabetic ketoacidosis, or myocardial infarction) until proved otherwise.

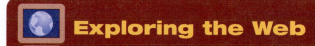

BREATHING PATTERNS

Eupnea is the term for normal breathing and is indicated by a normal respiratory pattern. **Dyspnea**, or difficulty breathing, is indicated by an abnormal respiratory pattern. When a patient is not breathing in a normal pattern, problems with oxygenation, diffusion, and perfusion can develop quickly. There are several types of irregular breathing patterns (see Figure 12-3) that can provide clues to the condition of the patient.

Tachypnea is rapid shallow breathing, and the rate is age related. Tachypnea is an early sign of respiratory distress. It is associated with compensating shock, cardiac problems, and diseases that can cause metabolic acidosis (e.g., diabetic ketoacidosis).

Hyperventilation is a respiratory rate greater than that required for normal body function. It is the result of increased respiratory rate or depth, or both. Hyperventilation causes an excessive intake of oxygen and an excessive elimination of carbon dioxide (**hypocapnia**). This disturbs the normal blood acid-base balance by increasing the pH. These pH changes can interfere with the normal function of other body systems. Both acute and chronic hyperventilation are associated with abnormal values for arterial partial pressures of carbon dioxide ($PaCO_2$) and sometimes with abnormal values for the partial pressure of oxygen (PO_2). Hyperventilation can result from many conditions, including:

- Asthma
- Chronic obstructive pulmonary disease (COPD)
- Acute myocardial infarction (AMI)
- Pulmonary edema (PE)

- Spontaneous pneumothorax
- Congestive heart failure (CHF)
- Hypoxia
- Increased metabolism (e.g., as caused by exercise, fever, or infection)
- Central nervous system lesions (e.g., stroke, encephalitis, head injury, meningitis)
- Accumulation of metabolic acids in the body (e.g., kidney failure, diabetic ketoacidosis, or alcohol poisoning)
- Drugs (e.g., cocaine, amphetamines, aspirin, epinephrine)
- Psychogenic factors (e.g., acute anxiety or pain)

Bradypnea is slow breathing and is common during normal sleep. In the sick child, however, it is an ominous sign indicating that he is too tired to breathe. Anything that can depress the central nervous system (e.g., narcotics, trauma, or disease) can cause bradypnea.

Hypoventilation is an irregular and shallow pattern that may occur at any respiratory rate. Hypoventilation is associated with asthma and diseases characterized by bronchial obstruction. It can also result from central nervous system depression. Both acute and chronic hypoventilation are associated with abnormal $PaCO_2$ values and sometimes with abnormal PO_2 values.

Biot's respirations are an irregular but cyclic pattern of increased and decreased rate and depth of breathing with periods of **apnea** (cessation of breathing). They are associated with various brain injuries and heatstroke.

Cheyne-Stokes respirations are a rhythmic pattern of gradually increased and decreased rate and depth of breathing with periods of apnea. They are associated with severe CHF, intracranial pressure, drug overdose, and meningitis and are the normally occurring sleep pattern of infants and the elderly. Cheyne-Stokes respirations are associated with neurological insult from either disease or trauma that affects the forebrain control of ventilatory stimulation.

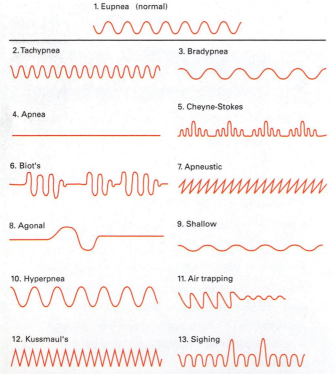

FIGURE 12-3 Respiratory patterns.

Clinical Carat

- Assuming that a hyperventilating patient only has anxiety hyperventilation is dangerous. As is done in up triaging, assume that the most serious possibility is happening and treat accordingly with oxygen and appropriate monitoring.

Kussmaul's respirations, or air hunger, is a distressing dyspnea occurring in paroxysms and is associated with diabetic acidosis, coma, and other causes of too much acid in the blood.

Agonal respirations are the dying breaths, characterized by irregular and progressively slowing gasps of air. Often, the layperson will report that the patient is still breathing when agonal respirations are present. These shallow gasps for air really do not count as breathing because typically no gases are exchanged in the lungs. This patient needs ventilatory assistance or, if an advance directive such as a Do Not Resuscitate order (DNR) is in place, needs to be made comfortable.

FEATURES OF DYSPNEA

The causes of chronic dyspnea with exertion are either pulmonary or cardiac. Patients with exertional dyspnea from pulmonary causes tend to recover more quickly with cessation of exercise than those with cardiac causes. The common causes of dyspnea without exertion include anemia, chest trauma, acute myocardial infarction (AMI), pulmonary embolism, and spontaneous pneumothorax.

Common factors that may exacerbate respiratory conditions include exercise or stress, infection, allergens, tobacco smoke, chemicals, or other irritants. These are referred to as triggers because they can set off a sequence of responses that create airflow obstruction. Drugs such as beta-blockers affect the ability of the sympathetic nervous system to cause bronchodilation and may provoke or worsen obstructive lung disease.

Examination of the patient in respiratory distress may reveal abnormal physical findings, in addition to an abnormal respiratory effort or pattern, that can provide useful information about the present event and the patient's medical history. A portion of the general population will have an asymmetrical thorax (e.g., kyphosis) that is normal for them and is not caused by any form of trauma. A large number of these patients will be elderly. For the EMS provider, the significance of this finding is related to the positioning of the patient. Whenever practical, let the patient help decide how he will be positioned for transport. The following is a list of abnormal physical findings that may be present in the patient presenting with acute dyspnea:

- Poor perfusion. This is indicated by cyanosis, pallor, or diaphoresis. A finding of central cyanosis (around the lips) is more reliable and useful than peripheral cyanosis (nail beds). Central cyanosis indicates hypoxemia, whereas peripheral cyanosis can be associated with cold ambient temperatures, poor circulation, smoking, and other conditions.

- Edema. Peripheral, central, or pulmonary edema may be seen.

- Clubbing. Enlarged fingertips or toes (Figure 12-4) may be associated with heavy smoking, COPD, lung cancer and fibrosis, chronic heart disease, and many other illnesses.

- Pulsus paradoxus. This is a marked decrease (10–20 mm Hg or more) in systolic blood pressure that coincides with inspiration and is associated with asthma, pulmonary embolism, tension pneumothorax, cardiac tamponade, and hypovolemic shock.

- Barrel chest. An enlarged chest with a rounded cross section (Figure 12-5A) is associated with COPD and sometimes asthma.

- Funnel chest (pectus excavatum). This is characterized by compression of the lower part of the sternum (Figure 12-5B).

- Pigeon chest (pectus carinatum). This is characterized by a protruding sternum (Figure 12-5C).

Pediatric Pearl

- In children, acute dyspnea most often occurs because of asthma, bronchiolitis, croup, or upper airway foreign body airway obstruction.

Geriatric Gem

- In the elderly, chronic dyspnea is often caused by COPD or heart failure.

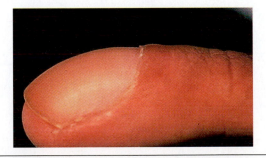

FIGURE 12-4 Clubbing. (Courtesy of Robert A. Silverman, MD, Pediatric Dermatology, Georgetown University)

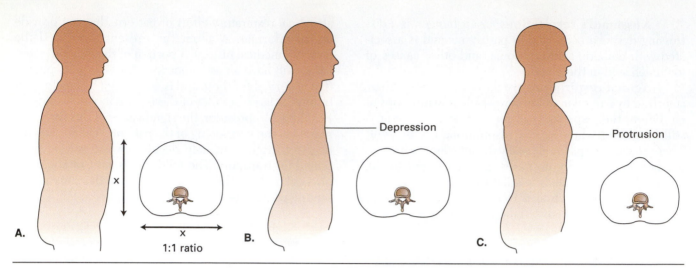

FIGURE 12-5 (**A**) Barrel chest. (**B**) Funnel chest, or pectus excavatum. (**C**) Pigeon chest, or pectus carinatum.

- Kyphosis (hunched back). This is an abnormal curvature of the spine associated with congenital disorders or disease (Figure 12-6A). In the elderly patient, kyphosis impedes the movement of respiratory muscles and can easily compromise the ventilation process, creating chronic states of hypoxia.
- Scoliosis. This is a lateral curvature of the spine (Figure 12-6B) due to a variety of causes, including accelerated growth rate and congenital, neuromuscular, and idiopathic problems.
- Lordosis. This is a forward curvature of the lumbar spine (Figure 12-6C) that is common in toddlers and small children and in obese and pregnant people. It is also associated with kyphosis, muscular dystrophy, and rickets.

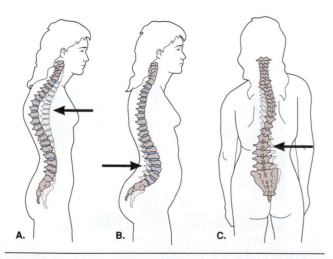

FIGURE 12-6 (**A**) Kyphosis. (**B**) Scoliosis. (**C**) Lordosis.

COMMON ACUTE RESPIRATORY CONDITIONS

The pathophysiology associated with respiratory conditions includes abnormalities that affect ventilation, diffusion, perfusion, or any combination of those. The most common causes of acute dyspnea include asthma, COPD, CHF, and anxiety. Subacute causes include obesity and poor physical condition.

Asthma, or Bronchospasm

Asthma is a form of reversible obstructive lung disease that is characterized by constriction of the bronchi, wheezing, and dyspnea. The patient experiencing a severe asthma attack, or bronchospasm, will appear to be in obvious distress with loud and rapid breathing. Wheezing may be heard with and without a stethoscope. As the condition worsens and the patient tires from the labored breathing, the respirations will become quiet; wheezing may not be heard even with a stethoscope. This state is critical and the patient is near respiratory arrest!

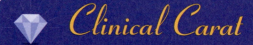

Clinical Carat

- A major warning sign is a quiet-sounding chest in a patient who is obviously tachypneic and short of breath. The patient is "too tight to wheeze"; respiratory failure may be imminent.

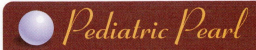

● Asthma is the leading cause of chronic and recurrent illness in children in the United States.

● Upper respiratory infections from any cause (e.g., tonsillitis, sinusitis) and pneumonia are common precipitants of acute exacerbations of asthma and COPD.

Allergies and Anaphylaxis

An **allergy** is a reaction from the body after an exposure to a foreign substance (allergen), and **anaphylaxis** is the most severe reaction to an allergen. Symptoms of an allergic reaction or anaphylaxis may occur within seconds of exposure to an allergen or may be delayed up to an hour or longer. Local and systemic responses affect the respiratory and the cardiovascular systems. Bronchial constriction and smooth muscle contraction, increased mucus production, and inflammatory changes in the bronchial walls resulting in mucosal edema are the three specific responses that lead to dyspnea for the patient. Edema and swelling may occur in any part of the upper or lower airways. Associated signs and systems vary and may include chest tightness, hoarseness, wheezing, stridor, nausea, abdominal cramps, diarrhea, chills, diaphoresis, flushing, progressive urticaria (hives), and **angioedema** (cutaneous swelling most often affecting the face, neck, head, and upper airways).

Airway Obstruction

Foreign body airway obstruction (FBAO) is most common in pediatric and elderly patients. A partial obstruction can quickly become a full obstruction resulting in apnea and cardiac arrest when not managed appropriately. Symptoms of FBAO include acute dyspnea, stridor, wheezing, signs of poor perfusion, and apnea.

Chronic Obstructive Pulmonary Disease

Chronic obstructive pulmonary disease (COPD) is any form of obstructive lung disease that is progressive and irreversible. Patients can have a combination of emphysema and chronic bronchitis, which is characterized by the slow insidious appearance of dyspnea and hypersecretion over several decades of disease. These patients maintain their respiratory system at various levels, compensating for deficiencies resulting from their disease. These levels can easily be disrupted, causing an acute decompensation (a failure to maintain or work properly); this is known as acute exacerbation of COPD. Upper respiratory infections and pneumonia are common precipitants of acute exacerbations of asthma and

COPD. Exertional dyspnea, orthopnea, and tachypnea are the classic symptoms, including accessory respiratory muscle use and pursed-lip breathing. Lung sounds can vary throughout the chest, ranging from wheezing to coarse crackles in the upper airways to wet or absent (consolidation) sounds in the bases. This variation may make it difficult for the EMS provider to differentiate COPD from acute pulmonary edema. Associated findings include changes in mental status and cyanosis due to poor perfusion, chronic productive cough, and weight loss.

Acute Pulmonary Edema

Acute pulmonary edema (APE) is a rapid onset of fluid in the alveoli and interstitial tissue of the lungs for any number of reasons, such as CHF, AMI, narcotic overdose, high altitude, near drowning, or exposure to hazardous materials. The clinical presentation is acute dyspnea, with or without pink-tinged sputum, tachycardia, jugular venous distension (JVD), and signs of poor perfusion. There is a distinct sensitivity to body positioning. Recumbent positioning increases venous return, creating a pressure backup into the lungs and worsening the condition; the effects of recumbent positioning explain why many EMS calls due to **paroxysmal nocturnal dyspnea (PND)** occur in the early hours of the morning.

Pulmonary Embolism

Pulmonary embolism (PE) is a serious condition caused by a foreign body (e.g., a clot) that lodges in the pulmonary capillary bed. Pulmonary embolisms develop from the deep venous system of the legs and pelvis. They are a common cause of death in the United States. Predisposing factors of PE include pregnancy and recent delivery, use of oral contraceptives, surgery, prolonged sitting (long automobile or airplane rides) or recumbency, healing leg or pelvic fracture, history of phlebitis, and a history of heart disease or cardiac dysrhythmias such as atrial fibrillation. The clinical presentation is often a complaint of chest pain that is pleuritic in nature and has persisted for several days; in addition, the patient may feel weak and faint. Dyspnea is often acute, but the periods may be brief. Abnormal lungs sounds are not always present but may include localized wheezes, rhonchi, or crackles. As the condition worsens, the patient may exhibit anxiety, agitation, or apprehension and will often appear to look severely ill, with peripheral cyanosis.

Pneumothorax

A **pneumothorax** is collection of air or gas in the pleural space of the chest causing one or both lungs to collapse. Predisposing factors to a spontaneous pneumothorax include rupture of a congenital defect (called a bleb), lung disease, and COPD. Spontaneous pneumothorax occurs most often in young, tall, thin males and menstruating women aged 20–30 years and usually affects the right lung. The clinical presentation is acute dyspnea with progressive worsening, sharp localized chest pain, decreasing breath sounds on the affected side, and an increasing respiratory rate. As the condition progresses, the patient becomes anxious, agitated, or apprehensive and complains of increasing dyspnea. A simple pneumothorax is not a life threat, but even the smallest pneumothorax can rapidly progress to a larger size, progressing to a tension pneumothorax. A **tension pneumothorax** is a life-threatening condition characterized by increasing respiratory distress, significantly decreased breath sounds on the affected side, the presence of JVD, a weak pulse, tachycardia, and other signs of poor perfusion. The key to assessing the patient with a pneumothorax is serial examinations with close attention to the lung sounds.

Pneumonia

Pneumonia is an inflammation of the lungs commonly caused by bacteria. Parts of the lungs become plugged with fluid. The fluid becomes thicker and may develop into pus as the disease progresses. Common predisposing factors for pneumonia include alcoholism, cigarette smoking, prolonged exposure to cold, extremes of age (very young and elderly), and depressed immune system. Typical clinical findings associated with pneumonia include acute onset of fever or chills, productive cough, pleuritic chest pain, and pulmonary consolidation. Atyp-

Exploring the Web

- Search the Web for information on each of the disorders discussed in this chapter. Create an index card for each disorder. Each card should contain the signs and symptoms of the disorder, assessment clues, and management techniques. Use these cards to review and study assessment of the disorder.

ical findings include nonproductive cough, sore throat, headache, muscle ache, fatigue, nausea, vomiting, and diarrhea. The elderly patient with pneumonia may have a normal or subnormal temperature due to decreased function of the thermoregulatory system.

CONCLUSION

Management of the patient with a respiratory problem includes prompt assessment and recognition of immediate life-threatening conditions and prompt intervention and resuscitation when appropriate. When the condition is unstable or critical, these steps take priority over a detailed assessment. However, the focused history and physical examination are always a high priority and should never be overlooked because the information obtained guides the course of treatment. Ask the most pertinent questions first without further exhausting the patient. Be alert for signs of rapid deterioration and quick to formulate a plan to intervene. Remember that many patients with a complaint of shortness of breath (SOB) or difficulty breathing are having a cardiac problem. The assessment process is dynamic, and the EMS provider must modify the focused history and physical examination to include more than one body system.

REVIEW QUESTIONS

1. When obtaining the focused history from a patient with a respiratory problem, the EMS provider should:

   a. determine the patient's age first.

   b. ask for the most pertinent information right away.

   c. medicate the patient so he will feel comfortable talking to you.

   d. determine whether the patient is having chest pain and nausea.

Geriatric Gem

- Elderly patients with pneumonia may have a normal or subnormal temperature.

2. All of the following are examples of acute respiratory problems except:

   a. acute pulmonary edema.

   b. upper airway obstruction.

   c. COPD.

   d. bronchospasm.

3. An indication of an immediate threat to the life of a patient experiencing respiratory distress would be:

   a. cyanosis of the fingers.

   b. an elevated pulse rate for more than 10 minutes.

   c. an SpO_2 value of 97.

   d. the inability to speak in full sentences.

4. A patient in severe respiratory distress, who is still conscious, will most likely be found in the _____ position.

   a. semi-Fowler's

   b. Trendelenburg

   c. tripod

   d. sniffing

5. The distension of the jugular veins may be found in any of the following conditions except:

   a. massive pulmonary embolism.

   b. left or right ventricular failure.

   c. cardiogenic shock.

   d. hypovolemic shock.

6. A shaking vibration of the chest wall during breathing is called:

   a. tactile fremitus.

   b. the PMI.

   c. an adventitious sound.

   d. a pulsatile mass.

7. A measurement of how rapidly a patient can exhale is called:

   a. capnography.

   b. electrocardiogram.

   c. peak flow.

   d. pulse oximetry.

8. The normal _____ reading is between 36 and 44 mm Hg and can be measured randomly or continuously depending on the device used.

   a. capnography

   b. electrocardiogram

   c. peak flow

   d. pulse oximetry

9. A continuous whistling sound caused by a narrowing of the lower airways that is usually heard at the end of exhalation is called a:

   a. rale.

   b. rhonchi.

   c. wheeze.

   d. stridor.

10. Pursed-lip breathing in the patient with lower airway disease is a reflex designed to:

    a. warm the air.

    b. provide PEEP.

    c. filter the air.

    d. decrease carbon dioxide retention.

CRITICAL THINKING QUESTIONS

1. Explain the differences in presentation of shortness of breath in an adult, pediatric, and geriatric patient. What may present assessment challenges in the pediatric and geriatric patients? Why?

2. You are assessing an 8-year-old child presenting with pneumonia-like symptoms. The child has a history of episodes of pneumonia, and the parents called EMS because this episode seemed to be the worst yet. The child's temperature shot up; he was complaining of pain on the left side; and his breathing was labored. What personal protective equipment should you be wearing to assess this patient? What type of lung sounds do you expect to hear? What care should be taken in palpation of the chest and thoracic area?

3. You respond to a call for a man who is having difficulty breathing. Upon your arrival, you see a man sitting on his front porch in the tripod position. You also notice a lawnmower in the middle of the lawn. He is clearly short of breath and is able to speak only two or three words with each breath. He is not able to give you an accurate history, and there are no family members around. What could have caused this man's difficulty breathing? What clues are available to help you determine the nature of the man's illness? What types of lung sounds do you expect to hear upon auscultation? What is this patient's priority?

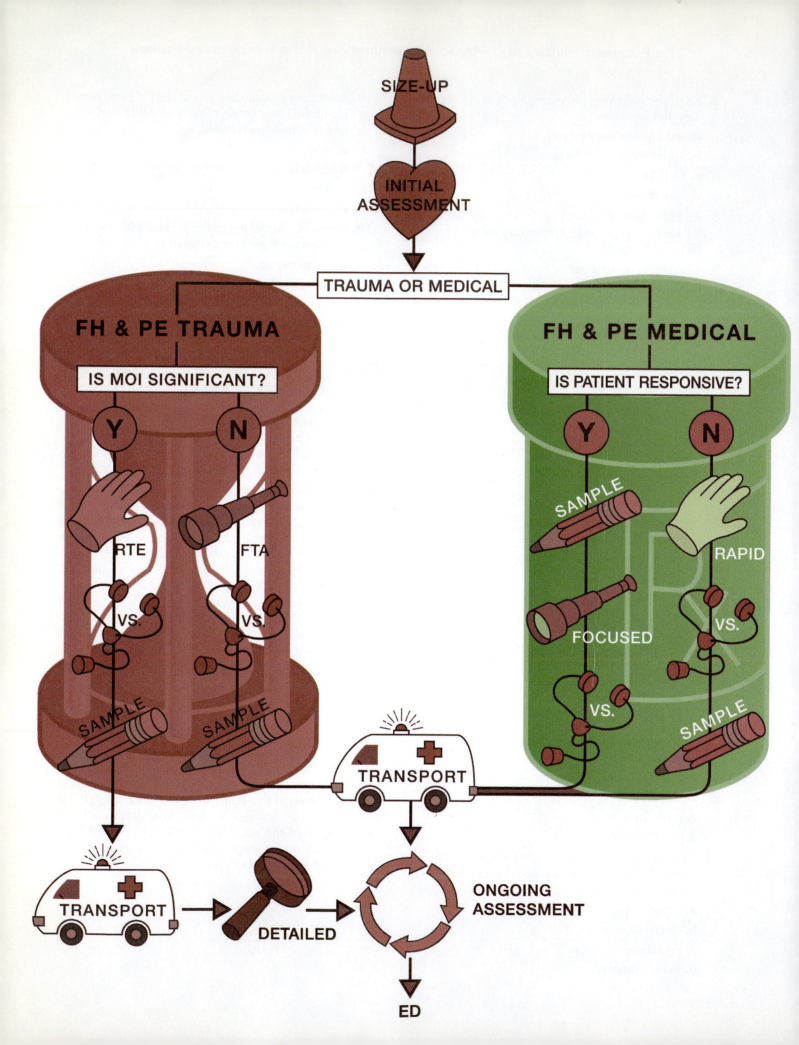

Chapter 13

The Focused History and Physical Examination of the Cardiac Patient

OBJECTIVES

Upon completion of this chapter, the reader should be able to:

- Describe some of the most common cardiovascular chief complaints found in the prehospital setting.
- Describe why the patient's history is so important when making a field impression of acute coronary syndrome.
- List several ways to ask a patient whether she is experiencing chest pain.
- List several causes of chest pain that are not cardiac related.
- Explain why *rule out* is not an acceptable term for the EMS provider when making a field impression of a patient.
- Using OPQRST, describe specific information pertaining to the focused history of the patient with a complaint of chest pain.
- Using SAMPLE, describe specific information pertaining to the focused history of the patient with a complaint of chest pain.
- Describe the significance of jugular venous distension in a patient with chest pain.
- Describe possible abnormal lung sounds that may be detected in a patient with chest pain or dyspnea.
- Describe the normal heart sounds S1 and S2.
- Describe the abnormal heart sounds S3 and S4.
- Describe the location of the point of maximal impulse and its significance.
- List abnormal features that may be found on the chest of a patient with a cardiac history.
- Describe the locations on the body that the EMS provider may examine to detect dependent (peripheral) edema.
- List the diagnostic tools the EMS provider may use to assess the patient with a possible acute coronary syndrome.

(continues)

OBJECTIVES *(continued)*

● List nine types of medications that may cause a syncopal event.

● List the three broad classes of rhythm disturbances found in pediatric patients.

● Describe the possible findings associated with a silent myocardial infarction.

● Describe why dyspnea is commonly associated with myocardial infarction.

● List the causes of noncardiac syncope.

KEY TERMS

acute coronary syndrome (ACS)

field impression

orthostatic changes

paroxysmal nocturnal dyspnea (PND)

pleuritic pain

point of maximal impulse (PMI)

rule out

S1

S2

silent myocardial infarction (MI)

Stokes-Adams syndrome

syncope

tilt test

INTRODUCTION

Many of the patients seen in the field have chest pain or other cardiac-related complaints. The EMS provider performs the focused history and physical examination on the cardiac patient after determining the patient's chief complaint and performing the initial assessment. This chapter discusses history taking unique to the patient with an **acute coronary syndrome (ACS)** as well as specific clinical signs, symptoms, and features of chest pain. A Skill Sheet for Cardiac Assessment is included in Appendix C.

The suspicion of ACS is based primarily on the patient's history. The physical examination and the use of diagnostic tools such as electrocardiography, pulse oximetry, capnography, and drawing blood samples for laboratory evaluation are helpful to determine the patient's current cardiovascular status, but a complete history is the most helpful in assessing cardiac problems.

When a patient complains of chest pain, the EMS provider needs to work quickly and efficiently, whether to treat a life-threatening dysrhythmia, to relieve chest pain, to treat congestive heart failure, or to transport the patient to the most appropriate facility. Efficiency depends on the ability to distinguish early in the assessment between urgent conditions such as acute myocardial infarction (AMI) and congestive heart failure (CHF) and less urgent conditions such as pneumonia, pleurisy, and anxiety reactions. Some of the most common cardiovascular chief complaints found in the prehospital setting appear in Table 13-1.

TABLE 13-1
Common Prehospital Cardiac Chief Complaints

● "I have chest pain."

● "I have a burning sensation in my chest."

● "I have a burning sensation in my stomach."

● "I don't remember passing out, but I feel OK now."

● "I feel weak."

● "I feel tired."

● "I don't feel right."

● "My heart is racing."

● "I feel palpitations."

● "My chest feels tight."

● "I feel a heaviness on my chest."

● "I can't breathe."

● "I get short of breath when I get up and walk."

● "I don't believe this is happening."

THE FOCUSED HISTORY

Obtaining a patient history is a key step to the identification of a patient's problem and the formulation of a rational course of treatment. The EMS provider's approach to history taking must be orderly. A random approach often results in missing important information and could lead to an unsuccessful patient outcome.

Order or sequence, however, does not imply rigidity. The same symptom may be interpreted in a different way from one individual to another. Often a patient will deny pain but will admit to having pressure or discomfort or will assume a position that suggests pain (Figure 13-1). Questioning or interviewing is a tool, and the EMS provider will need to develop skill in using it. Be deductive and learn to ask the same question in a variety of ways. For example, if the patient denies having chest pain but looks distressed, try asking the question in one of the following ways:

- Do you feel any pressure in your chest or abdomen?
- Does your chest feel tight?
- Can you take a deep breath without any pain?
- Are you short of breath?
- Are you feeling any discomfort?
- Can you show me where it hurts?

While attentively collecting information, give careful consideration to the obvious symptoms and clinical signs, and be sensitive to the subtle clues that are almost always to be found in the focused history or physical examination. The ability to obtain information distinguishes the good EMS provider.

The EMS provider obtains the history of the present illness by using the mnemonic OPQRST and the acronym SAMPLE. While obtaining the focused history from a patient with chest pain, the EMS provider should consider the many causes of chest pain, including those other than cardiac (see Table 13-2). The EMS provider begins to form a **field impression** (working diagnosis) of the patient's condition by considering the potential causes of chest pain. While carefully listening to the

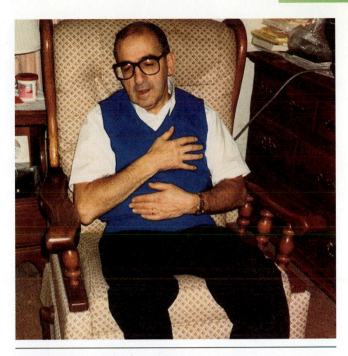

FIGURE 13-1 Some patients deny having pain yet hold their chest, as this man is doing.

TABLE 13-2
Differential Diagnosis of Acute Chest Pain

- Suspected acute myocardial infarction (AMI)
- Cardiogenic shock
- Acute pulmonary edema (APE)
- Unstable dysrhythmias
- Pulmonary embolism
- Pneumothorax
- Aortic dissection
- Esophageal rupture
- Thoracic aneurysm
- Anxiety reactions
- Esophageal reflux
- Musculoskeletal pain
- Pneumonia
- Pleurisy
- Costochondritis (inflammation of rib cartilage)

Clinical Carat

- A random approach often results in missing important information and could lead to an unsuccessful patient outcome.

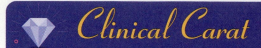

Clinical Carat

● "Rule out" is not acceptable as a diagnosis for most insurers!

patient as she describes the pain, discomfort, or distress, the EMS provider notes the tone of voice (is there anxiety, avoidance, fear, or panic?) in order to appreciate the patient's level of distress.

The EMS provider does not diagnose a specific ACS, nor does he use the words "rule out." **Rule out** is an admission dignosis to the cardiac care unit (CCU). They will be doing a test to determine if an MI has occurred. Through the assessment process, the EMS provider begins to differentiate the information obtained and discuss the patient's problem as a field impression.

The OPQRST History

In most cases the patient interview will be conducted simultaneously with the physical examination. Table 13-3 outlines questions using OPQRST to obtain specific information pertaining to the focused history of the patient with a complaint of chest pain. The EMS provider needs to remember two key points: (1) because so many conditions, some of which are life threatening, can cause chest pain, the EMS provider should consider that pain anywhere from the navel to the jaw is cardiac ischemia until proved otherwise, and (2) not all cardiac patients have the classic substernal chest pain. Many patients, including women, the elderly, and those with diabetes or neuropathic conditions, have atypical signs and symptoms during an MI. Such a case is called a **silent MI**. Findings such as weakness, mild dyspnea, and a complaint of "I just don't feel right" may be the only indication of a cardiac problem and are considered cardiac related until proved otherwise.

TABLE 13-3
OPQRST for the Cardiac Patient

Information	Questions	Remarks
Onset	How did the symptoms begin? Did the pain occur suddenly or over a period of time?	The pain from a myocardial infarction (MI) is often acute, whereas pain from pneumonia typically develops over a period of days and worsens gradually.
Provocation	What were you doing when the pain began? Were you at rest, for instance sleeping or watching television, when the pain began? Were you exerting yourself when the pain began, for instance playing basketball?	Pain from an MI is often brought on by physical or emotional stress, a large meal, or extreme temperatures. Pain from unstable angina occurs at rest without any stressors.
Quality	What does the pain feel like? Have you had any similar experiences? Is the pain constant, or does it come and go?	It is important to have the patient explain in her own words the type of pain or discomfort in order to form a field impression. If there a cardiac diagnosis (e.g., angina or previous heart attack), have the patient compare the present event with any previous events to determine the severity. Ask what was done to resolve the previous episode (e.g., rest or taking nitroglycercin brought relief); this may be the treatment to use today.

(continues)

TABLE 13-3 *(continued)*

Information	Questions	Remarks
Region, **R**adiation, **R**elief, **R**ecurrence	Please point to where you are experiencing pain. Please take a deep breath. Is the pain better, worse, or the same? Please cough. Is the pain better, worse, or the same? Please tell me whether the pain is worse as I feel your chest and abdomen. Do you have pain in any other areas? Does the pain appear to move from one area to another?	Increased pain with movement such as deep breathing, coughing, or even palpation tends to be pleuritic or musculoskeletal pain; pain that does not change with movement resembles more serious conditions such as a cardiac problem, pulmonary embolism, pneumothorax, or esophageal problems. Radiating pain is what the patient describes when experiencing pain from one point of the body toward another. Classic cardiac chest pain often is described as a substernal chest pain with pain radiating to the left arm, shoulder, or neck. Pain is distributed in this way because, during embryonic development, the heart and arms originated in the neck. Therefore, these structures transmit pain through nerve fibers from the same spinal cord segments. Not all patients with cardiac pain have radiating pain, but radiating pain helps to make a distinction.
	Have you done anything or taken anything to try to relieve the symptoms? Is there a particular position that you are more comfortable in? Have you ever had a similar event? How long did it last?	The patient may have attempted to relieve the pain or discomfort. Recurrence of the pain or discomfort is often the reason the patient calls EMS.
Severity	How would you rate the pain on a scale of 1 to 10, with 1 being no pain and 10 being the worst pain you have ever had?	Use this subjective scale to compare how the patient felt at the initial onset of pain, when it was the most intense, with how the patient felt after any self-treatment or EMS interventions.
Time	How long have you been experiencing pain?	Even when the onset is acute, a call for help is often delayed owing to denial or atypical cardiac pain. Because "time is (myocardial) muscle," it is paramount to determine the duration of pain in this type of patient.

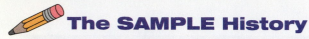

The SAMPLE History

Use the acronym SAMPLE (Table 13-4) to obtain additional information that is relevant and recent about the patient's medical history. Examples of relevant information include a cardiac diagnosis, recent surgery, illness, immobilization, or trauma; a change in mental status, physical ability (e.g., weakness, fatigue), medications, or daily living activities; or a family history similar to the current event.

TABLE 13-4
SAMPLE for the Cardiac Patient

Information	Questions	Remarks
Signs and **s**ymptoms	Can you describe how you are feeling today?	The patient may describe chest pain, pressure, tightness, squeezing; heartburn; palpations; radiating pain to stomach, arm, neck, jaw, back; shortness of breath; indigestion; nausea; vomiting; dizziness; light-headedness; anxiety, a feeling that something is wrong; weakness; fatigue; altered mental status; near fainting or syncope; sweating (diaphoresis); tingling or numbness; swelling in the feet, legs, hands (peripheral edema)
Allergies	Do you have any allergies? Are you allergic to any medications?	It is important to determine whether the patient is allergic to any medications the EMS provider may use to treat a cardiac problem (e.g., dilitiazem or lidocaine for dysrhythmias).
Medications	Are you currently taking any medications? What are you taking? Have you taken any over-the-counter medications or used any herbal remedies? Has the dosage of your medication changed recently?	The EMS provider needs to be able to recognize common medications prescribed for cardiac, respiratory, and hypertension disorders. When the patient is unable to explain what conditions the medications are for, the EMS provider will be able to make the association between the medicine and the condition. Even apparently minor changes in a medication schedule may be a factor in the current problem.
Pertinent past medical history	Do you have any heart conditions? Have you had any surgeries (e.g., pacemaker, abdominal surgery)? Do you have any breathing problems? Are you being treated for or taking medications for blood pressure? Have you ever fainted or passed out?	Be persistent and thorough because many patients will say they have no medical history until asked very specific questions. Although any person can have a cardiac event, examples of high-risk factors for an acute coronary syndrome include hypertension, obesity, smoking,

(continues)

TABLE 13-4 *(continued)*

Information	Questions	Remarks
Pertinent past medical history *(continued)*	When was your last visit to the doctor? Have you ever been to the hospital? If so, why and for how long? Do you smoke? Does any one in your family have a cardiac history?	family history of heart problems, diagnosed cardiac history (e.g., MI, CHF, or angina), age, diabetes.
Last oral intake	When did you last eat or drink? When did you last take your medication or an over-the-counter remedy?	If surgery or advanced diagnostic treatments are necessary in the emergency department, this information will be important.
Events leading up to this incident	What brought on the pain?	It is important to distinguish between exertional and nonexertional symptoms.

PHYSICAL EXAMINATION

In most cases, the flow of the exam will entail simultaneously interviewing the patient while continuing to assess the patient's mental status and level of distress. When more hands are available, oxygen saturation, serial vital signs (blood pressure, heart and respiratory rate), end-tidal carbon dioxide, and ECG monitoring can be performed at the same time.

During the initial assessment of the patient, the EMS provider should suspect cardiac-related conditions if any of the following are found:

- AMS. An altered mental status may indicate decreased cerebral perfusion due to poor cardiac output.
- Skin color, temperature, and condition. The general appearance of the skin is pale or diaphoretic (signs of shock). Warm or hot skin may indicate fever, infection, or sepsis.
- ABCs. Watch for signs of dyspnea that are mild, moderate, or severe or that worsen with exertion (possibly indicating heart failure) and for any abnormal breathing pattern or adventitious breath sounds.
- Abnormal distal pulses. A weak or absent pulse may indicate pump failure or cardiogenic shock.

An unequal pulse may be due to a pulse deficit occurring with various dysrhythmias. An irregular pulse is often suggestive of some sort of dysrhythmia, most commonly atrial fibrillation or premature ventricular contractions (PVCs), which can be caused by hypoxia, ischemia, or digitalis toxicity. Tachycardia persisting while at rest might indicate mild heart failure or stress from cardiac chest pain. Bradycardia in a patient who looks ill is abnormal and sometimes associated with inferior wall AMI or beta-blocker use.

The next step is to perform a physical examination giving special attention to the cardiovascular and respiratory systems. Assess the patient from head to toe. Look at the neck to assess the presence of jugular venous distension (JVD) as shown in Figure 13-2. To properly assess for the presence of JVD, the EMS provider should place the patient's head in a neutral position and elevate the torso approximately 45 degrees (semi-Fowler's). The presence of JVD indicates back pressure in the systemic venous system associated with acute or chronic heart failure. This sign is commonly due to left heart failure, pulmonary edema, and cor pulmonale (right heart failure). However, if the patient is hypovolemic for any reason, this sign may not be present.

Next listen to lung sounds and heart sounds and visually inspect and palpate the chest and abdomen.

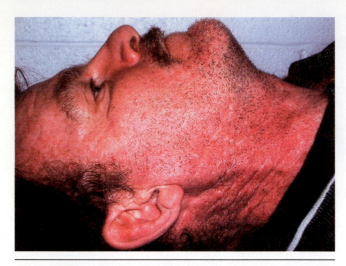

FIGURE 13-2 Assess for the presence of jugular venous distension.

The Lung Sounds

Reassess the respiratory rate and breathing pattern. Place the stethoscope on the skin to minimize external noises. Begin by listening to the apices of the lungs at the top of the chest (second intercostal space at the midclavicular line). Listen and compare one side of the chest with the other while moving down the chest and laterally in the fifth intercostal space midaxillary line to the bases of the lungs. Listen to the front (anterior) and the back (posterior), describing any differences from one side to the other (e.g., "the left lower lobe is diminished compared with the right lower lobe"). For a detailed description of lung sound assessment, see Chapter 21. The finding of abnormal lung sounds may include any of the following:

- Crackles, or rales. Wet and diffuse sounds indicate pulmonary congestion (edema)
- Rhonchi. Wet and fine sounds may indicate acute pulmonary edema, or coarse sounds may indicate an infection.
- Wheezes. Cardiac wheezing may be heard on inspiration; however, inspiratory wheezes by themselves suggest a foreign body. Expiratory wheezing is due to constriction of the bronchioles, as with complications of asthma.
- Decreased. Fainter sounds at the bases may indicate consolidation of pneumonia or the presence of pulmonary edema; at the apices, they indicate a pneumothorax.
- Absent. The absence of sounds on one side may be due to increased consolidation, decompensated

COPD, a complete foreign body obstruction, a collapsed lung, or surgical removal of a lung (pulmonectomy).

- Pleural friction rub. This is not a lung sound but is heard in the chest as a grating sound over the area that is painful for the patient, indicating an infection.

For a detailed description of abnormal breath sounds and breathing patterns, see Chapter 12.

The Heart Sounds

The two normal heart sounds to auscultate for are **S1** and **S2**, or the "lub-dub" sound. S1 is the first heart sound and is produced by the atrioventricular (AV) valves, both the tricuspid and mitral valves, closing during ventricular contraction. The second heart sound, or S2, is produced when the semilunar valves, both the pulmonic and aortic valves, close during ventricular diastole. Abnormal heart sounds are extra sounds. The S3, or a ventricular gallop, might be heard in CHF, and the S4, which is heard just before S1, is associated with an extra atrial contraction. (For a detailed description of listening to heart sounds, see Chapter 21.)

Heart sounds are rarely evaluated in the prehospital phase for two reasons. First, it is difficult to hear heart sounds unless you are in a controlled environment under ideal conditions. Second, the results of listening to heart sounds do not significantly change treatment. Even though assessing for heart sounds is rarely done in the prehospital setting, it is helpful to know how to do it. Using a stethoscope, lightly place the bell of the stethoscope over the **point of maximal impulse (PMI)** on the left anterior chest at the fifth intercostal space at the midclavicular line. This location is referred to as the mitral area, and the S1 sound, often described as the "lub" sound, can be heard best here. The S2 sound, often described as the "dub" sound, can be heard at the aortic and pulmonic areas.

Abnormal heart sounds are heard in the mitral and tricuspid areas as gallop sounds such as the S3, with its "ken-tuc-ky" sound, and the S4, with its "ten-nes-see" sound. Murmurs of either the aortic or pulmonic valves are usually heard at the location known as Erb's point, which is the third intercostal space to the left of the sternum. The landmarks for listening to the heart sounds are shown in Figure 13-3.

Visual Inspection and Palpation of the Chest and Abdomen

Look at the chest and abdomen and note the use of accessory muscles or retractions. Keep in mind that res-

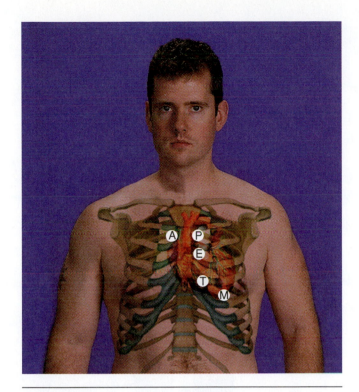

FIGURE 13-3 The landmarks for listening to heart sounds: (A) aortic area, (P) pulmonic area, (E) Erb's point, (T) tricuspid area, (M) mitral area.

piratory and cardiac problems are concurrent findings. Note the presence of any surgical scars, including those indicating a pacemaker, defibrillator, cardiac surgery (e.g., a coronary artery bypass graft, or CABG, would have midline chest and leg scarring), and any abdominal surgeries. Look for the presence of transdermal patches. Transdermal patches are used to deliver many types of medication (e.g., nitroglycerin, pain medication, nicotine). Is the abdomen distended from bloating, ascites, or dependent edema (indication of heart failure)? Abnormal findings associated with the chest and abdomen are outlined in Table 13-5.

Now palpate the chest and abdomen. Ask the patient to point to the exact location of the pain or discomfort, then palpate that area to determine whether the pain changes. Ask the patient to take a deep breath to determine whether the movement causes any change in pain or is reproducible with movement. Increased pain on palpation or with movement most likely is not cardiac pain. Do not completely exclude a cardiac cause, but look closely for another possible cause. Palpate the PMI (the point on the chest where the impulse of the left ventricle is felt most strongly) in the normal location on the left anterior chest at the fifth intercoastal space at

TABLE 13-5
Abnormal Physical Findings to Evaluate in the Chest and Abdomen

- Use of accessory muscles or retractions
- Surgical scars: pacemaker, defibrillator, cardiac surgery (e.g., coronary artery bypass graft, CABG, midline chest and leg scarring), any abdominal surgeries
- Abdominal distension, bloating, or dependent edema
- Transdermal patches: nitroglycerin, pain medication, nicotine
- Reproducible pain on inspiration or palpation
- Midline pulsation: aortic aneurysm

the midclavicular line. When the PMI is detected in another location, note the finding. Palpate the abdomen clockwise in four quadrants and note the presence of pain or tenderness, rigidity, masses, bloating, and distension; assess the midline for prominent pulsations. Prominent pulsations from the midline may indicate an aortic aneurysm; do not press on large midline pulsations! Dependent edema is an abnormal accumulation of fluid that settles within the intracellular spaces of the body with the help of gravity. It may be felt around the sacral area. The presence of edema, whether pitting or not, is significant. Pitting edema, however, is more likely to represent a significant heart, lung, or kidney problem. Pitting edema is recognized by the indentation left on a site after the site is pressed with a finger.

Assess the extremities for peripheral edema as a sign of heart failure. Cardiogenic edema can range from mild (nonpitting) to severe (pitting). Edema is most easily seen and felt in dependent areas such as the lower legs, the ankles, and the feet, also referred to as pedaledema (Figure 13-4). Edema can also collect in the presacral area for patients who are bedridden or limited to a recumbent position. Causes of peripheral edema other than cardiac may include chronic back pressure and similar etiologies or poor circulation.

Use of Diagnostic Tools

The three primary components that are used to diagnose an MI are the medical history, including the

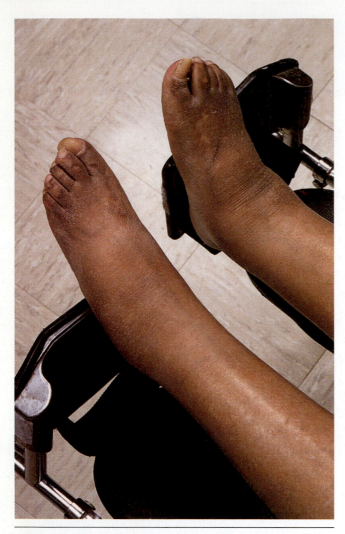

FIGURE 13-4 All patients with cardiac complaints should be examined for pedal edema. These ankles are obviously swollen.

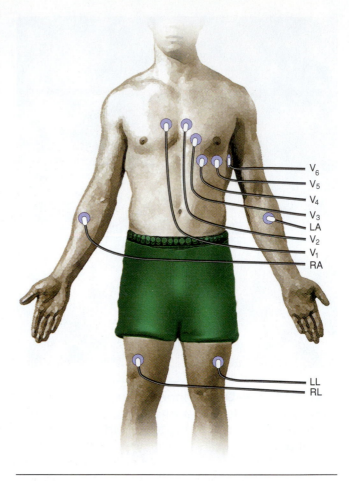

FIGURE 13-5 The proper positioning of the 10 electrodes used to obtain a 12-lead ECG.

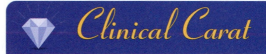
Clinical Carat

- A normal ECG test *does not* mean a patient is not experiencing a cardiac event.

patient's chief complaint or primary symptom; ECG changes or abnormalities; and cardiac enzyme analysis. In a significant percentage of cases, it is still difficult to diagnose AMI.

The ECG

An ECG alone cannot diagnose or exclude an AMI, but it can be helpful as a guide to treatment in the prehospital setting. A normal ECG test *does not* mean a patient is not experiencing a cardiac event. When an AMI is occurring, a 12-lead ECG may help identify the location of the infarction and help the EMS provider anticipate development of events. Table 13-6 provides examples of ECG findings and their possible associated cardiac conditions. Figure 13-5 illustrates the classic 12-lead electrode placement on the body.

Pulse Oximetry

Pulse oximetry is a noninvasive technique in which an electrode is placed on the patient's fingertip and an infrared light beam measures the oxygen saturation of the blood (SpO_2). Pulse oximetry may be of value, but it is not consistently reliable, especially in the patient with respiratory distress. Visual inspection for perfusion status should never be deemphasized or disregarded for a meter reading. The normal reading is 95% or greater. Patients whose saturation values are below 90% usually need supplemental oxygen.

TABLE 13-6
ECG Findings and Possible Acute Coronary Syndromes

Abnormal ECG Findings	Possible ACS
T waves	Abnormal T waves may be unusually tall, peaked, or inverted depending on the location of ischemia. They are often associated with ST depression and return to normal quickly when caused by angina but are often prolonged or permanent when due to an acute myocardial infarction (AMI).
Q waves	Abnormal Q waves are considered an indication of irreversible myocardial necrosis in the development of an AMI. A Q wave is considered significant if it is ≥0.04 second wide or one-third the height of the R wave. If neither of these conditions is met, the Q waves are not diagnostic of infarction. Abnormal Q waves usually begin to appear about 2 hours after the onset of the AMI, reaching maximum size in about 24–48 hours. They may persist indefinitely or disappear in months or years.
ST segments	Seen in ECGs during an AMI, indicating myocardial injury, and a variety of other causes (e.g., hyperkalemia, pericarditis, ischemia). The segments may be elevated or depressed, with an elevation or depression of ≥1 mm (≥0.1 mV) above or below baseline, measured 0.08 second (two small boxes) after the end of the QRS segment.
ST elevation	Often a sign of severe myocardial injury. Other common causes of ST elevation that may be confused with AMI are coronary vasospasm (Prinzmetal's angina) and acute pericarditis.
ST depression	Often a manifestation of myocardial ischemia. Other common causes of ST depression include left and right ventricular hypertrophy, left and right bundle branch block, and digitalis use.
Tachydysrhythmias include: • Sinus tachycardia (ST) • Atrial tachycardia (AT) • Atrial fibrillation (A-fib) • Atrial flutter (A-flutter) • Supraventricular tachycardia (SVT) • Ventricular tachycardia (VT) both paroxysmal and nonparoxysmal	Common finding during an AMI and with no specific cardiac condition.

(continues)

TABLE 13-6 *(continued)*

Abnormal ECG Findings	Possible ACS
Ventricular ectopy: • Premature ventricular contraction (PVC) • PVCs of 6 or more per minute • PVCs grouped • Multifocal or multiform PVCs • Accelerated ventricular • Idioventricular	Common finding during an AMI, indicating irritability of the heart
Bradydysrhythmias. In the development of an AMI, the rate varies with location and extent of the infarction.	Often indicative of an inferior wall infarction
Brady-tachy syndrome (BTS). Seen when tachydysrhythmia components are present intermittently during a slow rhythm.	Acute coronary syndrome (ACS)
Sick sinus syndrome (SSS) is not drug induced and the symptoms include near syncope, syncope, dizziness, chest pain, palpitations, and worsening CHF.	A term used to describe a variety of electrical conduction abnormalities due to a dysfunctioning sinoatrial node in the heart
Chest pain, abnormal Q waves, changing ECG, and cardiac enzyme elevation	Acute transmural infarction
Chest pain, abnormal ST segment and T waves, changing ECG, and cardiac enzyme elevation	AMI (probable subendocardial)
Chest pain, abnormal ECG, and nonspecific cardiac enzyme changes	ACS

(continues)

TABLE 13-6 *(continued)*

Location of Infarction by Leads	
Anterior wall infarction	Leads V_1, V_2, V_3, V_4
Inferior wall infarction	Leads II, III, aVF
Lateral wall infarction	Leads I, aVL, V_5, V_6
Septal wall infarction	Leads V_1, V_2
Right ventricular infarction	Leads, V_4R, V_5R, V_6R

Capnography

Capnography measures the level of carbon dioxide exhaled by the patient. End-tidal carbon dioxide ($EtCO_2$) is the concentration of carbon dioxide (CO_2) exhaled at the end of exhalation. The reading obtained can help determine whether a patient is breathing effectively or whether an airway adjunct is properly inserted. The normal reading is 36–44 mm Hg, and this can be measured randomly or continuously depending on the device. For a detailed discussion of capnography, see Chapter 6.

Blood Tests

Blood samples are taken on all potential cardiac patients as early as possible. Troponin and myosin are components of the myocardium and are released into the blood during ischemia. Even in patients who turn out not to have suffered an AMI, elevated troponin levels may identify high-risk patients for life-threatening dysrhythmias. Measurements of troponin, myosin, and CK-MB (creatine kinase–muscle; brain) over a 12–24 hour period are currently the tests of choice for the diagnosis of AMI.

Orthostatic Changes

Orthostatic changes may be seen when a patient sits up from a lying position (**tilt test**) or stands up to be repositioned on the stretcher. These movements result in an increase in heart rate and a decrease in blood pressure. A significant change in both of these vital signs indicates hypovolemia or dehydration. The patient may become dizzy or lose consciousness. If you suspect the patient is having an AMI, do not attempt a tilt test because she may go into cardiac arrest.

Pediatric Pearl

- It is uncommon to see the same cardiac problems in children that are seen in adults. With the exception of children with congenital heart problems, most children have not yet developed coronary artery disease, ischemia, and other associated abnormal conditions such as heart blocks or dysrhythmias. The American Heart Association in its Pediatric Advanced Life Support course (PALS) classifies cardiac rhythm disturbances for children into three broad classes: bradycardias, tachycardias, and absence of pulse. See Table 13-7.

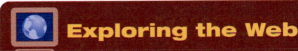

Exploring the Web

- Search the Web for information on the risk factors, signs, and symptoms of cardiovascular disease. Create index cards that list common risk factors, signs, and symptoms. Look at the differences in presentation between men and women. Also consider the differences in presentation among different ethnic groups.

TABLE 13-7
Pediatric Cardiac Arrhythmias

Rhythm	Infant	Child
Bradycardia	Heart rate <60 bpm and poor systemic perfusion	Heart rate <60 bpm and poor systemic perfusion
Wide- and narrow-complex tachycardia with adequate perfusion	Heart rate >220 bpm	Heart rate >180 bpm
Wide- and narrow-complex tachycardia with inadequate (poor) perfusion	Heart rate >220 bpm	Heart rate >180 bpm
Asystole, pulseless electrical activity (PEA); ventricular fibrillation and pulseless ventricular tachycardia (VT)	No pulse	No pulse

FEATURES OF CHEST PAIN

Chest pain can be caused by many disease processes as well as ACS. It is important to ask the right questions, know the signs and symptoms associated with these processes, and interpret irregularities in the patient's physical findings in order to narrow down the possibilities and arrive at an accurate working diagnosis.

To help determine the origin of chest pain, focus on the following key points: onset, duration, precise quality of the pain, any radiation, and any associated findings. The most distinguishing symptom of acute myocardial infarction is a sudden painful sensation of pressure. It is often described as a "heaviness or squeezing pain" in the chest, not sharp or stabbing. Sometimes

Clinical Carat

- Rather than making a field impression of AMI versus angina, most EMS providers now use the term *acute coronary syndromes* because it can sometimes be impossible to differentiate early on.

the pain radiates to the arms, shoulders, neck, or back, and it usually lasts more than 20 minutes. The patient may complain of associated symptoms such as sweating, nausea, and vomiting. In most cases of severe AMI, the patient looks sick and feels extremely apprehensive or anxious. Positioning usually does not change the intensity of the pain, nor is the patient able to find a comfortable position, as shown in Figure 13-1 in which the patient is clutching his chest. This position is also known as Levine's sign.

The type of chest pain that often changes with positioning, breathing, or palpation is associated with pleurisy, pneumothorax, pericarditis, pneumonia, or musculoskeletal problems. Any condition that causes inflammation of the lungs or heart can extend to the pleural surfaces of the lung and produce chest pain referred to as **pleuritic pain**. This is the reason that chest pain associated with pneumonia is sometimes pleuritic in nature. Patients with pericarditis will frequently describe their chest pain as being worse on inspiration or when they lie supine and relieved by sitting up or leaning forward.

When assessing chest pain of this type, look for signs of infection such as increased temperature, chills, increased sputum, or coughing. Patients who have limited mobility (e.g., stroke, bedridden, nonambulatory, severely disabled patients) or restricted older patients are at an increased risk for aspiration, pneumonia, and respiratory infections. Pain that is described as a tearing sensation in the chest, abdomen, or back or as referred pain into the back is suggestive of aortic dissection. It is not restricted to either the young or old patient and may present as a sudden cardiac arrest due to the rapid significant blood loss.

COMMON CARDIAC CONDITIONS

Cardiovascular disease is the single leading cause of death in the United States. The American Heart Association reports that each year more than 480,000 adult Americans die of heart attack or related complications. High blood pressure accounts for most of these cases, but other cardiovascular conditions also contribute to the high number of cardiac-related deaths each year. EMS providers are often called for cardiac-related events. The following section presents an overview of the common cardiac conditions the EMS provider may experience in the field.

The Silent Myocardial Infarction

A significant number of individuals experience an MI without the typical signs and symptoms; this is called the silent MI. The elderly, patients with diabetes, women, and those with neuropathic conditions can experience AMI with atypical symptoms that may be very subtle. Any one or a combination of the following may indicate the presence of an AMI:

- Altered mental status, confusion, or syncope
- Weakness or fatigue
- Dyspnea that is mild to severe or occurs with exertion
- Epigastric, back, or neck pain

Shortness of Breath

Dyspnea, or shortness of breath, is a very common symptom associated with MI and may be the primary or only symptom of acute heart failure, especially in the elderly or diabetic patient. Shortness of breath, exertional dyspnea, and **paroxysmal nocturnal dyspnea (PND)** strongly suggest a cardiac problem; PND is an attack of dyspnea that occurs during the night due to advanced heart failure. Like chest pain, however, dyspnea may have many noncardiac causes. If the patient has dyspnea with or without other associated cardiac signs and symptoms, obtain a history based on a complaint of respiratory distress. Ask about duration, details of onset, relief, COPD history, recent infections, fever, cold, productive cough, and cardiac history. The focused history for the respiratory patient is discussed in detail in Chapter 12.

Anxiety is a common finding associated with dyspnea and chest pain. The patient will often appear to be stressed, and the anxiety level may increase enough to produce associated symptoms such as hyperventilation, dizziness, and tingling of the mouth, lips, or hands but not the typical nausea, vomiting, or diaphoresis that may be present with cardiac pain. Anxiety symptoms are especially common in younger women or when the patient is in a stressful work environment. The patient may not volunteer information about her stress but, if asked, often will talk. Inquire about stress at work, at home, or with a family member or significant other. Supportive listening may help reduce a patient's stress or anxiety and thus reduce or eliminate symptoms.

Congestive Heart Failure

A past medical history of heart disease is important to differentiate congestive heart failure (CHF) from an acute exacerbation of COPD. Shortness of breath with or without pink-tinged sputum, the presence of JVD, peripheral edema, chest discomfort, cardiac dysrhythmia, and inspiratory crackles in the base of the lungs are associated findings. Look for diuretics in the patient's medication list and for a recent change in medication schedule. Even minor changes with medications can precipitate CHF.

Cardiac Syncope

The lay-man's term for **syncope** is fainting or passing out. Cardiac syncope is caused by a sudden decrease in cardiac output and a transient decrease in cerebral perfusion. The event may be transient or prolonged. A syncopal event in the elderly patient is especially important because it may be the only clinical sign of a cardiac problem. Syncope is a sign that should not be missed; therefore, question

Pediatric Pearl

- Clinical signs of heart failure are subtle in infants. Be suspicious when a sudden change in feeding or color occurs. Classic signs to look for include dyspnea or tachypnea, tachycardia, jugular venous distension, and hepatomegaly (enlargement of the liver). In older children, look for a sudden onset of dyspnea and tachypnea with air hunger.

the patient about fainting even if there was no obvious loss of consciousness reported. Causes of cardiac-related syncope include the following:

- Heart blocks
- Dysrhythmias such as bradycardia SVT, **Stokes-Adams syndrome**, or sick sinus syndrome
- Aortic stenosis
- AMI and angina

Many causes of syncope are not cardiac in nature. It is important to discern pre- and postsyncope information, such as the position of the patient. Syncope in a supine patient is serious and most likely cardiac in nature, whereas syncope occurring after a patient stands up may be cardiac in origin but more often indicates orthostatic changes as seen in noncardiac syncope. Try to determine whether there have been any previous similar episodes. Ask about associated cardiac symptoms before the syncope (e.g., chest pain, shortness of breath, palpitations) and symptoms after it. Causes of noncardiac-related syncope include the following:

- Orthostatic syncope or postural hypotension. This type of fainting occurs when a patient rises up from a supine or seated position. This event is suggestive of significant volume depletion and may be caused by hypovolemia, dehydration, prolonged bed rest, or autonomic dysfunction. Many types of medications can cause this type of response.
- Medications. Examples of medications that may cause syncope include beta-blockers, diuretics, antihypertensives, narcotic analgesics, antiarrhythmics, nitroglycerin, digitalis, ACE (angiotensin-converting enzyme) blockers, and psychiatric medications (especially tricyclics).
- Vasovagal faint. A parasympathetic response from stimulation of the vagus nerve (coughing, shaving, bowel movement, removing a contact lens) can slow the heart down enough to cause a syncopal event.
- Vasodepressor syncope. This is the most common type of fainting and may be caused by pain, emotional stress, mild volume loss, anemia, or fever.

Duration of the loss of consciousness is a helpful clue. Cardiac and neurological syncope usually occur without warning and can last a few minutes. Recovery is often slow and is accompanied by confusion, headache, dizziness, orthostatic changes, or local dysfunction. Noncardiac syncope often occurs in patients with no underlying disease; it is usually brought on by a stressor such as pain, emotion, or medication, lasts only briefly, and has a quick recovery period. If recovery from fainting is not quick, the patient should be transported for further

Exploring the Web

- Search the Web for additional information for each of the cardiovascular-related disorders discussed in this chapter. What are the signs and symptoms of each? What assessment tools are useful for each? Are there prevention methods that will help patients alleviate risks for the disorders?

evaluation of a possible cardiac event. However, a brief recovery phase in the patient with a cardiac history does not preclude a cardiac event.

CONCLUSION

The standardized approach for assessment of a patient experiencing cardiac problems begins with the ability to recognize cardiac-related symptoms, obtain a focused history, and perform an appropriate physical examination. The etiology of chest pain is often difficult to determine in the prehospital setting. Formulate a field impression from the focused history using OPQRST and SAMPLE. Be alert for the subtle clues of atypical cardiac symptoms while considering the obvious clinical signs and symptoms. Finally, remember that the history, not the presence of ECG changes, is the most important factor in formulating the field impression of an acute coronary syndrome.

REVIEW QUESTIONS

1. The suspicion of an acute coronary syndrome is primarily based upon:
   a. the 12-lead ECG.
   b. a series of blood tests.
   c. the patient's history.
   d. the patient's SpO$_2$ value.
2. If a patient denies chest pain but looks distressed, the EMS provider should ask the patient:
   a. Does your chest feel tight?
   b. Can you take a deep breath without any pain?
   c. Do you feel any pressure in your chest or abdomen?
   d. all of the above

3. An increase in the heart rate and a decrease in the blood pressure when a patient rises from a supine or sitting position is called:

   a. orthostatic changes.

   b. a positive Levine's sign.

   c. a negative Rothberg's sign.

   d. PND.

4. Of the following, which is considered a normal heart sound?

   a. S4

   b. S3

   c. a diastolic murmur

   d. S2

5. Back pressure in the systemic venous system associated with acute or chronic heart failure may be suspected when a patient exhibits:

   a. weak distal pulses.

   b. distended neck veins.

   c. ascites or yellow skin.

   d. rhonchi or wheezes.

6. Wet and fine sounds that may indicate acute pulmonary edema are called:

   a. a wheeze.

   b. rhonchi.

   c. rales.

   d. a pleural rub.

7. The heart sound that is loudest at the PMI is the _____ sound.

   a. lub

   b. dub

   c. ken-tuc-ky

   d. ten-nes-see

8. An aortic murmur is usually heard at the _____ location.

   a. PMI

   b. Erb's point

   c. second rib

   d. V_1

9. Chest pain that is associated with the movement of the lungs from the breathing process is called _____ pain.

   a. ischemic

   b. sharp

   c. pleuritic

   d. referred

10. Patients who are at high risk for silent MI include:

   a. the elderly.

   b. diabetics.

   c. those with neuropathic conditions.

   d. all of the above.

CRITICAL THINKING QUESTIONS

1. You are called to the home of a 75-year-old man who is experiencing chest pain. Upon arrival, you note that he is paralyzed on the left side. What do you suspect about this patient? What types of questions do you need to ask this patient?

2. You are dispatched to a local park where a woman has fainted. It is sunny and warm, with midday temperatures in the eighties. The woman is in her mid-forties and had been playing softball in a tournament. She tells you she hasn't eaten since breakfast, and it is now 3 P.M. Do you suspect the origin of the fainting to be cardiac in nature? What other factors could have contributed to her fainting?

3. Cardiovascular disease is the leading cause of death in the United States. What are the risk factors for cardiovascular disease? Why do you think it is such a problem in the United States? How would you prepare a discussion on the prevention of cardiovascular disease?

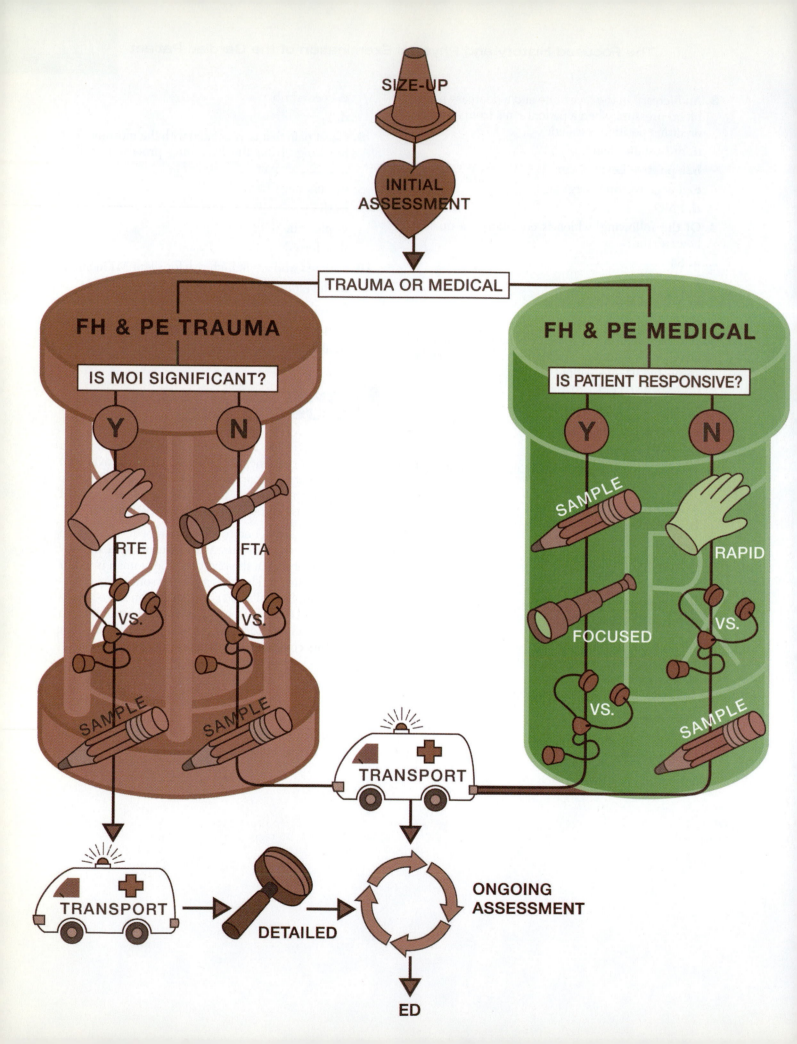

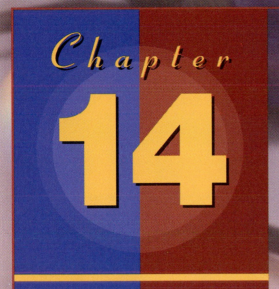

Chapter 14

The Focused History and Physical Examination of the Patient with a Neurological Problem

OBJECTIVES

Upon completion of this chapter, the reader should be able to:

- List the most common neurological emergencies EMS providers encounter.
- Describe why the duration of symptoms is helpful in making a field impression of a neurological event.
- List some of the reasons why getting a focused history for a patient with a neurological problem may be difficult.
- Give examples of clues the EMS provider should look for in the SAMPLE history of a patient with a neurological problem.
- List the six components of the neurological examination.
- Describe the key factor in the assessment of the patient with a neurological emergency.
- Describe the functions of the 12 pairs of cranial nerves.
- Describe how to assess the cranial nerves.
- Describe two ways to assess a patient's coordination.
- List the diagnostic tools that are useful in performing a neurological examination.
- Describe the two prehospital ministroke tests developed to help in the assessment of a suspected stroke patient.
- Explain the mnemonic AEIOUTIPS in the assessment of the patient with altered mental status.
- Describe three types of seizures.
- List the two most common causes of headache.
- List six other causes of headache.
- Describe the four general categories of head injury.
- Describe the three phases of brain herniation syndrome.

KEY TERMS

absence seizure

accommodation

acuity

AEIOUTIPS

affect

anisocoria

aphasia

ataxia

aura

Babinski's reflex

cerebrovascular accident (CVA)

Cincinnati Prehospital Stroke Scale

consensual light reflex

contrecoup

coup

cranial nerves

Cushing's triad

dermatomes

diffuse axonal injury (DAI)

diplopia

dysarthria

dysphagia

dysphasia

epidural hematoma

extraocular muscles (EOMs)

festination

field of vision

focal head injury

generalized seizure

ictal phase

Los Angeles Prehospital Stroke Screen (LAPSS)

neurogenic shock

nystagmus

partial seizure

plantar reflex

pre-ictal phase

pronator drift

proprioception

spastic hemiparesis

steppage

subdural hematoma

transient ischemic attack (TIA)

traumatic brain injury (TBI)

INTRODUCTION

The nervous system is the most complex of all body systems, yet the EMS provider can easily assess and test the individual components of the nervous system to form a reasonable field impression. This chapter covers a systematic method of performing the focused neurological examination and the causes of the most common neurological emergencies. A Skill Sheet for the Neurological Assessment is included in Appendix C.

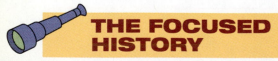

THE FOCUSED HISTORY

Obtaining the focused history using OPQRST and the SAMPLE history for a patient experiencing a neurological emergency can be challenging for the EMS provider. A patient having a neurological emergency may have difficulty communicating. The patient may not be able to form words, speak clearly, or say what is being thought even when he can understand what is happening. Altered mental status or unconsciousness may also limit the EMS provider's ability to verify the patient's baseline condition and medical history. Any of these factors make getting a history difficult. Whenever possible, verify information with family, caretakers, or coworkers.

The OPQRST History

When a patient is conscious and able to communicate, the interview is conducted simultaneously with the physical examination. For the unconscious or AMS (altered mental status) patient, the EMS provider should proceed to the rapid physical examination and then obtain the focused information from family or bystanders. When more responders are available, these tasks can be completed simultaneously. Using the OPQRST acronym, Table 14-1 outlines specific information pertaining to the focused history of the patient with a neurological emergency.

TABLE 14-1
OPQRST for the Neurological Patient

Information	Questions	Remarks
Onset	What were the circumstances when this event began? Did this come on fast or gradually? Did you have a headache, seizure, or fainting spell with the onset of symptoms?	It is important to determine how the event began and whether there are any factors that precipitated the event.
Provocation	Is there anything making the condition worse or better? Have you changed anything you have eaten or ingested recently? Have you had a change in prescription or dosage of medication? Have you been ill or had any other discomforts before this episode?	The EMS provider needs to determine any preexisting factors (e.g., change in medication schedule, alcohol or substance abuse, headache, fever, infection, diabetes, or other concurrent disease processes) that may have brought on the event.
Quality	Are you experiencing pain with this episode? Do you have any numbness or paralysis? Is this a new problem, or has this been ongoing with a history of similar events?	With a neurological problem, it is important to establish just what type of problem is occurring (e.g., severe headache, acute paresthesia).
Region, **R**adiation, **R**elief, **R**ecurrence	How have the symptoms progressed? Have you taken anything to try to relieve the symptoms? Do you have any other medical problems?	Often, concomitant medical factors such as hypertension, recent infection, diabetes, or substance abuse problems result in neurological emergencies.
Severity	Please rate your pain on a scale of 1 to 10, with 1 being no pain and 10 being the worst pain you have ever experienced. Is this event similar to any previous episodes? If so, how does this event compare with prior events?	It is important to determine whether the patient has lost any abilities to function as a result of this event (e.g., walking, talking, swallowing, vision).
Time	How long has this event been going on? When were you last symptom free? Did you call for EMS right away, or did you wait to see whether the symptoms would go away?	This information is especially important for the stroke or trauma patient. Strokes often occur during the night, and symptoms are not realized until the morning.

The SAMPLE History

Use the SAMPLE acronym, shown in Table 14-2, to obtain additional information that is relevant and recent about the patient's past medical history. Look for clues that may suggest that the presenting condition is related to another problem, such as a change in medications or severe infection, which can cause an altered mental status, depression, or psychosis. Patients with chronic neurological conditions are often using prescription medications. Table 14-3 lists the most common medications used to treat neurological disorders. It will be important for the EMS provider to determine the medications the patient is taking.

TABLE 14-2
SAMPLE for the Neurological Patient

Information	Questions	Remarks
Signs and **S**ymptoms	Why did you call EMS today? What are you experiencing? Please describe what you are feeling. Have you had any illnesses or injuries recently?	Obtain the patient's current complaints, problems, and symptoms. Associated symptoms that may be present with a neurological emergency include headache, memory loss, confusion, motor disturbance (e.g., acute or progressive loss of mobility), neck or back pain, paralysis, paresthesia, paresis, speech disturbances, stiff neck, syncope, vertigo, vision disturbances, weakness, and loss of bladder or bowel control. There are many medical problems that can cause or worsen a neurological illness. Be alert for other explanations for what may, at first, appear to be an obvious behavioral problem (e.g., AMS, unresponsiveness, coma, abnormal respiratory pattern, hypo- or hyperglycemia, and hypo- or hyperthermia). Consider using AEIOUTIPS to remember the many causes of AMS (see Table 14-7).
Allergies	Do you have any allergies? Are you allergic to any medications?	An allergic reaction can cause loss of neurological function. Many medications have side effects that may alter neurological functioning and cause a neurological emergency.
Medications	Are you currently taking any medications? Has your dosage or medication changed recently?	Look for any changes in the medication schedule, especially noncompliance. Investigate the possible use of over-the-counter (OTC) medications, herbals, homeopathic therapies, or use of

(continues)

TABLE 14-2 *(continued)*

Information	Questions	Remarks
Medications *(continued)*	Have you taken any over-the-counter products to relieve your symptoms?	someone else's medication. Table 14-3 contains some of the more common medications prescribed for neurological problems.
Pertinent past medical history	Have you ever experienced anything like this before? Do you have any other medical conditions you are currently being treated for?	Does the patient have a history of this type of condition or a condition that may cause the current emergency (e.g., uncontrolled hypertension leading to stroke or an insulin-dependent diabetic having a hypoglycemic event)?
Last oral intake	When did you last eat? When did you last have anything to drink? Have you taken any medications or tried any home remedies to alleviate the symptoms?	Be specific about medication doses, alcohol, and meals (e.g., hypoglycemia may be involved).
Events leading up to this incident	What were you doing when you began experiencing the problem? Have you had any recent illnesses or injuries?	Make inquiries about associated conditions that may have precipitated this condition such as noncompliance with medications, new illness, new or recent trauma, and any changes in the patient's daily living environment.

TABLE 14-3
Common Medications for Neurological Disorders

Disorder	Medications
Alzheimer's disease	donepezil, ergoloid, nalozone, selegiline, tacrine, Aricept
Parkinson's disease	amantadine, atropine, benztropine, biperiden, bromocriptine, carbidopa, levadopa, diphenhydramine, pergolide, pramipexole, procyclindine, selegiline, trihexyphenidyl
Seizure	lamotrigine, mephenytion, methsuximide, Nurontin, Dilantin, phenobarbital, Tegretol, tiagabine, Topomax, Zarontin
Migraine headache	Maxalt, Immitrex, Tegretol

THE PHYSICAL EXAMINATION

The neurological examination evaluates the following six components: mental status (MS), cranial nerves (CN), motor response, sensory response, coordination, and reflexes. Assessing for symmetry is one of the objectives of the exam, and asymmetrical findings are abnormal until proved otherwise. In some people asymmetry is normal. They may have had a previous insult or injury, such as a stroke or trauma, or they were just born that way. The EMS provider must always ask the patient, "Is this normal for you?"

Obtain a baseline assessment and, whenever possible, verify findings with a family, friend, coworker, or caregiver to determine changes in mental status and any acute or recent changes of neurological functions. Perform and record serial assessments to determine whether the baseline findings are changing and in which direction.

Mental Status

One of the best indicators of nervous system dysfunction is the finding of subtle changes that may be occurring in a patient's mental status. In the initial assessment, the mnemonic AVPU is used for the minineuro exam, followed by the Glasgow Coma Scale (GCS), which is performed in the focused examination. AVPU is quick and easy to perform and provides a gross estimation of the neurological status of the patient. Review Chapter 4 for more details on the procedure of assessing and using AVPU.

The GCS is also easy to perform and provides a more quantitative level of disability. The test was devel-

Clinical Carat

- Assessing for symmetry is one of the objectives of the exam, and asymmetrical findings should be considered abnormal until proved otherwise.

Clinical Carat

- Serial assessments are a key factor to determine whether changes in neurological status are occurring. It helps to determine whether the patient's condition is improving or deteriorating.

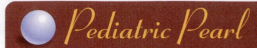

Pediatric Pearl

- There is a pediatric version of the GCS, known as the Modified Glasgow Coma Scale for Infants (see Table 14-4).

oped as a tool to assess trauma patients but is routinely used on medical patients and as a triage tool for making transport decisions. GCS uses three components—eye response, verbal response, and motor response—to develop a score for the best response by the patient. The higher the score, the better the patient's neurological status. Fifteen is the best possible GCS rating. Review Chapter 5 for more information on the GCS.

Mental status evaluation also takes into consideration the patient's **affect** (emotional reaction), behavior, cognition, and memory (recall and short- and long-term memory). The EMS provider considers the patient's

TABLE 14-4
Modified Glasgow Coma Scale for Infants

Activity	Best Response	Score
Eye opening	Spontaneous	4
	To speech	3
	To pain	2
	None	1
Verbal	Coos, babbles	5
	Irritable cries	4
	Cries to pain	3
	Moans to pain	2
	None	1
Motor	Normal spontaneous movements	6
	Withdraws from touch	5
	Withdraws from pain	4
	Abnormal flexion	3
	Abnormal	2
	None	1
Total GCS score		3–15

affect, behavior, and cognition throughout the interview process. Recall and short- and long-term memory are evaluated by the following test and questions:

- Recall. Instruct the patient to remember the name of an object (e.g., red door, blue ball), and then ask the patient to recall that object at 5-minute intervals.
- Short-term memory. What day of the week is it? When did you eat last? When did you take your last dose of medication?
- Long-term memory. What is your date of birth? What is your Social Security number? What is your address?

Cranial Nerve Assessment

Assessing the cranial nerves provides clues to the possible location of insult or injury. The examination can be performed only if the patient is willing and able to follow a few simple commands. When the patient is unable to follow commands (e.g., is unconscious), testing reflexes is appropriate. There are 12 pairs of **cranial nerves** (CN) that innervate mostly the head and face; they control sensory and motor functions. Cranial nerve I is the olfactory nerve and is not routinely tested in the prehospital setting. Cranial nerves II through VII are the most significant in the prehospital setting, and IX through XII are of little value in the field. The testing of cranial nerves is described in Table 14-5.

TABLE 14-5
Testing the Cranial Nerves

CN		Function	Technique
I	olfactory	Smell	Not routinely assessed in the prehospital setting
II	optic	Vision	Acuity, accommodation, field of vision
III	oculomotor	Extraocular muscles (EOMs)	Cardinal positions of gaze, consensual light reflex, pupils
IV	trochlear	EOMs	Cardinal positions of gaze, down and inward eye movement
V	trigeminal	Facial sensation, speech, chewing	Abnormal speech (aphasia, dysphasia, dysarthria), drooling, move jaw against resistance
VI	abducens	EOMs	Cardinal positions of gaze, lateral eye movement
VII	facial	Facial movement	Ask the patient to smile at you and show teeth, then frown and raise the brows.
VIII	acoustic, vestibulocochlear	Hearing	Acute hearing loss
IX	glossopharyngeal	Gag reflex, palate	Insertion of an oropharyngeal airway (OPA) during unresponsiveness; observe the palate as the patients says "aah"
X	vagus	Gag reflex, swallowing, heart rate	Insertion of an OPA during unresponsiveness
XI	spinal accessory	Shoulder shrug, head turning	Shrugging shoulders against resistance
XII	hypoglossal	Tongue movement	Ask the patient to stick out the tongue.

Note: Facial symmetry is tested in active motion.

Assess the pupils for size, shape, and reaction to light. Assess acuity, accommodation, field of vision, and movement of **extraocular muscles (EOMs)**. Extraocular muscles produce movement of the eyes. The pupils should be equally round and about 3–5 mm in diameter (Figure 14-1). A difference of more than 1 mm is abnormal. The term **anisocoria** means unequal pupils and may indicate a central nervous system disease or traumatic injury; however, a small percentage of the population has anisocoria normally. Ask the patient whether this is normal!

The pupils should constrict as a normal reaction to a light source. When the ambient light is bright, the EMS provider should use her hand to block out the light source and observe for dilation. When a light is shone into one eye, the pupils of both eyes should constrict as a normal response; this is called the **consensual light reflex** and involves CN III.

Assess visual **acuity** by asking the patient if he needs glasses to read and have the patient use them to read your name tag or count the number of fingers you are holding up. **Accommodation** is the ability of the eyes to adjust to focus on variations in distance (Figure 14-2). Normally the eyes move apart (diverge) as they focus on a distant object. As the object comes closer to the face, the eyes should move toward each other

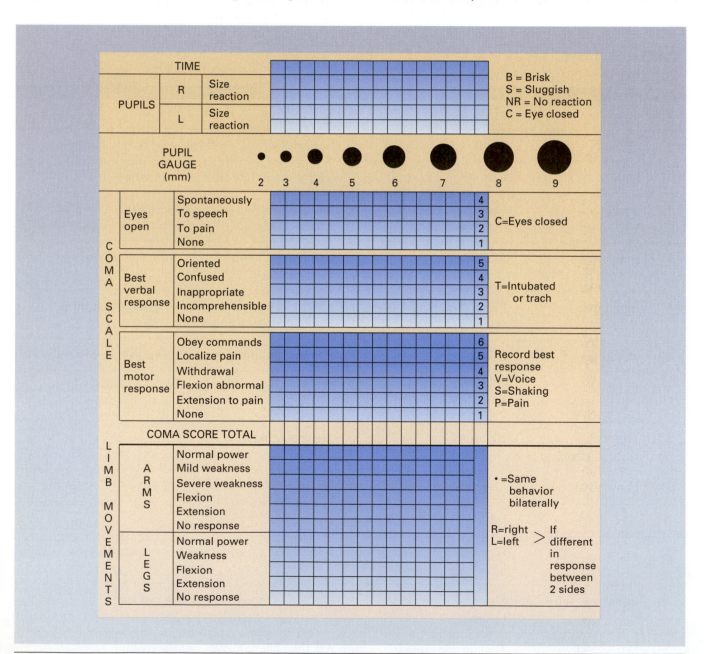

FIGURE 14-1 The pupil gauge as it is incorporated into a neurological flow sheet.

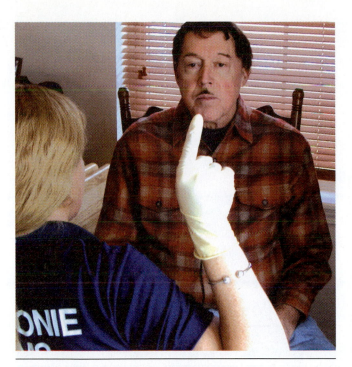

FIGURE 14-2 Testing a patient for accommodation helps to evaluate cranial nerve II.

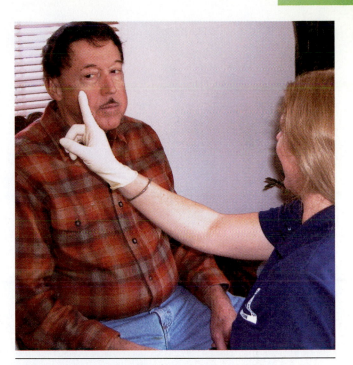

FIGURE 14-3 Testing the extraocular muscles by having the patient follow your finger through the "H" motion helps to evaluate cranial nerves III and IV and VI.

(converge), and the pupils should constrict. Ask the patient to first focus on a distant object then to focus on your finger as you hold it in front of the face and watch for accommodation and constriction. Convergence involves CN II and III.

Assess the **field of vision** (peripheral vision). Ask the patient to cover one eye, stand back a couple of feet, and look directly at you while you stretch out your arm with your index finger pointing up. Then ask the patient to tell you when he can see your finger as you bring it to the center from the periphery. He should see your finger at the same time you do. The field of vision involves CN II.

Three cranial nerves are involved in the innervation of the extraocular muscles (EOMs). Checking EOMs is the single best method for measuring brain stem integrity, specifically the pons and midbrain. Assess the six cardinal positions of gaze (Figure 14-3) by asking the patient to look at your finger while you hold it up in front of his face. Tell the patient not to move his head but to follow your finger only with his eyes. Slowly move your finger up and down and side to side in the shape of the letter H. The inability to move one or both eyes may indicate a neurological deficit involving CN III, IV, and VI. Paralysis of a lateral gaze is an early sign of rising intracranial pressure (ICP), and paralysis of the upward gaze may indicate an orbital fracture.

During the assessment of the eyes, **nystagmus**, a fine motor twitching of the eyeball, may be noted and is normal during extreme lateral gaze but not in any other

position. This condition may be caused by heavy alcohol intoxication, multiple sclerosis, brain lesion, or disease in the ear canal.

For recording purposes, the letters PERRLA are commonly used to document normal findings with the eyes. They represent *p*upils *e*qually *r*ound, *r*eactive to *l*ight and *a*ccommodation.

Facial movement and sensation are assessed by asking the patient to smile at you and show his teeth, then frown, and raise the brows. Drooping on one side of the face is an abnormal finding of CN VII that is associated with paralysis as seen in a cerebrovascular accident (CVA) or a transient ischemic attack (TIA). Assess the palate, and CN X, by asking the patient to open his mouth and say "aah"; the soft palate should rise in the middle and the uvula should be midline. Ask the patient to stick out his tongue to assess CN XII. The tongue should be midline when sticking out. The tongue's turning to one side or the other would indicate paralysis toward the deviated side (Figure 14-4). The gag reflex is assessed on unresponsive patients by attempting to insert an oropharyngeal airway (OPA). If the patient gags during the attempt, he has a good gag reflex and you have assessed CN IX and X. An absent gag reflex is a bad sign and indicates deep unconsciousness.

Note any abnormal speech: for example, **aphasia** (defect or loss of the power of speech), **dysphasia** (abnormal speech due to lack of coordination), or

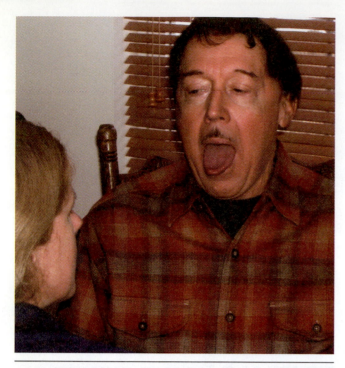

FIGURE 14-4 Assessing the patient's tongue movement helps to evaluate cranial nerve XII.

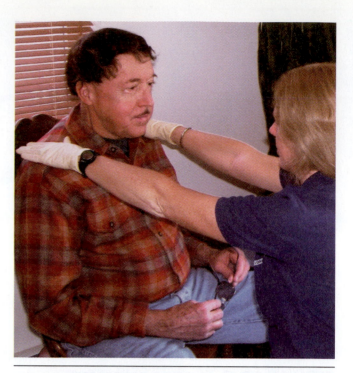

FIGURE 14-5 Assessing the patient for a shoulder shrug against your resistance helps to evaluate cranial nerve XI.

dysarthria (abnormal speech due to a disturbance in muscle control). Also note difficulty swallowing (**dysphagia**) or chewing and drooling. To assess CN V, ask the patient to move the jaw from side to side while you place resistance with your hands; note any unilateral weakness. A sudden loss of hearing is a significant finding, often involving CN VIII. Otherwise, hearing is not further assessed in the prehospital setting.

Test the strength and symmetry of the shoulder shrug (Figure 14-5) by positioning yourself in front of the patient, placing your hands on his shoulders, and then asking him to shrug his shoulders against your resistance. This motion helps to evaluate CN XI.

Exploring the Web

● Search the Web for functioning of the cranial nerves and techniques to use to assess function. Create index cards for each nerve, indicating what the nerve innervates, how to assess for that function, and the alterations in functions to look for. Concentrate your attention on cranial nerves II through VII.

Assessment of Motor Response

Testing of motor responses is performed to assess muscle strength, tone, symmetry, and paralysis. Assess for equality in both upper and lower extremities. For the testing of motor responses to be valid, the EMS provider must determine whether the patient has any preexisting conditions or deficits. When pain or injury is present, do not test the affected extremity.

To test the upper extremities, test grip strength and assess for a **pronator drift**. Have the patient grasp both of your hands and squeeze while you feel for equality of grip strength. Next ask the patient to extend both arms out in front of him with the palms up and have him close both eyes (Figure 14-6). If one arm "drifts" lower or the palm turns downward, this is considered a deficit or indicator of focal weakness.

If the EMS provider suspects the patient is feigning unconsciousness, the "drop test" may be used. Lift the patient's arm over his face and let the arm drop. When the patient is feigning, the arm will drop more slowly than normal or will fall with exaggerated speed away from the face. This test is usually successful provided the patient does not know the test.

Assess the lower extremities by asking the patient to push and pull his feet against the resistance of both of your hands simultaneously. Assess for unilateral weakness. When appropriate, assess the patient's gait by

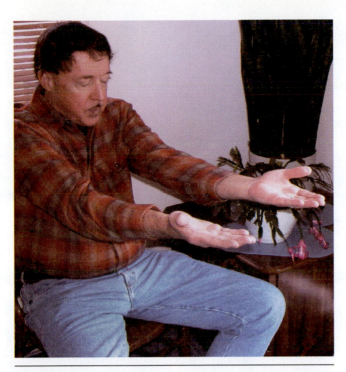

FIGURE 14-6 Assessing the patient for pronator drift is done with the palms up and patient's eyes closed.

having him take a few steps (e.g., walking to the stretcher). A deficit would be an imbalance while walking. If the patient's gait is abnormal, ask whether this way of walking is normal for him.

Assessment of Sensory Response

The sensory response component of the neurological exam is useful in the patient who is conscious or has a suspected spinal cord injury (SCI); otherwise, it may be the least exact component. **Dermatomes** (Figure 14-7) are the areas on the surface of the body that are innervated by afferent nerve fibers from one spinal root. Dermatomes can be used to estimate a rough correlation to the level of a spinal injury. For the suspected SCI patient with loss of sensation or paralysis, begin at the head and work down the neck and torso to find the line of demarcation for loss of sensation. For the non-SCI patient, assess for distinction between sharp and dull touch on the skin of the face and extremities. Ask the patient to close his eyes while you alternately touch the skin with a sharp and a dull object, such as the point and eraser on a pencil. Have the patient tell you where and which type of touch he feels. Light touch is lost before dull, and dull touch can remain intact even in severe SCI. In the unconscious patient, assess for deep pain response by using a sternal rub or pinching the nail beds.

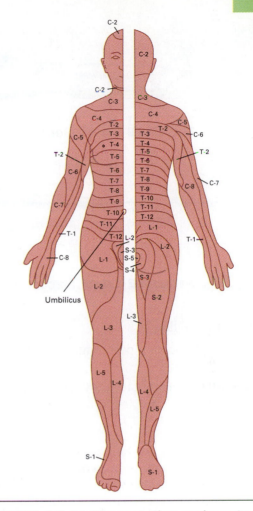

FIGURE 14-7 The anterior and posterior dermatome distributions.

Assessment of Coordination and Reflexes

Testing balance and the ability of fine movements assesses cerebellar function of the brain. Observing the patient's gait assesses motor responses and coordination. Some examples of an abnormal gait would be **ataxia** (wobbly and unsteady as when one is intoxicated or heavily medicated), **festination** (uneven and hurried as seen in Parkinson's disease), **spastic hemiparesis** (unilateral weakness and foot dragging), and **steppage** (the person appears to be walking up steps when on an even surface). Fine movements are assessed by asking the patient to touch his finger to his nose. Fine movements can also be assessed by having the patient close his eyes and then touch his two index fingers together.

Reflexes are also tested to determine the possibility of SCI. In the prehospital setting, the assessment of reflexes is primarily used in the unconscious or unresponsive patient. The level of reflex response from good to bad is listed as follows:

- Purposefully withdrawing from pain

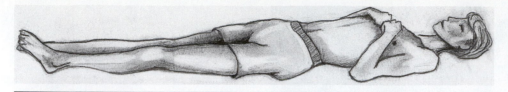

FIGURE 14-8 Decorticate or flexion posturing.

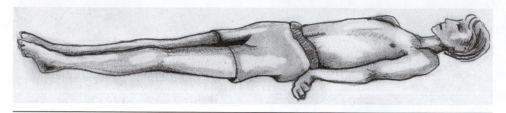

FIGURE 14-9 Decerebrate or extension posturing.

- Absent gag reflex
- Flexion (decorticate posturing, as shown in Figure 14-8)
- Extension (decerebrate posturing, as shown in Figure 14-9)
- No response

The **plantar reflex** is assessed on both conscious and unconscious patients with suspected SCI. With the end of a capped pen, draw a light stroke up the lateral side of the sole of the foot and across the ball of the foot, like an upside-down letter J. The normal response is plantar flexion of the toes and foot. The abnormal response is dorsiflexion of the big toe and fanning of all the toes. This is a positive **Babinski's reflex** (Figure 14-10) and

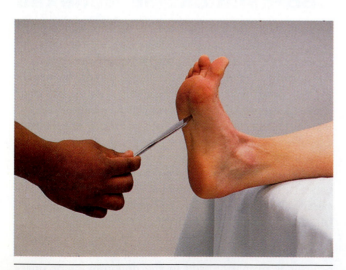

FIGURE 14-10 In a positive Babinski's reflex, the big toe turns upward when a blunt stimulus is applied to the sole of the foot.

Pediatric Pearl

- In pediatrics a positive Babinski's reflex is normal until the spinal cord and nerves mature at approximately 18 months.

indicates a disturbance in the motor response of the central nervous system.

Use of Diagnostic Tools

The diagnostic tools used during the neurological exam should include:

- Glucometer/dexistrip. A blood sugar reading should be taken on every patient with an AMS to exclude the possibility of hypo- and hyperglycemia.
- Thermometer. Hypo- and hyperthermia, especially in the very young and the elderly, are causes of neurological problems.
- ECG. An electrocardiogram reading can alert the EMS provider to the presence of cardiac dysrhythmias, which can provoke neurological problems.
- Pulse oximetry. Hypoxia is a cause of AMS, and pulse oximetry to determine oxygen saturation (SpO_2) may be of value. However, visual inspection for perfusion status should never be deemphasized or disregarded for a meter reading.
- Capnography. The level of end-tidal carbon dioxide ($EtCO_2$) can help determine whether a patient is breathing effectively or whether an airway adjunct is properly inserted.

FEATURES OF A NEUROLOGICAL EMERGENCY

Some of the most common neurological emergencies include stroke, altered mental status (AMS, e.g., dementia, Alzheimer's disease, alcohol overdose), seizure, headache, and **traumatic brain injury (TBI)**. One of the features helpful in making a field impression of a neurological event is the duration of onset. Pathologies that are vascular in nature are more likely to be acute in onset (e.g., seconds to minutes). Some vascular pathologies may come with a warning sign, such as a **transient ischemic attack (TIA)** before a **cerebrovascular accident (CVA)**. A TIA is a temporary interruption of blood flow to the brain, and a CVA is a stroke that involves an interruption of blood flow to the brain. Rapid changes that have occurred over 2 or 3 days may be due to dehydration, central nervous system (CNS) infection, subdural hematoma, a medication problem, or other toxic metabolic conditions. Degenerative or chronic neurological diseases are those that progressively worsen over weeks or years. A patient with Alzheimer's or Parkinson's disease can have mental status changes that vary from day to day, with good and bad days.

COMMON NEUROLOGICAL CONDITIONS

Neurological emergencies occur as a result of an injury by trauma or insult by illness or disease to the nervous system. Assessment of a patient with a neurological emergency includes evaluation of the nervous system, cerebral hemispheres, cerebellum, brain stem, spinal cord, and peripheral nerves. This section briefly discusses the most common neurological emergencies found in the field, including patients who present with signs and symptoms of stroke, AMS, seizures, headache, traumatic brain injury, or neurogenic shock. In all cases, the EMS provider should administer oxygen early to treat hypoxia and obtain a blood glucose reading quickly to exclude hypo- or hyperglycemia as causes of the current emergency.

Stroke

Cerebrovascular accident (CVA) is an acute loss of blood flow to the brain, and transient ischemic attack (TIA) is an acute temporary loss of blood flow to the brain. Both conditions are associated with easily recognizable symptoms and neurological deficits, as listed in Table 14-6.

The American Heart Association has recognized two prehospital ministroke tests to help in the assess-

TABLE 14-6
Symptoms and Neurological Deficits Associated with Cerebrovascular Accident and Transient Ischemic Attack

Symptom

- Acute or persistent severe headache with no apparent cause
- Acute vision disturbance; blurred or decreased vision in one or both eyes
- Difficulty with speech or understanding simple statements
- Numbness, weakness, or paralysis of muscles in the face, arm, or leg—especially on one side of the body
- Loss of balance or coordination—especially when combined with another one of the symptoms listed above

Deficits

- Visual: **diplopia** (double vision), loss of peripheral vision, loss of half of the visual field
- Motor: ataxia (unsteady gait), dysarthria (difficulty forming words), dysphagia (difficulty swallowing), hemiparesis (one-sided weakness), hemiplegia (one-sided paralysis)
- Sensory: paresthesia (tingling or numbness of body parts), difficulty with **proprioception** (perceptions concerning movements and position of the body)
- Verbal: expressive aphasia (can understand but cannot utter the words), receptive aphasia (cannot understand spoken, written, or tactile speech), global aphasia (total aphasia involving all functions of communication)
- Cognitive: short- and long-term memory loss, decreased attention span and ability to concentrate, poor judgment and reasoning

ment of a suspected stroke patient. They are the **Cincinnati Prehospital Stroke Scale** (Figure 14-11) and the **Los Angeles Prehospital Stroke Screen**

Facial droop (have the patient show his teeth or smile):

- Normal: the two sides of face move equally
- Abnormal: one side of face does not move as well as the other

Arm drift (patient closes eyes and holds both arms straight out for 10 seconds):

- Normal: both arms move the same or both arms do not move at all (other findings, such as strength of grip, may be helpful)
- Abnormal: one arm does not move or one arm drifts down compared with the other

Abnormal speech (have the patient say, "You can't teach an old dog new tricks"):

- Normal: patient uses correct words with no slurring
- Abnormal: patient slurs words, uses the wrong words, or is unable to speak

Interpretation: If any one of these three signs is abnormal, the probability of a stroke is 72%.

FIGURE 14-11 The Cincinnati Prehospital Stroke Scale. (Reprinted with permission from the *Annals of Emergency Medicine*, 33, 273–278, 1999. St. Louis, MO: Mosby)

(LAPSS) (Figure 14-12). These scales are easy to apply and beginning to gain widespread use. The EMS provider should be alert for facial asymmetry, such as abnormal facial droop or difficulty with speech. Be sure to assess grip strength and pronator drift in the field examination of the suspected stroke patient.

Altered Mental Status

Altered mental status (AMS) has numerous causes and varying degrees of severity. The mnemonic **AEIOUTIPS** (Table 14-7) is used to remember the many possible reasons a person may experience an altered mental state. These may be as subtle as confusion or agitation or as

Exploring the Web

- Search the Web for each of the causes of altered mental status (AMS) in Table 14-7. Create an index card for each, listing the signs and symptoms of AMS for each condition, assessment findings you can expect, and treatment priorities.

TABLE 14-7
AEIOUTIPS for Causes of Altered Mental Status

Alcohol: acute or chronic abuse, intoxication, or overdose

Epilepsy, **e**ndocrine, **e**xocrine, or **e**lectrolytes

Infection: local or systemic

Overdose: accidental or intentional

Uremia: due to renal failure, hypertension, or traumatic injury

Trauma: new or old; **t**emperature: hypo- or hyperthermia

Insulin: hypo- or hyperglycemia

Psychosis: various conditions

Stroke: hemorrhagic or ischemic; **s**hock, **s**pace-occupying lesion, or **s**ubarachnoid bleed

obvious as unconsciousness or coma. Use AEIOUTIPS to begin a differential diagnosis and exclude causes such as trauma, hypoxia, and hypoglycemia during the focused history and examination. While obtaining vital signs, include taking a body temperature and a blood glucose reading, as these are common causes of AMS especially in the very young and the elderly.

Seizure

During the focused history, the specific information to ask about seizures is whether this is a first-time seizure or whether there is a history of seizures. Once it has been determined that the seizure is the patient's first seizure, the EMS provider should ask about recent head trauma, illness, or infection. For the patient with a history of seizures, ask about changes or compliance with antiseizure (anticonvulsant) medication and the use of alcohol or substance abuse. Also determine whether today's seizure was different in any way from the patient's previous seizure pattern because a difference may be a clue to a new underlying problem.

Seizures occur in all age groups, and their causes vary slightly with each group. Regardless of the causes, the EMS provider should manage the ABCs and be prepared for another seizure during the assessment and management of the patient. Consider treatable causes first, such as hypoglycemia and hypoxia. For most seizure calls, the seizing will have stopped by the time EMS arrives and the patient will be in the post-ictal phase (period following the seizure activity). The post-

1. Patient name: _____   _____
                        (last name)   (first name)

2. Information/History from:

    [ ] Patient
    [ ] Family member   _____   _____
    [ ] Other   (last name)   (first name)

3. Last known time patient was at baseline or deficit free and awake:

    _____   _____
              (military time)   (date)

SCREENING CRITERIA

	Yes	Unknown	No
4. Age >45	[ ]	[ ]	[ ]
5. History of seizures or epilepsy absent	[ ]	[ ]	[ ]
6. Symptom duration less than 24 hours	[ ]	[ ]	[ ]
7. At baseline, patient is not wheelchair bound or bedridden	[ ]	[ ]	[ ]

	Yes	No
8. Blood glucose between 60 and 400	[ ]	[ ]

9. Exam: **LOOK FOR OBVIOUS ASYMMETRY**

	Normal	Right	Left
Facial smile/grimace	[ ]	[ ] Droop	[ ] Droop
Grip	[ ]	[ ] Weak grip [ ] No grip	[ ] Weak grip [ ] No grip
Arm strength	[ ]	[ ] Drifts down [ ] Falls rapidly	[ ] Drifts down [ ] Falls rapidly

Based on exam, patient has only unilateral (and not bilateral) weakness:

Yes	No
[ ]	[ ]

10. Items 4, 5, 6, 7, 8, 9 all YESs (or unknown)—LAPSS screening criteria met:

Yes	No
[ ]	[ ]

11. If LAPSS criteria for stroke met, call receiving hospital with a "code stroke." If not, then return to the appropriate treatment protocol. (Note: the patient may still be experiencing a stroke even if the LAPSS criteria are not met.)

For more information, contact Chelsea S. Kidwell, MD, Department of Neurology, UCLA Medical Center, Reed NRC, 710 Westwood Plaza, Los Angeles, CA 90095 or email ckidwell@ucla.edu.

FIGURE 14-12 The Los Angeles Prehospital Stroke Screen (LAPSS). (Reprinted courtesy of Chelsea S. Kidwell, MD, Department of Neurology, UCLA Medical Center, Los Angeles, CA)

Clinical Carat

● Change matters! Recent seizure activity may be a clue to a new problem, such as a child who is growing out of her needs.

ictal phase varies in duration for each individual. Most patients will be exhausted from the event, and many will be confused initially but will progressively improve over several minutes.

Seizures can be broken down in three phases: **pre-ictal phase** (before), **ictal phase** (seizure attack), and post-ical phase (after). There are several types of seizure, and each has classic findings before, during, and after the seizure. These findings can help identify which type of seizure the patient may have experienced or help to identify a second or third should it occur before arriving at the emergency department. If the EMS provider did not witness the seizure, she should question persons who did.

Partial seizures occur in a particular area of the brain, so the patient remains conscious and the effects are apparent only in a specific area of the body. Partial seizures are further classified as simple, complex, and partial with secondary generalization. A simple partial, or focal, seizure may appear as a shaking in only one arm or leg. A complex partial seizure briefly impairs the mental status and may include an aura. An **aura** is a subjective sensation (e.g., voices, a specific smell, or colored lights) experienced just before the attack. The AMS may be confusion or personality changes with outbursts and fits of rage. Partial seizure with secondary generalization is easily recognized by the description; it begins in one local area and spreads throughout the entire body. This type of seizure is sometimes called Jacksonian march.

Generalized seizures involve the entire brain and are classified as complete motor seizure, absence seizure, and atonic seizure. The complete motor seizure (formerly called grand mal) may include an aura followed by a loss of consciousness and muscle contractions (tonic phase) and continuing on with alternating muscle spasms (clonic phase). During the tonic phase, normal respirations are briefly disrupted, and the disruption may cause hypoxia. In the clonic phase, the classic tongue biting and incontinence (usually urine) may occur. The post-ictal phase will be apparent, with disorientation, confusion, fatigue, and sometimes headache.

Absence seizures, once called petit mal seizures, are common in children, and the patient is described as staring off into space or daydreaming. This type of seizure usually comes without warning or an aura, and the post-ictal phase is usually brief. Atonic seizures, common in children, arise with a complete loss of pos-

tural control, causing the patient to collapse and possibly sustain secondary injuries from the fall.

The Patient Complaining of a Headache

Headaches in and of themselves are a common neurological complaint and often are an associated symptom of other medical complaints. They can also be a side effect of medications such as nitroglycerin. The most common causes of headache in adults and children are tension or muscle contraction and sinusitis. Less common types include vascular (including migraine) and cluster headaches and those caused by temporal arteritis, subarachnoid bleed or leak, increased intracranial pressure, glaucoma, eyestrain, meningitis, or systemic problems (e.g., anemia, uremia, brain tumors or infection).

During the focused history, determine whether the headache is acute, recurrent, or chronic. The type of headache, severity, and location of pain are important information in the differentiation of its causes.

Types and Severity

Tension headaches are associated with stress (emotional or physical), anxiety, long periods of intense concentration, and depression. Sinus headaches tend to begin in the morning and worsen progressively throughout the day. Often there is increased pressure with coughing or sneezing.

Migraine headache pain is severe and throbbing initially, then changes to a persisting dull pain. The pain increases rapidly and steadily and can last for hours or days. Associated symptoms include light sensitivity, nausea, and vomiting. Some patients describe experiencing an aura before a migraine headache. Cluster headaches are very severe, with stabbing and burning sensations. They occur in patterns such as starting at the same time each day but lasting for shorter durations.

Location of the Head Pain

The location of a headache does not always indicate the cause, but there are certain conditions that present with somewhat consistent associated findings. Hypertension, for example, together with severe headache may indicate subarachnoid hemorrhage. Headache accompanied by fever may indicate meningitis, encephalitis, or brain abscess. Additional examples of findings associated with headaches are shown in Table 14-8.

Additional associated signs and symptoms that may be present with headache include nausea, vomiting, photophobia (sensitivity to light), dizziness, hypertension, acute neurological deficits such as vision or speech disturbance, loss of balance or coordination, weakness, or paralysis.

It is often difficult to determine the specific cause of a headache, especially in the prehospital setting. Do

TABLE 14-8
Findings Associated with Headaches

Cerebral aneurysm: localized unilateral pain

Cluster: unilateral and periorbital

Glaucoma: eye pain

Meningitis: pain in the back of the head

Migraine: unilateral or bilateral pain

Subarachnoid hemorrhage: worst headache ever experienced

Temporal arteritis: pain of temporal artery

Tension: pain could be anywhere in the head

Temporomandibular joint (TMJ) syndrome: pain upon jaw movement

Trauma: pain could be anywhere in the head

Trigeminal neuralgia (tic douloureux): facial pain

not try to make a specific diagnosis in the field; rather, exclude as many possible associated findings and report your information to the emergency department.

The Patient with a Traumatic Brain Injury

During the initial assessment, a head injury is identified as open or closed, depending on the presence of penetration (e.g., hole from a gunshot wound or depressed skull). A careful scene size-up will help reveal the mechanism of injury (MOI). One or more of the four general categories of head injury—focal, diffuse axonal, coup, and contre-coup—may result from TBI. The MOI should alert the EMS provider to suspect such an injury. Assessment findings might strengthen those suspicions, but a computerized axial tomography (CAT) scan, in the emergency department, is needed to help make the specific diagnosis.

Focal Injury

A **focal head injury** results in brain lesions such as a cerebral contusion, intracranial hemorrhage, or epidural hematoma. Assessment findings associated with a cerebral contusion (Figure 14-13) may include confusion or unusual behavior, complaint of a worsening headache, photophobia (fear of bright light), loss of short-term memory (repetition of the same phrases), and signs and symptoms of rising ICP (AMS, decreased Glasgow Coma Scale, vomiting, changes in pupils, decreased pulse rate, and increased blood pressure). Assessment findings associated with intracranial hemorrhage include those seen with cerebral contusion as well as neurological posturing, paralysis of one side of the body, or seizure activity.

Diffuse Axonal Injury

Diffuse axonal injuries (DAIs) occur as a result of rapid acceleration or deceleration on the brain, as occurs in some motor vehicle collisions. The classic injury seen is the concussion (Figure 14-14). A concussion results in a transient episode of neuronal dysfunction with a rapid return to normal neurological activity.

The forces exerted cause bruising of the brain tissue with or without bleeding. Assessment findings may include persistent confusion, disorientation, and amnesia of the event or amnesia of moment-to-moment events. The patient may have a focal deficit, an inability to concentrate, and periods of anxiety or mood swings.

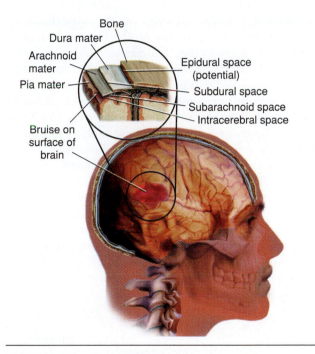

FIGURE 14-13 The contusion injury.

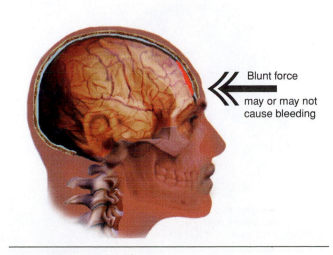

FIGURE 14-14 The concussion injury.

A more severe injury may cause unconsciousness, posturing, and signs of ICP.

Coup and Contrecoup Injuries

Coup injuries develop directly beneath the point of impact, and **contrecoup** injuries develop on the opposite side of the point of impact. When the two occur in the same event, the injury is called coup-contrecoup (Figure 14-15).

Deterioration of a Brain Injury

Deterioration of a mild injury to a severe injury and death has a predictable pattern of signs and symptoms. Mild to severe head injuries cause AMS, amnesia of the event, confusion, disorientation, combativeness, or focal neurological deficits. Pressure on the hypothalamus causes vomiting, and pressure on the brain stem causes the blood pressure to rise. The elevated blood pressure is a normal compensatory response that is needed to perfuse the injured tissues.

Severe injuries may continue to put pressure on the brain stem, causing the vagus nerve (CN X) to stimulate bradycardia and posturing such as flexion or extension (see Figures 14-8 and 14-9). Because pressure on the oculomotor nerve (CN III) causes unequal or unreactive pupils, the presence of unequal pupils should not be considered an early indication of head injury. The earliest indication of head injury would be a significant MOI and the presence of subtle changes in the mental status. Pressure on the respiratory center causes irregular respirations, leading to carbon dioxide retention, brain swelling, and hypoxemia in the brain tissue.

Intracranial Hemorrhage

When bleeding in the brain (intracranial hemorrhage) occurs as a result of injury, the type of intracranial hemorrhage is identified by its location (Figure 14-16) in relation to the layers of the meninges: epidural hematoma, subdural hematoma, subarachnoid hemorrhage, and intracerebral hematoma. The neurological deficits that may develop will depend on the area of the brain involved, the size of the hemorrhage, whether the bleeding continues with subsequent brain herniation, and associated injuries.

Epidural hematoma (Figure 14-17) is rare and almost always involves an arterial tear, usually from the middle meningeal artery. It is the rationale for the use of batters' helmets in baseball to protect the side of the head exposed to the pitch. An understanding of the classic presentation of an epidural hematoma can help save a patient's life. These injuries usually involve a blow to the temporal skull followed by a period of unconsciousness. The patient often regains consciousness and has a lucid interval. Then, within a short time, the patient's condition rapidly deteriorates to coma. By recognizing this classic presentation, deciding to rapidly remove the patient to a trauma center, and informing the emergency department personnel while en route that an epidural

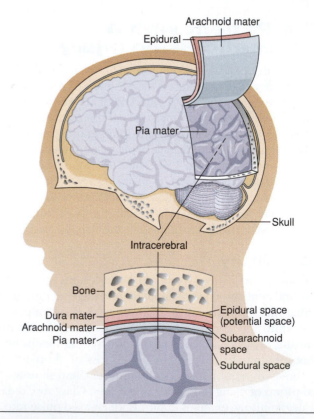

FIGURE 14-16 The anatomy of the scalp, meninges, and brain defines the location of a hematoma, such as epidural, subdural, subarachnoid, and intracerebral.

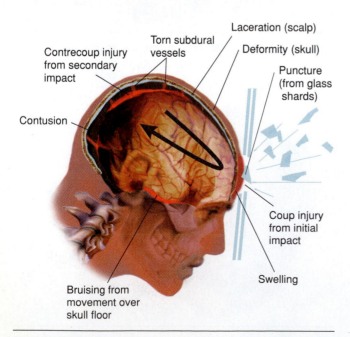

FIGURE 14-15 The coup-contrecoup injury.

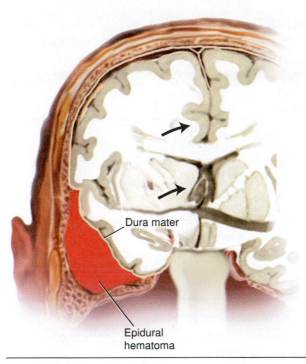

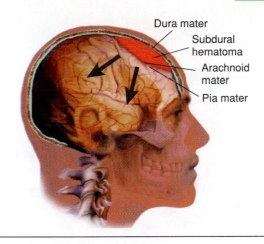

FIGURE 14-18 The subdural hematoma. Note the shift of the midline structures.

FIGURE 14-17 The epidural hematoma. Note the shift of midline structures (small arrows).

hematoma is likely, the EMS provider can dramatically increase the patient's chance for survival.

Subdural hematoma (Figure 14-18) is bleeding from the rupture of bridging veins between the cortex (neural tissue that covers the brain) and dura mater. Subdural hematomas can be acute, chronic, or delayed. This injury is very common, especially in the elderly and chronic alcoholics, who frequently fall down and hit their head. Subarachnoid hemorrhage usually results from rupture of an aneurysm in the 35 to 65 year age group. The patient will complain of having the worst headache ever experienced and may rapidly develop stupor progressing to coma. Intracerebral hematoma occurs from small deep intracerebral hemorrhages

within the brain substances and is associated with other brain injuries. The deficits will be reflective of the specific location of the bleeding.

The skull is hard and nonexpandable, so when bleeding in the brain occurs and continues there is little room for both the blood and the brain. When bleeding and/or swelling continues, the pressure inside the skull increases (rising intracranial pressure, or ICP) and the brain is pushed out (herniated) of the skull through the only opening, the foramen magnum at the base of the skull (Figure 14-19).

Brain herniation syndrome has three phases (Table 14-9): early, late, and terminal. In the moments just before death, a recognizable pattern of falling blood pressure, bradycardia, and irregular breathing patterns will appear as the late stage, which lasts only 4 to 6 minutes.

Neurogenic Shock

Neurogenic shock, a form of shock often called fainting or syncope, is due to disorders of the nervous system with an absence of sympathetic response. Three assessment findings that, when displayed together, indicate

Clinical Carat

- Recognize Cushing's triad when examining the head-injured patient. **Cushing's triad** is three assessment findings that, when displayed together, indicate increasing intracranial pressure (ICP). They are rising blood pressure, decreasing pulse rate, and changes in the respiratory pattern.

Exploring the Web

- Search for additional information on each of the types of brain injury discussed in this chapter. What are the significant findings in each? What assessment techniques can be used to alert you to the signs and symptoms of brain injury? What are the consequences if you miss the possibility of a brain injury?

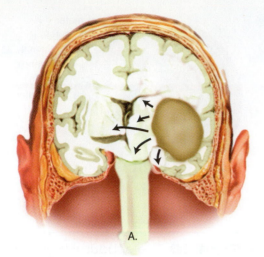

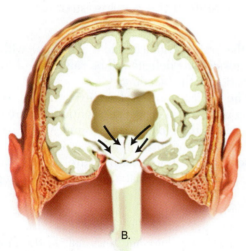

FIGURE 14-19 Brain herniation causes increased intracranial pressure and brain stem compression. An uncal herniation (**A**) occurs in one hemisphere, and a central herniation (**B**) occurs in both hemispheres, as shown by the arrows in the diagram.

TABLE 14-9
Three Phases of Brain Herniation Syndrome

Early

- Altered mental status
- Focal neurological deficits such as facial droop or unilateral weakness
- Increased blood pressure
- Nausea or vomiting or both
- Pupils reactive
- Normal response to pain stimuli

Late

- Increasing blood pressure
- Irregular respirations such as Cheyne-Stokes or ataxic breathing
- Wide pulse pressure
- Bradycardia
- Pupils sluggish, unequal, or nonreactive
- Decorticate posturing (flexion) followed by decerebrate posturing (extension)

Terminal

- Ataxic respirations (erratic or absent)
- Irregular pulse rate with great swings in rate
- Blown pupil on the side of injury
- Flaccid muscle tone
- ECG with QRS, ST, and T wave changes

neurogenic shock are decreasing blood pressure, normal or slightly slow pulse rate, and decreasing respiratory rate. Causes of neurogenic shock include injury or transection of the spinal cord (also referred to as spinal shock), central nervous system injury, anaphylactic reaction, insulin overdose, septicemia from bacterial infection, and Addisonian crisis (a disorder of the adrenal glands).

CONCLUSION

The key aspect of a neurological examination for the EMS provider is to determine whether the patient's baseline assessment findings are changing and in which direction. The EMS provider should perform serial assessments and document the findings of the mental status using AVPU and the Glasgow Coma Scale (GCS), respiratory pattern, vital signs, cranial nerves, and sensory and motor responses. In this way, the EMS provider will be able to get an early indication of the subtle changes occurring in the patient's neurological status. The use of additional diagnostic measures such as blood sugar, ECG, temperature, oxygen saturation (SpO$_2$), and end-tidal carbon dioxide (EtCO$_2$) readings is necessary to find and correct immediate life-threatening conditions such as hypoglycemia and hypoxia. The patient having difficulty communicating often understands what is happening and is frightened. The EMS provider must realize that the inability to speak or write coherently does not necessarily mean that there is a loss of mental competence and therefore must provide psychological support as a part of patient care.

REVIEW QUESTIONS

1. An example of a degenerative or chronic neurological disease would be:
   a. dehydration.
   b. Alzheimer's.
   c. subdural hematoma.
   d. transient ischemic attack.

2. The neurological examination evaluates each of the following components except:
   a. degree of pain.
   b. reflexes.
   c. motor response.
   d. cranial nerves.

3. Of the following, which cranial nerve is tested and most useful to the EMS provider's field assessment?
   a. I
   b. III
   c. VIII
   d. XII

4. When you shine a light into one eye and both eyes constrict, this reaction is _____ and is called _____ .
   a. abnormal; accommodation
   b. abnormal; the conjungate gaze
   c. normal; the consensual light reflex
   d. normal; the field of vision

5. The extraocular muscles are innervated by cranial nerves:
   a. II, III, and V.
   b. I, III, and VI.
   c. IV, VII, and IX.
   d. III, IV, and VI.

6. Difficulty swallowing is referred to as:
   a. aphasia.
   b. dysphagia.
   c. dysarthria.
   d. neuralgia.

7. A rough estimate of the level of spinal cord injury can be determined by assessing the patient's:
   a. dermatomes.
   b. spastic hemiparesis.
   c. festination.
   d. steppage.

8. Common neurological emergencies seen in the field include all of the following except:
   a. seizure.
   b. stroke.
   c. TBI.
   d. hypoglycemia.

9. Of the following seizures, which is not classified as a generalized seizure?
   a. an absence seizure
   b. a tonic seizure
   c. a focal seizure
   d. a complete motor seizure

10. An epidural hematoma is most likely _____ bleeding from the _____ .
    a. venous; internal jugular vein
    b. arterial; cerebral artery
    c. arterial; middle meningeal artery
    d. venous; external jugular vein

CRITICAL THINKING QUESTIONS

1. You are dispatched to a residence for a 13-year-old boy who has been complaining of fatigue and has been difficult to arouse. Upon your arrival, the child is listless and unable to respond to questions. His mother tells you she picked him up from soccer practice about an hour ago. He head-butted a ball and passed out but came to quickly and said he felt fine. She says he hasn't been acting right in the last half hour. What do you expect may have happened in this case? What type of injury do you suspect? What priority is this patient?

2. You are dispatched to an office complex. A woman had a seizure, and her coworker called EMS. Upon your arrival, the woman is conscious but tired and lethargic. She is drinking a glass of orange juice. What questions should you ask this woman? What do you suspect may be the cause of her seizure?

3. You are called to a residence at 6 o'clock in the morning. A 70-year-old man woke up and was disoriented and slurring his speech. His wife became alarmed and called EMS. What questions should you ask in this situation? What do you suspect is happening to this patient? What is the priority for this patient?

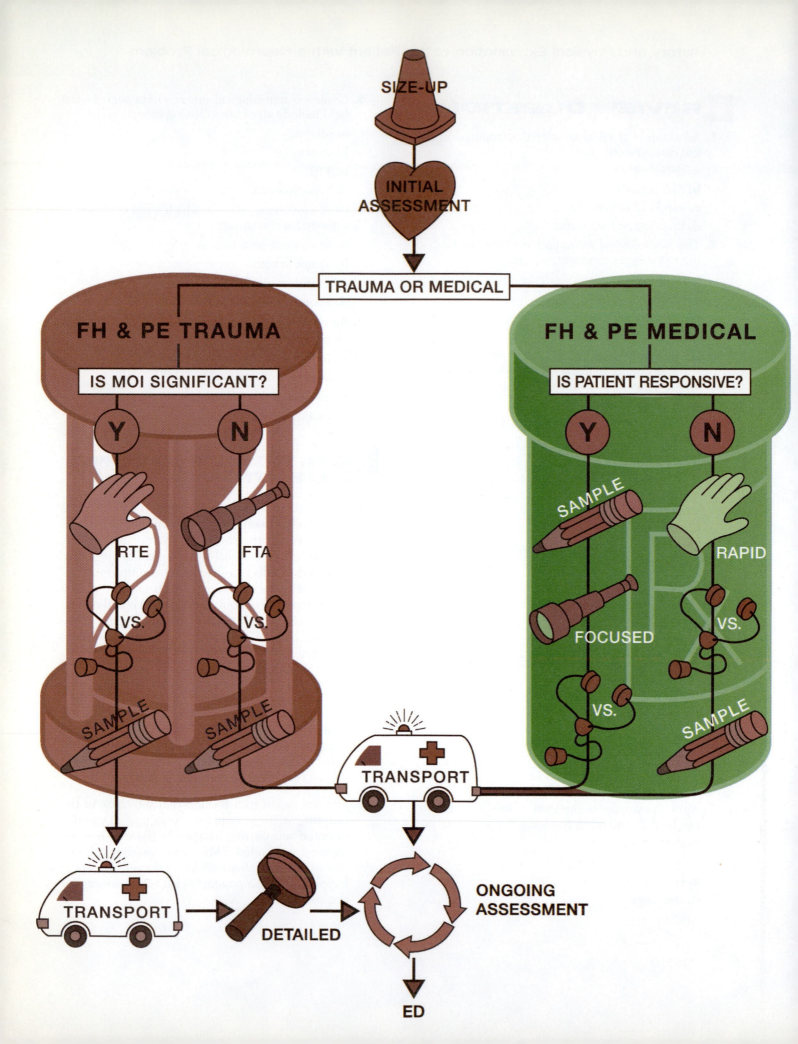

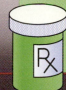

Chapter 15

The Focused History and Physical Examination of the Patient with Abdominal Pain

OBJECTIVES

Upon completion of this chapter, the reader should be able to:

- Describe specific information using OPQRST pertinent to the patient complaining of abdominal pain.

- Describe specific information using SAMPLE pertinent to the patient complaining of abdominal pain.

- Describe the steps to prepare a patient for physical examination of the abdomen.

- List the normal and abnormal features to observe about the abdomen.

- Describe the key feature of auscultation of bowel sounds for the EMS provider.

- Describe the steps for light palpation, deep palpation, and rebound tenderness of the abdomen.

- Describe the normal percussion tones of the abdomen.

- List the diagnostic tools the EMS provider may use during the examination of the patient with abdominal pain.

- List and describe the three distinctive types of abdominal pain.

- Describe why examination of the abdomen is different from that of other body parts.

- Describe three reasons why the patient with severe abdominal pain may be difficult to assess.

- List the most common causes of abdominal pain, including intra-abdominal, extra-abdominal, metabolic, and neurogenic causes.

- List the causes of acute abdominal pain requiring surgery.

- List the major gastrointestinal and genitourinary conditions the EMS provider may see in the prehospital setting.

- Describe the clinical features associated with the major gastrointestinal and genitourinary conditions.

KEY TERMS

Cullen's sign

dysuria

fluid wave test

Grey Turner's sign

McBurney's point

melena

pulsus differens

referred pain

scaphoid abdomen

somatic pain

striae

tympany

visceral pain

INTRODUCTION

There are many etiologies of acute abdominal pain, making it a frequent prehospital complaint. Most causes are not life threatening and require only supportive care. However, causes such as acute myocardial infarction are life threatening, and others such as ectopic pregnancy or acute appendicitis require emergency surgery. This chapter covers specific clinical signs, symptoms, and history taking unique to the patient with acute abdominal pain.

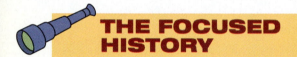

THE FOCUSED HISTORY

The information to obtain in the focused history of the patient with abdominal pain should include how and when the pain began (e.g., was it acute or gradual), the location and character of the pain, associated symptoms,

and any factors that irritate or alleviate the pain (e.g., stress, spicy or greasy food, milk, small and frequent meals). Be alert for clues to extra-abdominal causes of acute abdominal pain such as acute myocardial infarction (AMI) and ectopic pregnancy.

The OPQRST History

Using OPQRST, Table 15-1 highlights specific information pertaining to the focused history of the patient with abdominal pain.

The SAMPLE History

Use SAMPLE to obtain specific information pertaining to the focused history of the patient with abdominal pain. Table 15-2 highlights the types of questions to ask. Table 15-3 lists symptoms associated with abdominal pain and their possible causes.

TABLE 15-1
OPQRST for the Patient with Abdominal Pain

Information	Questions	Remarks
Onset	When and how did the pain begin? Did it develop suddenly or over a period of time?	It is important to determine when the pain started and whether it was acute or gradual.
Provocation	What were you doing when the pain began? Have you had any recent injuries? Are you having any difficulty breathing? Are you having any chest pain? What have you had to eat or drink today?	Obtain the details of the present episode. Determine what the patient was doing at the time of onset, and try to differentiate trauma as a cause. Always ask about associated shortness of breath or chest pain. Abdominal pain with or without typical chest pain is a common symptom of an acute myocardial

(continues)

TABLE 15-1 *(continued)*

Information	Questions	Remarks
Provocation *(continued)*	Have you had any problems moving your bowels or urinating?	infarction (MI). Ask about recent meals and recent changes in bowel movements because these are commonly associated factors that may have provoked this incident. Ask about **melena** (blood in stool), **dysuria** (difficulty urinating), pain with urination or bowel movements (BMs), and when the last BM was.
Quality	What does the pain feel like, and where is it located? Are you able to move without making the pain worse? Have you ever had an episode like this before?	It is important to determine whether the patient is describing visceral, somatic, or referred pain. Look to see whether the patient is guarding. Determine whether the patient can move without further provoking the pain. Ask about abnormal BMs and the quality of stool such as the color, consistency, and odor of the stool. A very dark or black tarry stool indicates digested blood, suggesting an upper gastrointestinal (GI) bleed; bright red blood suggests a lower GI bleed or upper GI bleeding with rapid transit or bleeding hemorrhoids; dark red blood is usually bleeding from the ileum to the right colon; clay stool is associated with gallbladder obstruction; yellow stools may be seen with many malabsorption syndromes; silver stool is associated with obstruction and GI bleed. Examples of abnormal consistency of stool are excessive diarrhea (which can quickly lead to dehydration and electrolyte imbalance, especially in the young and elderly) and pellet-sized stool, which is a common finding with irritable bowel syndrome. The odor of stool from a GI bleed is unmistakably foul and can be detected upon entry into the patient's room. The EMS provider will easily recognize the odor after having experienced it once.

(continues)

TABLE 15-1 *(continued)*

Information	Questions	Remarks
Region, **R**adiation, **R**elief, **R**ecurrence	Can you point to where the pain is located. Have you done anything to try to relieve the pain? Are there positions that are more comfortable than others? Have you ever experienced anything like this before?	Radiating pain is common with abdominal pain. See Table 15-4 for examples of abdominal pain that radiates to another location in the body. Determine whether the patient did anything to try to relieve the pain (e.g., maintain a position of comfort, take an antacid, belch). Ask the patient whether this episode is a recurrence of a similar event. If it is, ask more questions about the prior events: When was it? What did you do for relief then? Did you go to the hospital?
Severity	Rate your pain on a scale of 1 to 10, with 1 being no pain and 10 being the worst pain you have ever felt. How does this episode compare with previous episodes that are similar?	Obtain a baseline assessment followed by serial assessments in order to determine whether the condition is improving. If there is a history of similar events, ask the patient to compare the severity with the prior event(s).
Time	How long has the pain been present?	The onset may have been acute; however, a call for help is often delayed because the patient believes the problem will go away. Unfortunately, by the time EMS is called, the patient is often in a critical state.

TABLE 15-2
SAMPLE for the Patient with Abdominal Pain

Information	Questions	Remarks
Signs and **S**ymptoms	Please describe what you are feeling. Please show me where the pain is. What other symptoms are you experiencing?	Determine what type of abdominal pain the patient is presenting with: somatic, visceral, referred, or any combination. Ask about any associated symptoms. Examples of associated symptoms with abdominal pain that may provide clues to a particular cause are listed in Table 15-3. If the patient has been vomiting or has diarrhea, ask how many times and

(continues)

TABLE 15-2 *(continued)*

Information	Questions	Remarks
Signs and **S**ymptoms *(continued)*		what the color and consistency was for either. Observe the patient's position of comfort for clues to help determine the patient's level of distress. A patient lying still and flat is usually guarding from peritoneal pain, whereas a patient who is writhing in pain and unable to find a position of comfort often has an obstruction or a kidney stone.
Allergies	Do you have any allergies? Are you allergic to any medications?	It is important to determine allergies to medications that might be used to treat the pain.
Medications	Are you currently taking any prescribed medications? Have you tried any over-the-counter products or home remedies to relieve the pain? Have you recently changed medications or a dose of medication?	Ask about all medications taken. Look for medications commonly used for stomach disorders, such as stool softeners, medications that affect gastric acid secretion, and cancer treatment drugs. Also look for recent or sudden changes in dosages or for discontinued medications. Include prescribed, over-the-counter (OTC), homeopathic, and herbal medications, recreational drugs and the use of someone else's medication.
Pertinent past medical history	Have you ever had this type of pain before? Are you currently being treated by a doctor for any illnesses? Have you had any recent injuries? Have you had any surgery? Are you on dialysis or any special treatments for a kidney disorder? Is there a possibility that you are pregnant?	Determining whether the patient has had any surgery is a question often overlooked in the prehospital setting, yet it is important in assessing acute abdominal pain. The patient complaining of lower right quadrant abdominal pain, is an obvious candidate for appendicitis unless the patient has had an appendectomy. A diagnosis of cancer is another question often omitted from the history taking, but it is a common cause of abdominal pain, either from the cancer itself or from the treatment and medications taken for the cancer. A history of dialysis is significant and often a cause of severe abdominal pain from the complications associated with

(continues)

TABLE 15-2 *(continued)*

Information	Questions	Remarks
Pertinent past medical history *(continued)*		dialysis. Ask women of childbearing age about pregnancy and any previous ectopic pregnancies; always assume pregnancy is a possibility until ruled out in the emergency department. A history of alcohol abuse is a red flag for abdominal disorders such as cirrhosis and acute pancreatitis. Also ask about any preexisting urologic conditions because they can also precipitate abdominal pain.
Last oral intake	What and when did you last eat or drink? Have you taken any medications?	Certain foods may cause abdominal pain, and most patients know which foods they are sensitive to. Ask about the last fluids and medication taken, if any home remedy was tried, the last bowel movement, and vomiting. Specifically, ask whether any of these alleviated or further aggravated the condition.
Events leading up to this incident	What were you doing when you began having the pain? Did it come on suddenly, or has it worsened over time? Has there been any change in eating habits or medication regimes? Have you had previous episodes?	Make inquiries about associated conditions that may have precipitated this condition such as recent trauma, cardiac history, possible pregnancy, changes in bowels, or new or changed treatments for preexisting conditions.

TABLE 15-3
Symptoms Associated with Abdominal Pain and Their Possible Causes

Associated Symptoms	Possible Cause
Dyspnea, weakness, nausea, diaphoresis	Cardiac
Fever or chills	Infection
Nausea, vomiting, decreased oral intake, change in bowels	Gastrointestinal problem such as an obstruction or blockage
Anxiety, agitation, or confusion	Shock

PHYSICAL EXAMINATION

The physical examination of the patient with abdominal pain is the same as that for any patient in that the mental status and ABCs are evaluated and managed first. Next, inspect the skin color, temperature, and condition (CTC) for signs of poor perfusion. A patient in distress from an abdominal condition will most likely have autonomic nervous system reactions such as tachycardia and diaphoresis. Signs of dehydration are common in chronic cases. Look for poor skin turgor (Figure 15-1) or a furrowed tongue (Figure 15-2). After the initial assessment, the focus of the exam can be directed to the chief complaint, the abdominal pain.

The abdomen is an oval cavity that contains many organs. The locations of the various organs within the abdominal cavity are described by dividing the abdomen into four quadrants (Figure 15-3): two imaginary lines run perpendicular, with the umbilicus being in the center. In some advanced texts, the same area is described as being divided into nine sections, but for the EMS provider the four-quadrant method is the standard description.

Examination of the abdomen begins with observation, followed by auscultation and then palpation and percussion. Have the patient lie on her back and try to get her to relax the abdomen. The EMS provider wants to avoid having the patient tense the abdominal muscles during the examination. Sometimes, having the patient bend the knees helps the abdominal muscles to relax. The EMS provider should warm his hands before touching the patient's stomach or should palpate through thin clothing when his hands are cold. Asking questions related to the patient's history might distract the patient,

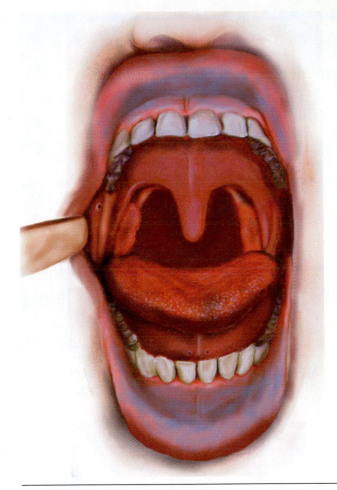

FIGURE 15-2 The tongue should be examined for cyanosis and a furrowed or dry, cracked appearance, which may indicate dehydration.

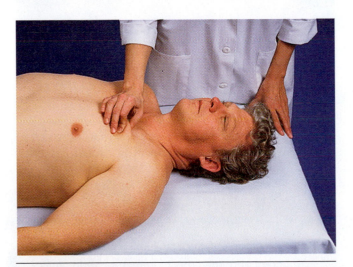

FIGURE 15-1 Skin turgor is assessed to observe the speed with which the skin returns to its original contour when released. Poor skin turgor may indicate dehydration.

thereby enhancing compliance with the exam. Palpate any painful areas last. Watch the patient's face for signs of pain or distress.

Observation

Observe the abdomen for symmetry and even skin tone. Note the presence and size of any masses, bulges, surgical scars (Figure 15-4), rashes or lesions, transdermal patches, and colostomy attachments. Some patients may have abdominal **striae**, which are atrophic lines or streaks from a rapid or prolonged stretching of the skin. The striae pattern may have been caused by an abdominal tumor, obesity, ascites, or, more commonly, pregnancy (Figure 15-5). Masses and bulges are abnormal and are often caused by hernias. Abnormal skin conditions include redness, indicating localized inflammation, and a yellowish hue, associated with jaundice. Rashes and lesions are caused by a number of conditions; glistening and taut skin is seen with ascites, and contusions

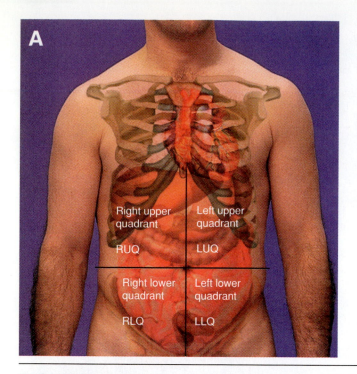

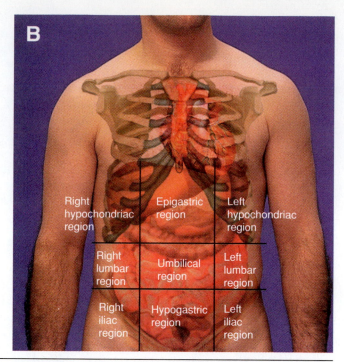

FIGURE 15-3 Comparison between the (**A**) four-section system and the (**B**) nine-section system of abdominal region mapping.

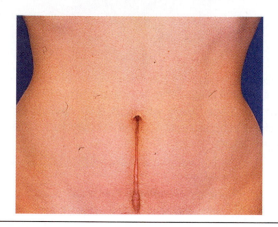

FIGURE 15-4 An abdominal scar from a hysterectomy.

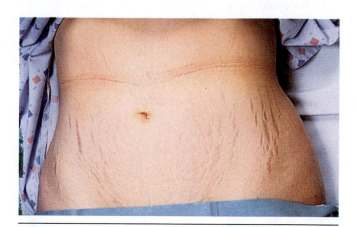

FIGURE 15-5 Abdominal striae are caused by a rapid or prolonged stretching of the skin.

or ecchymosis in the periumbilical region (around the belly button) is **Cullen's sign**. When the flanks also have ecchymosis, this is **Grey Turner's sign**. Both signs are remarkable late signs indicating internal bleeding. Presacral edema may be observed in patients with limited mobility, particularly when there is a cardiac history.

Pulsations from the abdominal aorta in the epigastric area are a normal finding in thin persons. Pulsations from masses or bulges are not normal findings. Respiratory movement is normal in infants, toddlers, and small children and is seen more often in men than in women. Always ask the patient about distension and bloating. Distension or bloating is not normal and is not

an obvious finding unless the EMS provider knows the patient well. Distension develops when an obstruction is present and causes a backup of intestinal contents.

Pediatric Pearl

● Infants, toddlers, and small children have a protuberant abdomen due to immature abdominal muscles, and they are primarily belly breathers.

Scaphoid abdomen is the opposite appearance of distension, characterized by a sinking, concave abdomen. Scaphoid abdomen is associated with some serious disorders.

Auscultation

Bowel sounds are not usually auscultated in the prehospital setting because of noise and time constraints. To listen properly takes a little time (2–5 minutes to auscultate accurately for absent bowel sounds). If the EMS provider has the time to listen for bowel sounds, this assessment technique should be performed before any palpation because physical manipulation can increase peristalsis, and the increase would give a false evaluation of bowel sounds. Auscultate for the presence or absence of bowel sounds in each quadrant. Normal bowel sounds occur irregularly from 5 to 30 times a minute. For the EMS provider, the most significant finding in the auscultation of bowel sounds is the absence of sounds, and this should be noted. This finding indicates obstruction

or inflammation of the peritoneum. The procedure of listening to bowel sounds is described in Chapter 21.

Palpation

The next step is to palpate the abdomen for tenderness, temperature, and presence of abnormal structures. The abdomen should be soft to the touch without any tenderness for the patient. There should be no masses or bulges. When muscle spasm in the abdomen is noted, the EMS provider must attempt to determine whether the spasms are voluntary (caused by nervousness) or involuntary (causes of guarding). The EMS provider performs this test by placing one hand on the abdomen and depressing it slightly and gently. Next, ask the patient to take in a long breath. During this maneuver, the muscle will relax if only voluntary spasm is present. In true spasm (involuntary guarding), the muscle remains taut.

Two organs that normally should not be felt during examination but may be appreciated with deep palpation when enlarged are the liver, in the upper right quadrant, and the spleen, in the upper left quadrant. To enhance the feel of these two organs, use one hand placed on the patient's side at the lowest ribs to support while palpating with the other. Deep palpation with one hand or a second hand for patients with a rigid muscular abdomen or obese patients is shown in Figure 15-6.

There are three types of palpation used to examine the abdomen: light touch, deep palpation, and a technique to assess for rebound tenderness. Begin with light palpation in a quadrant area away from the painful area and move through all four quadrants, saving the painful area for last. Light palpation (Figure 15-7) is performed using one hand to palpate approximately 1 cm (less than 1 inch) in depth. Note any tenderness and heat or coldness and, if guarding is present, try to distinguish between voluntary muscle guarding and involuntary rigidity.

Next perform deep palpation (2–3 inches) in the same path. For the obese patient, use the two-handed technique by placing one hand over the other and pushing down on the hand that is assessing. When a mass is identified, note the size, shape, location, and presence of tenderness or pulsations. Do not use deep palpation on any mass detected.

Rebound tenderness is assessed by palpating one quadrant of the abdomen then quickly removing the hand and releasing the pressure on the abdomen. Pain felt immediately after the release of pressure is called rebound tenderness and indicates peritoneal irritation. Any maneuver that jars the inflamed peritoneal cavity (e.g., bumps in the road during the ambulance transport) should result in rebound tenderness. Assessment for rebound tenderness can cause severe pain and rigidity, so it should always be done last.

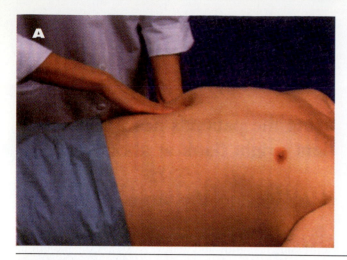
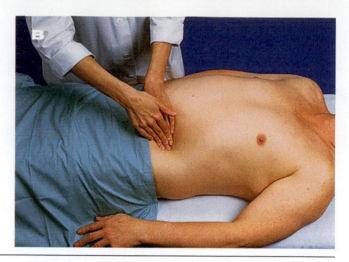

FIGURE 15-6 (A) A one-handed method of deep palpation of the right upper quadrant. **(B)** A two-handed method of deep palpation is used if there is muscular rigidity or for an obese patient.

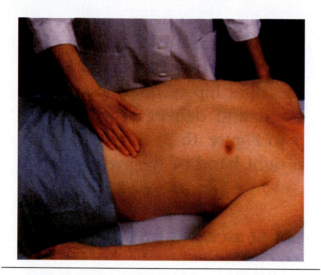

FIGURE 15-7 Light palpation of the abdomen.

sound that is loud and sounds like a drum. This sound is called **tympany**. Percussion over dense organs, such as the liver or spleen, will normally sound dull and produce a sound like a muffled thud. When the abdomen is distended, percussion is most helpful to distinguish the presence of fluid from gas or adipose tissue.

Percuss the abdomen by placing the nondominant hand firmly on the patient's abdomen, with the middle finger hyperextended. Use the middle finger of the dominant hand to strike the top of the middle finger of the nondominant hand. Quickly bounce the middle finger off the stationary finger and repeat. Move to a new area and repeat while keeping the technique even. The technique is mostly in the wrist action, and the wrist should be relaxed. The skill is not difficult but does take a little practice to master. The method of palpating the abdomen for ascites when the patient is lying facedown is shown in Figure 15-8.

Percussion

Percussion may be performed next; however, this assessment skill is not often used in the prehospital setting owing to time constraints. Percussion is done by touching and tapping the fingertips on various body parts and listening to determine the size, position, and consistency of underlying structures. Various areas of the body have what is called normal percussion tone. Think of this as the normal sound when "tapped." Diseases, such as the accumulation of fluid in the lungs, provide a dull (hyporesonant) or flat tone. Abnormal collections of air, such as a pneumothorax, make the percussion tone louder, or hyperresonant. The abdomen has two normal percussion tones. Percussion over an air-filled viscus, such as the stomach or intestine, normally provides a

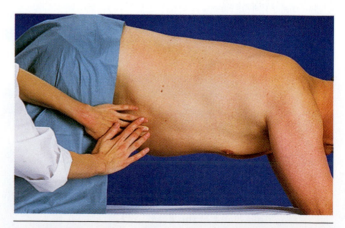

FIGURE 15-8 Percussion of the patient's abdomen when he is lying facedown.

One additional special procedure that is performed on the abdomen to test for ascites is the **fluid wave test**. This is accomplished by having the patient or a partner press the side of her hand firmly on the midline of the patient's stomach. The EMS provider uses the right hand to support the left flank and, with the left hand, swiftly strikes the right flank. If impulses to the right hand are easily detected, then suspect ascites (Figure 15-9). This test will be positive if there are large amounts of ascitic fluid, which is associated with congestive heart failure, hepatitis, pancreatitis, cancer, cirrhosis, and portal hypertension.

Before completing the physical examination, assess for orthostatic changes because they may be associated with fluid loss, shock, and **pulsus differens**. Pulsus differens is a condition in which the pulses on either side of the body are unequal; it is sometimes seen in a patient with an aortic dissection.

Use of Diagnostic Tools

The EMS provider should obtain an ECG, pulse oximetry, and temperature reading. No other advanced diagnostic equipment is routinely used in the prehospital setting for abdominal complaints. An electrocardiogram

reading can alert the EMS provider to the presence of cardiac dysrhythmias. Pulse oximetry may be of value, but visual inspection for perfusion status should never be deemphasized or disregarded for a meter reading. Obtaining a temperature with a thermometer can help rule out hypo/hyperthermia. Infection is often associated with a fever.

TYPES OF ABDOMINAL PAIN

There are three distinctive types of pain associated with the abdomen: visceral, somatic, and referred pain. **Visceral pain** is caused by the stretching of nerve fibers surrounding either solid or hollow organs in the abdomen and is associated with conditions such as early appendicitis, bowel obstruction, and cholecystitis (gallbladder infection). Visceral pain is often poorly localized, diffuse, and difficult for the patient to describe. The patient may explain visceral pain as feeling crampy and gaseous and being intermittent, that is to say it comes and goes. The patient may be found guarding the abdomen by maintaining a particular position of comfort, such as keeping the legs flexed or lying perfectly still (as in Figure 15-10).

Somatic pain tends to be more localized to the area of pathology. It is caused by irritation of pain fibers in the parietal peritoneum. The patient can usually be specific about the location of pain and may describe it as being sharp and constant rather than diffuse and intermittent. Somatic pain is associated with conditions such as kidney stones or late appendicitis, which is localized with sharp pain in the lower right quadrant. This location is known as **McBurney's point** (Figure 15-11).

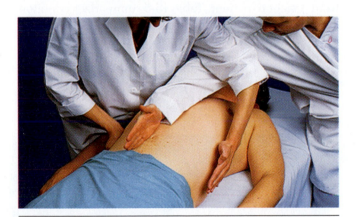

FIGURE 15-9 Palpation for ascites: the fluid wave test.

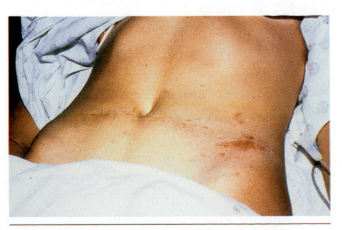

FIGURE 15-10 Some patients with abdominal pain may lie very still, "guarding" the painful area, and other patients may be found in a knees-flexed position. (Courtesy of Deborah Funk, MD, Albany Medical Center, Albany, NY)

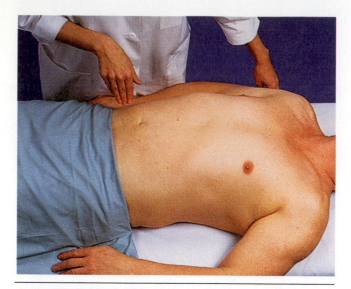

FIGURE 15-11 Pain in the right lower quadrant can indicate appendicitis. This location is known as McBurney's point.

McBurney's point, identified in the 1800s by Charles McBurney, a surgeon, is a landmark on the abdomen associated with the late pain of appendicitis. An imaginary triangle on the anterior lower right quadrant, McBurney's point runs from the navel out to the right superior iliac spine.

Referred pain is pain originating from one area of the body that is also sensed in another area. Referred pain is especially common with abdominal pain. There are a number of known referral patterns associated with specific pathologies. A list of some of these common referral patterns appears in Table 15-4.

TABLE 15-4
Referral Patterns of Abdominal Pain

- **Biliary pain:** radiates around the right side of the abdomen to the back and right scapula

- **Diaphragmatic irritation:** the upper abdomen and the top of the shoulder

- **Kidney stone:** most often unilateral on the affected flank but as the stones move they can also cause pain in the groin or external genitalia

- **Pancreas:** straight through to the lower thoracic area of the back

- **Ruptured or leaking aneurysm:** to the lumbosacral area and sometimes in the thighs

FEATURES OF ABDOMINAL PAIN

Examination of the abdomen is different from examination of other parts of the body for a few reasons. First, the location of pain is not always an accurate indication of the cause of pain. For this reason, life-threatening conditions, such as AMI and ectopic pregnancy, must be considered early in the field impression; then there should be a prompt effort to rule out these conditions in the emergency department. In the prehospital setting, the EMS provider should first suspect pain occurring anywhere from the umbilicus to the jaw as being the pain of an AMI. Abdominal pain of cardiac origin is often in the upper abdomen or epigastric area. In females of childbearing age (12–50), suspect and manage acute abdominal pain, with or without discharge, as an ectopic pregnancy until pregnancy is ruled out (e.g., by a pregnancy test in the emergency department or other medical facility). Assume it has already ruptured if she is in shock.

Certain disease processes typically cause pain in particular areas, although there is fairly extensive overlap between the causes of pain and the quadrants of the abdomen they may affect. This correlation may vary from patient to patient. Table 15-5 summarizes common causes of abdominal pain by their location.

The patient with severe abdominal pain may be difficult to assess because the pain and anxiety interfere with the patient's compliance. The patient's general appearance—especially facial expression, skin condition, and position of comfort—provides the first

Geriatric Gem

- Normal changes in aging result in a decreased sense of pain. The elderly patient's lack of abdominal pain in the presence of associated symptoms may hide the severity of the actual condition.

Clinical Carat

- Shock with an unexplained source (either medical or trauma) is considered internal bleeding until proved otherwise.

TABLE 15-5
Common Causes of Abdominal Pain by Location

Location	Possible Conditions
Upper right quadrant	Pancreatitis, pneumonia with pleurisy, cholecystitis, duodenal ulcer, pyelonephritis
Upper left quadrant	Pancreatitis, pneumonia, duodenal ulcer, pyelonephritis
Lower right quadrant	Appendicitis, ectopic pregnancy, diverticulitis, kidney stone, ovarian cyst, pelvic inflammatory disease
Lower left quadrant	Ectopic pregnancy, diverticulitis, kidney stone, ovarian cyst, pelvic inflammatory disease
Epigastric	Myocardial infarction, duodenal ulcer, gastroenteritis
Periumbilical	Appendicitis, pancreatitis, abdominal aortic aneurysm
Unlocalized	Bowel obstruction, food poisoning, neurological lesion, metabolic problem (e.g., diabetic ketoacidosis)

evidence of the level of distress the patient is in. The patient may be exhibiting guarding, be writhing in pain, or be so focused on the pain that any cooperation with the examination will be limited. Guarding of the abdomen is described as voluntary or involuntary. Voluntary guarding is tensing of the stomach muscles by the patient when tickled, touched unexpectedly, or touched with cold hands. Involuntary guarding is a constant rigidity of the stomach muscles and a protective mechanism associated with intra-abdominal pain. Another assessment finding that may be present only in the abdomen is rebound tenderness, which is associated with peritoneal inflammation. Rebound tenderness is discussed in the section on palpation.

COMMON CAUSES OF ABDOMINAL PAIN

The specific diagnosis of the condition causing the pain is difficult even in the emergency department and is not the objective for the EMS provider. The causes of abdominal pain are numerous and arise from intra-abdominal, extra-abdominal, metabolic, and neurogenic etiologies. Inflammation, obstruction, infection, hemor-

rhage, or any combination can cause abdominal pain. The following is a list of common causes of abdominal pain:

- Common intra-abdominal conditions: appendicitis, cholecystitis, cholelithiasis, diverticulitis, gastroenteritis, gastritis, intestinal obstruction (mechanical or neurogenic), irritable bowel syndrome, pancreatitis, peptic ulcer
- Extra-abdominal causes of acute abdominal pain: AMI, ectopic pregnancy, sickle cell anemia, pneumonia (particularly right lower lobe), diabetic ketoacidosis, muscle strain, dysmenorrhea, salpingitis, reflux esophagitis, esophageal disease
- Metabolic: diabetes, sickle cell anemia, lupus, scorpion and spider bites
- Neurogenic: herpes zoster and neural disturbance of normal peristalsis

Acute Abdominal Pain Requiring Emergency Surgery

Conditions that require surgical intervention include appendicitis, cholecystitis, ectopic pregnancy, perforated peptic ulcer or viscus, tumors, dissecting and ruptured aneurysms, and bowel infarctions.

Pain Associated with Gastrointestinal and Genitourinary Conditions

The major gastrointestinal (GI) and genitourinary (GU) conditions and clinical features for each are summarized in Table 15-6.

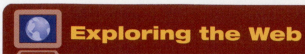

Exploring the Web

● Search the Web for five of the disorders listed in this section of the text. For each disorder, list the signs and symptoms of the disorder, assessment findings in patients with the disorders, and the priority of the patient presenting with these signs and symptoms. Which disorders present with the most critical problems?

TABLE 15-6
Major Gastrointestinal and Genitourinary Conditions

Condition	Clinical Features
Appendicitis	Appendicitis is in inflammation of the appendix due to the occlusion of the lumen by a small piece of stool. As the obstructed appendix distends, its blood supply is cut off. Simple appendicitis then progresses to gangrenous appendicitis, when tissue begins to die. Soon (usually within 24–48 hours from initial symptoms), the appendix ruptures, leading first to localized, then generalized, peritonitis. The classic presentation is periumbilical crampy pain that then localizes in the lower right quadrant. Nearly all persons with acute appendicitis have anorexia (markedly decreased appetite). Missed appendicitis is common in young children, elderly patients, and pregnant women because the symptoms are often atypical.
Bowel obstruction	Blockage of any portion of the large or small bowel leads to a bowel obstruction. Potential causes are numerous. The most common include tumors (especially in obstruction of the lower colon) and scar tissue from previous abdominal inflammation or surgery ("adhesions"). The clinical picture usually evolves over 24–72 hours as the bowel gradually distends and "backs up." The result is abdominal distension, nausea, vomiting, and an inability to pass stool. A twisting of a loop of bowel on itself (volvulus) may also occur, resulting in rapid distension and progression of symptoms (including pain). In this case, urgent surgery is usually required.
Cholecystitis	Cholecystitis is an acute inflammation of the gallbladder, usually due to gallstones. These are particles of variable size that block the lumen, interfering with bile flow. Distension of the gallbladder causes upper right quadrant pain that may radiate to the right shoulder area. Nausea and vomiting are common. Attacks may be accompanied by jaundice. The condition is not contagious, but clinical differentiation from acute hepatitis may be impossible.
Colitis	Colitis is a general term indicating inflammation of the colon for any of a number of reasons. The most common causes are infectious (viral), inflammatory disease (e.g., Crohn's disease, ulcerative colitis), and sexually transmitted disease (gonorrheal colitis).
Crohn's disease	Crohn's disease is a chronic condition resulting in inflammation, usually of the small intestine. Patients have recurrent exacerbations consisting of pain, diarrhea, and sometimes

(continues)

TABLE 15-6 *(continued)*

Condition	Clinical Features
Crohn's disease *(continued)*	lower GI bleeding. The initial presentation may mimic appendicitis, leading to emergency surgery and the correct diagnosis. Crohn's disease and ulcerative colitis, another inflammatory bowel disorder, are not contagious.
Diverticulitis	Diverticulosis is the presence of numerous small outpouchings in the colon, called diverticula. More than 70% of lower GI bleeding is from this source, yet only 3% to 5% of patients with diverticula ever bleed from them. Diverticula may also become inflamed, resulting in diverticulitis and abdominal pain (usually in the lower left quadrant).
Esophageal varices	Esophageal varices are dilations of the veins of the esophagus secondary to increased portal vein pressures. Alcoholic varices are secondary to cirrhosis caused by alcohol ingestion. Patients with alcoholic cirrhosis and varices may bleed from varices (40% of the time) but are as likely to have bleeding from gastritis, gastric ulcer (30%), or duodenal ulcer (20%). Patients with nonalcoholic cirrhosis and varices are four times as likely to bleed from varices as from peptic ulcer. Gastritis in these patients is rare.
Gastroenteritis	Gastroenteritis is a general term for the inflammation of any part or parts of the large or small intestine due to infection. The most common infection is due to viruses. These are usually self-limiting. Bacterial causes (e.g., salmonellosis) may be life threatening. Patients present with nausea, vomiting, diarrhea, general malaise, and variable degrees of dehydration. The maintenance of airway, breathing, and circulation (replenishment of fluid loss) is the best out-of-hospital approach, regardless of cause. Remember to observe body substance isolation (BSI) procedures—some of these agents are contagious.
Hemorrhoids	Hemorrhoids result from a dilation of veins in the lower portion of the colon (rectum). Though a common cause of lower GI bleeding, it is rarely hemodynamically significant. The most common symptoms are rectal itching and difficulty in defecation. Because hemorrhoids are nothing more than varicose veins of the rectum, they may occasionally clot (thrombosed hemorrhoid), leading to sudden and severe rectal pain. Though not life threatening, a thrombosed hemorrhoid requires prompt medical attention.
Hepatitis (acute)	Acute hepatitis refers to an inflammation of the liver for any reason. In common usage, it usually refers to viral hepatitis, an infection. Patients present with malaise, nausea, and vomiting. Often jaundice and upper right quadrant tenderness are present. Most forms of hepatitis are contagious.
Kidney stone	Kidney stones (urolithiasis) are small particles that form from a variety of substances. They are trapped in a portion of the kidney or ureter when the body attempts to pass them in the urine. The result is acute and severe pain, nausea, and often vomiting. The pain continues until the stone passes. Typically, patients have flank pain that radiates into the anterior lower quadrant on the involved side. People with kidney stones tend to writhe about in pain, unable to find any comfortable position. This fact may be helpful in diagnosis—people with inflammatory conditions (e.g., appendicitis) tend to lie quietly because movement usually aggravates their pain.

(continues)

TABLE 15-6 *(continued)*

Condition	Clinical Features
Reflux esophagitis	Esophagitis is caused by an erosion or irritation of the esophagus and may be a source of bleeding. The most common cause is acid reflux (backflow) from the stomach. The condition may be asymptomatic, may cause severe chest pain (mimicking AMI, thus the name "heartburn"), or any degree of symptoms in between. Even if a patient has a history of "heartburn," assume that chest pain is due to myocardial ischemia until proved otherwise.
Ulcers (peptic ulcer)	Peptic ulcer disease involves erosions of either the stomach or duodenum. Bleeding may occur, though pain and gastric distress are far more common. One out of six patients who bleed from a peptic ulcer has had no prior symptoms or history of ulcer disease. Gastritis presents in a similar fashion and is impossible to differentiate, in most cases, from peptic ulcer disease in the field. Acute gastritis results from erosions of the stomach lining, often caused by stress or a recent excessive ingestion of alcohol or salicylates.

CONCLUSION

Examination of the abdomen in the prehospital setting is performed to quickly identify any significant injury, potential hemorrhage, or need for surgery. The specific diagnosis of the condition causing the pain is difficult even in the emergency department and is not the objective for the EMS provider. The objectives are to obtain a focused history, perform a focused physical examination of the abdomen, and consider life-threatening conditions such as AMI and ectopic pregnancy early.

REVIEW QUESTIONS

1. Pain that is caused by the stretching of nerve fibers surrounding either solid or hollow organs in the abdomen is called _____ pain.
   a. guarding
   b. somatic
   c. visceral
   d. colicky

2. The name that corresponds with the location of late pain from appendicitis is called:
   a. McBurney's point.
   b. the left lower quadrant.
   c. the right upper quadrant.
   d. the visceral point.

3. Pain that originates in one area of the body yet is sensed in another area is called _____ pain.
   a. melena
   b. referred
   c. recurrent
   d. somatic

4. When a patient who has a maladaptive syndrome describes her stool, she is most likely to say it was:
   a. dark and tarry.
   b. bright red.
   c. yellow.
   d. silver.

5. When a patient who has an upper gastrointestinal bleed describes her stool, she is most likely to say it was:
   a. dark and tarry.
   b. blue.
   c. bright red.
   d. clay colored.

6. If a patient with an abdominal complaint is writhing in pain and unable to find a position of comfort, she may be experiencing:
   a. shock.
   b. a kidney stone.
   c. peritonitis.
   d. gallbladder disease.

7. Signs of dehydration may include any of the following except:

   a. tachycardia.

   b. a furrowed tongue.

   c. poor skin turgor.

   d. a bulging fontanelle.

8. Atrophic lines or streaks in the abdominal skin are called:

   a. striae.

   b. jaundice.

   c. a rash.

   d. transderms.

9. When examining a patient who has a history of hypertension, you find a pulsation from a bulge in her abdomen. What do you suspect?

   a. The patient has an enlarged heart.

   b. The patient may have an abdominal aortic aneurysm.

   c. The patient has ascites and needs to be drained.

   d. The patient may have overdosed on her medications.

10. What does rebound tenderness indicate?

    a. The patient may need abdominal surgery.

    b. The patient has ascites and needs a diuretic.

    c. The patient has an abdominal aortic aneurysm.

    d. It is a nonsignificant finding and rarely located.

CRITICAL THINKING

1. You are called to the scene of an auto accident. A woman lost control of her car in a parking lot and struck a light pole. The airbag did deploy, and she was wearing a seat belt. She is complaining of a headache and pain in her lower abdomen. The front driver's side of the car is damaged significantly. What assessment techniques might be useful in making a field impression of this patient? What type of injury might you suspect? Is this a high- or a low-priority patient?

2. You are called to a residence for a 14-year-old boy with severe abdominal pain. The boy's father brings you the child. The boy is holding his right side and grimacing. He does not want you to touch him; he is afraid it will hurt more. What assessment techniques can you use with this patient? What do you suspect the problem may be? Is this a high- or a low-priority patient?

3. You are assessing a 16-year-old girl with pain in her lower abdomen that radiates into her back. Her parents are present, and she is reluctant to answer questions. She is lying on the couch in a fetal position. She says this position relieves some of the pain. What assessment techniques can be used with this patient? How might you be able to get her to more openly answer your questions? What do you suspect may be the cause of her pain? Is this a high- or a low-priority patient?

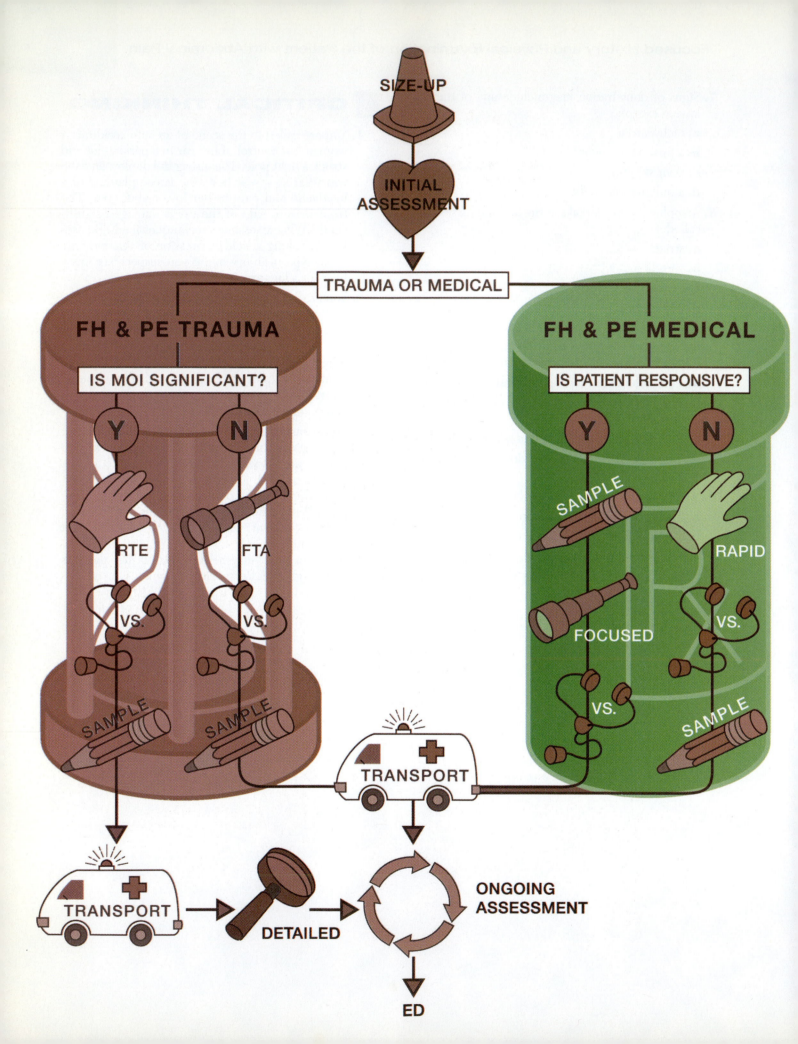

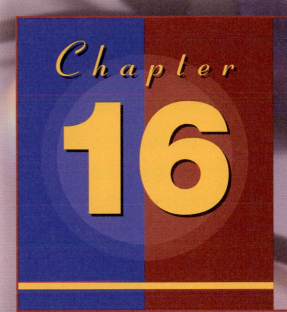

Chapter 16

The Focused History and Physical Examination of the Patient with a Behavioral Emergency

OBJECTIVES

Upon completion of this chapter, the reader should be able to:

- Describe the elements that lead up to a behavioral emergency.
- Describe the EMS provider's role in controlling the setting in a behavioral emergency.
- List 11 classifications of psychiatric disorders and provide an example of each.
- Provide examples of specific behaviors manifested by persons with emotional and psychiatric disorders.
- List a major misconception concerning behavioral emergencies.
- Describe examples of nonverbal communication.
- Describe specific risk factors the EMS provider should screen for during the focused history of a patient experiencing a behavioral emergency.
- Describe the components of the mental status examination.
- List the most common behavioral emergencies for which the EMS provider is called.
- List medical conditions that mimic behavioral disorders.
- List the possible signs and symptoms of ineffective or failing coping mechanisms of stress that may be seen in EMS providers.

KEY TERMS

affect   delusion
body language   hallucination
crisis   psychosis

INTRODUCTION

Every type of illness and injury will be accompanied by some type of emotional or psychological element, and behavioral emergencies often occur when people with or without a psychiatric history become stressed or overwhelmed or feel they are losing control of their life. A **crisis** occurs when a person's perception and interpretation of an acute distressing event results in an abnormal behavioral response. The crisis is an internal experience that can create reactions such as severe anxiety, panic, paranoia, or some other brief psychotic event.

The EMS provider will need to display confidence and take an active role in controlling the situation in a behavioral emergency. Crisis is often unpredictable, and the EMS provider must always consider personal safety first. It is essential the EMS provider avoid making any threatening actions, statements, or questions and make a clear, short, and calm statement of who she is and why she is there. When the call is obviously a behavioral problem at the onset and police, crisis intervention workers, or family members are on the scene, the following questions need to be asked before approaching the patient:

- What is the problem? Get a description of any unusual activities; ask about risk factors (e.g., previous suicide attempts or psychiatric care) and the possibility of alcoholism or substance abuse.

- How many people are involved? Get an idea about specific psychosocial stress factors.

- Is this a crime situation? Have there been previous or similar episodes with this patient, and what was the outcome?

COMMON CLASSIFICATIONS OF PSYCHIATRIC DISORDERS

Most EMS providers are not formally trained in crisis intervention or in making a field impression of psychiatric conditions. It is helpful to have an understanding of these conditions to better assess the common classifications of psychiatric disorders.

Mental, emotional, and behavioral disorders are organized under the umbrella of psychiatric disorders. It is estimated that these disorders affect as much as 20% of the U.S. population and incapacitate more people than all other health problems combined (American Psychiatric Association, 1994). A list of classifications of psychiatric disorders with examples is found in Table 16-1.

TABLE 16-1
Classification of Psychiatric Disorders

Disorder Type/ Classification	Examples
Anxiety	Anxiety attacks, panic attacks, phobias, posttraumatic stress disorders (PTSDs)
Cognitive	Dementia, delirium
Dissociative	Personality disorders, schizophrenia
Eating	Anorexia, bulimia
Factitious	Conscious or deliberate fabrications
Impulse control	Pyromania, kleptomania
Mood	Depression, bipolar
Personality	Maladaptive behavior and inability to function normally in society; paranoiac, antisocial, narcissistic, dependent, avoidant, compulsive, passive-aggressive, schizoid
Schizophrenic and psychotic	Paranoia, delusional disorders, hallucinations
Somatoform	Neurotic disorders characterized by physical complaints (e.g., paralysis or blindness) with no apparent physical cause
Substance	Intoxication, abuse, dependence, addiction (e.g., drugs or alcohol)

Exploring the Web

- For each of the classifications of psychiatric disorders listed in Table 16-1, search the Web for additional information on signs and symptoms patients with these disorders will exhibit. Try to find information on what would lead to a crisis or emergency resulting in the need to call EMS with these disorders. Is there information available to help EMS providers with tips and suggestions on how to handle an emergency call with a patient who has any of these disorders?

FEATURES OF EMOTIONAL OR PSYCHOLOGICAL DISORDERS

The key to recognizing a patient who is experiencing a behavioral emergency is to observe the patient's body language as well as verbal responses for clues. There are many types of psychological disorders, each with its own characteristics. The following is a list of general examples of recognizable behavior manifested by persons with various emotional and psychiatric disorders.

General Appearance

Some people will have a noticeable decline in or disregard for their own grooming and personal hygiene. The way they dress may be inappropriate for the present circumstances, ambient temperatures, or conditions (e.g., T-shirt and shorts for an evening party, multiple layers of clothing in the summer). Others may exhibit excessive or extreme attention to their appearance, as in the case of some obsessive-compulsive disorders. A person who ignores one side of the body may have a brain lesion.

Intellectual Function

Memory, concentration, judgment, and orientation should all be assessed. Short- and long-term memory and recall memory can all be affected by psychiatric disorders as well as other factors. Use simple recall questions to test and obtain a baseline assessment followed by serial assessments. Questions EMS providers might ask to assess memory include:

- Long term. What is your date of birth? What is your Social Security number?
- Short term. What medications have you taken in the past 24 hours? What have you eaten in the past 24 hours?
- Recall. Tell the patient to remember the name of three items (e.g., flower, rock, and water), wait a few minutes, and then ask the patient to repeat the three items. Then repeat this test a few minutes later.

The inability to concentrate is another clue to note. Judgment is assessed during the interview by what the patient communicates about the current situation, past medical history, or medication regimen. Orientation is the well-known assessment of the patient's understanding of person, place, and time. Disorientation to place and day are the most significant to note.

Thought Content

Thought content and perceptions should be logical, consistent, and connected with the current situation. Clues to note are the patient's inability to complete a thought; having thoughts that are illogical, unusual worries, **delusions** (false personal beliefs or ideas that are portrayed as true), **hallucinations** (perceptions, visual or auditory, of something that is not actually present); and making any threat of suicide or violence to another person.

Physical Complaints

Physical complaints are often vague and may include headache, muscle ache, stomachache, lack of energy, irritability, weight loss, sleeplessness, and loss of appetite. These symptoms may also be the vague symptoms of a communicable disease, so be sure to consider other causes before saying these have emotional origins.

Motor Activity

The EMS provider may see overt behavior in the posture of a person who may be tense or slumped and is not willing to get up. Other patients may be restless, pacing, wringing their hands, rocking, crying, fidgeting, or moving slowly. Always consider the possibility of drug intoxication, pain, blood sugar abnormality, or hypoxia when abnormal motor activity is present.

Speech and Language

Consider the word choice, quality, pace, and articulation of the patient's speech and language. Silence, rambling, mumbling, loudness, slowness, quiet, taking excessive pauses, or having difficulty in choosing words are associated with psychological disorders. Consider too that conditions such as stroke, tumors, or trauma can affect speech, causing aphasia, dysphasia, or dysarthria, so consider other factors in addition to a psychiatric disorder.

Body Language

Body language is the expression of thoughts or emotions by means of posture or gestures. Observe whether the body language is appropriate for the current situation and environment. Always stay alert to potential danger by watching for gestures, posture, or evidence of rage, elation, hostility, depression, fear, anger, anxiety, or confusion (Figure 16-1).

Mood

Clues about the patient's mood and **affect** (the emotional mind-set prompting an expressed emotion or behavior) can be seen in the facial expression and other body language as well as in how the patient responds to questions posed by the EMS provider. Observe the patient's mood and affect to determine whether they are appropriate for the current situation and change accordingly with topics in conversation. Overt behavior signals mood swings, depression, and intense anxiety. A person may become violent. Examples of attitudes that may be inappropriate for the circumstances and signaled by behavior are a lack of interest or detachment, paranoia, hostility, or rage or elation at an inappropriate time.

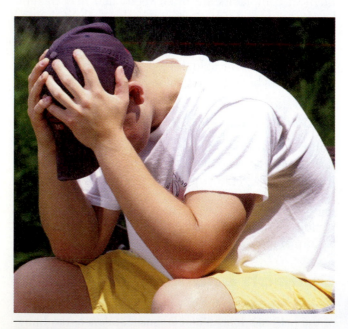

FIGURE 16-1 A patient's posture can offer clues to his state of mind.

ASSESSMENT OF THE PATIENT WITH A PSYCHOLOGICAL DISORDER

There are many misconceptions about dealing with the patient with a psychological disorder. It is important for EMS providers to approach the assessment of the patient exhibiting abnormal behavior in the same manner as they approach that of patients presenting with other problems. Treating a patient on the basis of preconceived notions and prejudices could put the patient, bystanders, and crew in danger. Focus on assessing the current situation, following all the steps in the assessment algorithm.

Scene Safety

A major misconception concerning behavioral emergencies is that all mental patients are unstable and dangerous. The truth is that many psychiatric patients are perfectly calm and never present any danger to themselves or to others. This does not mean that EMS providers should drop their guard when on the scene of a behavioral emergency.

EMS providers learn that personal safety is the highest priority in their job for many good reasons. Responding to the call that comes in as a suicide attempt or an act of violence intended to harm another person is a red flag to the responder to keep her guard up for signs of danger. However, many behavioral cases initially present as a medical problem such as an altered mental status or a cardiac or respiratory condition, and the signs of danger may not immediately be apparent.

The EMS provider's approach to the patient in most cases should be slow and purposeful, being alert for potential danger. Keep the following questions in mind: Are EMS providers in danger? Is the patient in danger? Consider the environment, traffic, and crowds and the presence of weapons or potential weapons. Additional details on scene size-up are discussed in Chapter 3. Observe the patient for overt behavior and body language. Be careful to respect the patient's personal space (approximately 3 to 4 feet) until a rapport is established with the patient. When appropriate, limit the number of people around the patient so as not to further overwhelm the patient.

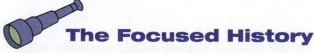 ## The Focused History

Obtaining information from a patient with a behavioral problem is often complicated. Either the information is unreliable or the patient is a poor historian or uncooperative. Family or caregivers may not be available or may distort information. Consider the use of police, dispatch, or crisis intervention services as a source for information about prior incidents.

There are predisposing risk factors for certain behavior problems, such as depression and suicide. Table 16-2 is a list of some of the risk factors that the EMS provider should screen for during the focused history taking in a behavioral emergency. The more risk factors present, the higher the level of suspicion of a possible behavioral disorder. The list is a guideline and it is important to note that not all patients will present with any specific risk factors.

The OPQRST History

Using OPQRST, Table 16-3 highlights specific information to obtain pertaining to the focused history of the patient with an emotional or psychological emergency.

TABLE 16-2
Risk Factors Associated with Behavioral Disorders

Depression	An unhappy event (death, divorce, or loss of friend or relative), prolonged or chronic illness, various medications (steroids, antihypertensives, tranquilizers), drug and alcohol intoxication and withdrawal; more frequent in women than in men and often associated with premenstrual syndrome, pregnancy (during and postpartum)
Pediatric and adolescent depression	Abuse or neglect, stress, smoking, chronic illness, loss of a parent or caregiver, attention disorder; twice as frequent in girls as in boys during adolescence
Elderly depression	Medications, organic brain disease, fever, infection, dehydration, electrolyte imbalance, hypoxia, hyponatremia, metabolic disorder, thyroid disease, decreased quality of life, loss of spouse or support system, fear of dying, decreased independence, financial insecurity, significant illness or injury
Suicide	Previous suicide gestures or attempts, irrational thinking, loss of spouse (separated, widowed, or divorced), excessive use of alcohol or drugs, major life event, lack of support system; most frequent in males <19 or >45 years old
Pediatric and adolescent suicide	Access to lethal weapons, drug and alcohol abuse, neglect, exposure to domestic violence or violence at school, loss of a loved one, breakup of a romance, inadequate support system
Elderly suicide	Loss of lifelong mate, loneliness or isolation, significant illness or injury, loss of independence, financial insecurity, decreased quality of life

TABLE 16-3
OPQRST for the Patient with a Behavioral Emergency

Information	Questions	Remarks
Onset	Where were you when you started to feel this way? Why did you call EMS?	It is important to determine how the event began and what led up to the incident. Determine who called EMS

(continues)

TABLE 16-3 *(continued)*

Information	Questions	Remarks
Onset *(continued)*	Did anything happen that led up to this episode?	and why. During a behavioral emergency, the police or crisis intervention may also be involved on the scene.
Provocation	What is the problem today? How many people are involved? Have you been under any stress recently? Have you been having any problems as the result of a life crisis? Have you had any alcoholic beverages to drink? Have you taken any drugs? Did you intend to hurt yourself?	Obtain the details of the current episode. Determine whether there is more than one patient and whether this is a crime scene (e.g., attempted suicide). Behavioral emergencies can be precipitated by stressful events such as recent changes in social, economic, employment, or health status. Substance abuse may bring about a behavioral emergency. It is also important to find out whether the patient actually intended to harm himself.
Quality	Describe how you are feeling. Have you ever felt like this before?	Determine the type of emergency or crisis the patient is experiencing (e.g., panic attack, hopelessness, severe depression, suicide attempt).
Region, **R**adiation, **R**elief, **R**ecurrence	Are you being treated for any illnesses or have you had any recent injuries? Are you under a doctor's care? Do you have a case manager? Has this ever happened before? Did this start suddenly, or has it been coming on gradually?	Determine whether there are any concomitant medical factors that may have precipitated this event. Determine whether the patient functions adaptively in society when not in crisis. If he does, ask about coping mechanisms (e.g., therapy, counseling, support group, pharmacologic treatment). Find out whether this has ever happened before and whether the condition is progressively worsening.
Severity	Is this event similar to any other episodes? How does this compare with past episodes?	If a similar event has happened before, try to contact the patient's doctor, family, or case manager. Determine the effect of the stressful event on the patient's overall functioning. If the patient has expressed suicidal thoughts or tendencies, explore further by asking about his exact plans and means of carrying them out.
Time	Have you had similar problems in the past? Is this the first time this has ever happened?	If the patient has a history of this type of problem, there may be information on how the crisis was alleviated and resolved in the past.

✏️ The SAMPLE History

The acronym SAMPLE is used to obtain specific information pertaining to the focused history of the patient with a behavioral crisis. Look for clues to organic causes (cardiac, respiratory, or neurological illnesses) of an apparent emotional or psychiatric illness. Also look for clues that may confuse the presenting condition, such as medications and severe infections, which can cause an altered mental status, depression, or **psychosis** (a serious mental disorder characterized by a loss of contact with reality). Table 16-4 highlights questions to ask during the SAMPLE history. Table 16-5 lists common psychotropic medications.

TABLE 16-4
SAMPLE for the Patient with a Behavioral Emergency

Information	Questions	Remarks
Signs and **S**ymptoms	Can you describe how you are feeling today?	Determine what type of crisis the patient is having. Obtain the patient's current complaints, problems, and signs and symptoms. Associated signs and symptoms to ask about include generalized symptoms, tachycardia, palpitations, anxiety, confusion, weakness, changes in appetite, excessive crying, and sleep disturbances. Many medical problems can cause or worsen a behavioral illness. Be alert for other explanations to what may at first appear to be an obvious behavioral problem.
Allergies	Do you have any allergies? Are you allergic to any medications?	Ask about allergies to medications as well as about known side effects to medications. Many psychotropic medications have powerful side effects and severe interactions with other medications.
Medications	Are you currently taking any medications? Have you taken any drugs or over-the-counter medications? Have you recently changed medications or dosages of medications?	The major classes of psychotropic medications that you may see prescribed are reviewed in Table 16-5. Ask about all medications taken and why they are taken. Medications commonly used for behavioral disorders are antidepressants. Some of these are used to treat other conditions such as migraines, seizures, and smoking, so do not assume anything. Look for recent or sudden changes in dosages or for discontinued medications. Many times patients stop taking their medications because they do not like the severe side effects. Investigate the

(continues)

TABLE 16-4 *(continued)*

Information	Questions	Remarks
Medications *(continued)*		possible use of over-the-counter (OTC) medications, recreational drugs, homeopathic therapies, or herbals or the use of someone else's medication.
Pertinent past medical history	Are you currently being treated for an illness? Have you had any recent injuries? Have you ever had an episode like this before?	If the patient has a history of this type of behavior, determine the degree of severity, treatment, and response (unstable or adaptable). A history of alcohol or substance abuse is a red flag for behavioral disorders because of the high use of addictive medications. A history of alcohol abuse and drug addiction is not uncommon and can worsen the underlying problem.
Last oral intake	When did you last eat? When did you last take your medication? When did you last drink anything? What did you drink?	Lack of eating could precipitate a behavioral emergency. It may also preceed or could bring about hypoglycemia, which may exhibit characteristics of a behavioral emergency.
Events leading up to this incident	What happened before you were feeling this way? Have you been under any stress at home or at work? Have you had any changes in social or work activities?	Make inquiries about associated conditions that may have precipitated this condition such as new stressors, changes in social status (e.g., loss of a significant other) or economic status (e.g., change or loss of a job), recent arguments or aggressive confrontations with family members, neighbors, or coworkers.

The Mental Status Examination

Assessment of a patient's mental status is not always a smooth process. Initially, the EMS provider should limit physical contact to necessary procedures while determining the presence of any immediate life threats or the need for rapid intervention. When no immediate life threat is apparent, attempt to establish rapport and, if the patient permits, continue the physical examination as appropriate for any physical complaints. Begin the physical examination by asking the patient for permis-

sion to take vital signs. Most patients will have no problem with the EMS provider's taking a pulse. Checking a blood pressure is a nonthreatening way of removing multiple layers of clothing and a good transition to further physical examination. Communication, both verbal and nonverbal, is a key skill for the EMS provider when dealing with a behavioral emergency. Tips and guidelines for verbal and nonverbal communication are reviewed in Table 16-6.

The mental status is inferred through assessment of the patient's behaviors. Pay particular attention to the patient's appearance, behavior, affect, speech, cognitive

TABLE 16-5
Common Psychotropic Medications

Antipsychotics (neuroleptics)

- Benzodiazepines — alprazolam, diazepam, traizolam
- Butyrophenones — haloperidol
- Phenothiazines — Thorazine, Trilafon, Prolixin
- Thiozanthines — Taractan, Daxolin

Antidepressants — amitriptyline, doxepine, Imipramine, nortriptyline, trazodone, Prozac, Wellbutrin

- Lithium — Eskalith, Lithan, Lithobid

MAO inhibitors — Nardil, Parnate

functions, and thought processes. A Skill Sheet for Mental Status Assessment is located in Appendix C.

Steps of the Focused Mental Status Examination

Obtain a baseline assessment and whenever possible verify findings with a family, friend, coworker, or caregiver.

- Appearance or presentation. Note the patient's physical position and posture, personal appearance and hygiene, and appropriateness of dress for climate, age, and gender.
- Affect. What feelings is the patient exhibiting?
- Behavior. What is the patient doing? Observe body language cues.
- Cognitive functions. Assess the patient's level of consciousness. Does the patient know where he is and what is happening now? Assess his memory, both long and short term. Check long-term memory by asking the patient about verifiable events such as his date of birth and historical events.

TABLE 16-6
Communication Tips

	Verbal	Nonverbal
Introduction: Take an active role in controlling the situation.	Make a calm, clear, short statement of who you are and why you are there.	Respect personal space and avoid staring, as this may be perceived as threatening.
Interview: Do not judge, make fun, or play into the patient's delusions.	Be confident but not overbearing. Do not hesitate to screen for suicidal or violent intentions: ask about risk factors and pertinent personal history. Center your questions on the immediate problem.	Act or intervene with formal expression. Be aware of your own facial expressions and posture. Listen actively and limit interruptions. Do not downplay or belittle the patient's complaint.
Act: Delaying is dangerous for the crisis patient.	Ask for permission to assess vital signs; this is a good transition to the physical exam. Tell the patient what is being done now and what is going to happen next.	Move with purposeful intent, but do not move so fast as to further overwhelm or frighten the patient.
Recap: The patient is often confused.	Be supportive and empathetic while explaining what has happened, what is being done now, and what is going to happen next.	Present yourself as a nonthreatening professional here to help.

Check short-term memory by asking what he has eaten in the past 24 hours. Assess mood and affect by observing verbal and nonverbal (facial expressions and body language) cues.

- Speech. Assess word choice, content, intonation, clarity, and pace.

- Thought processes. Determine whether his judgment is reasonable for the situation. Note whether the thought content and perceptions about what is happening currently are logical and consistent (e.g., is the patient experiencing visual, auditory, or other sensory phenomena?). Is the patient making rational decisions?

COMMON CALLS FOR BEHAVIORAL EMERGENCIES

According to the experts at the American Psychiatric Association, "20 percent of the ailments for which Americans seek a doctor's care are related to anxiety disorders, such as panic attacks, that interfere with their ability to live normal lives" (APA, 1997). All people, regardless of gender, income, and race, are susceptible to mental health disorders. Phobias are the most common, followed by depression. The key criterion in assessing a psychological disorder is the degree of impairment of normal functioning.

Depression

Depression is a common reaction to major life stresses. A depressed person has a dejected state of mind and feelings of sadness, discouragement, and hopelessness. Patients often exhibit a reduced activity level, an inability to function, and sleep disturbances. There are many risk factors for depression (see Table 16-2), and severe depression is a risk factor for suicide. Depression may present as another disease. Elderly people commonly

Geriatric Gem

- Depression is common in the elderly. Causes may be psychological (e.g., loss of support system or loss of independence) or physiological (e.g., medications, poor nutrition, dehydration, or organic brain disease).

appear to have an organic illness (e.g., a cardiac or respiratory condition) when, in reality, they are severely depressed.

Mental Illness

The pathophysiology of behavioral and psychiatric disorders is multifactorial. Some aspects of certain illnesses are clearly genetic. A person's surroundings and circumstances affect all disorders to some extent. Many of these disorders have been shown to occur not simply because of surroundings but also because of chemical alterations in the brain. Sometimes, the cause of the disorder is an organic illness. Chemicals called neurotransmitters normally serve to convey messages between different portions of the brain. Either an excess or, more commonly, a deficit of these transmitters results in various types of behavioral and psychiatric disorders, such as schizophrenia or depression.

Substance Abuse

Substance-related disorders include dependence, abuse, and intoxication. True addiction is both a psychological and a physical event. The patient has both a psychological and a physical craving for the drug as well as for its effect. Alcoholism is particularly insidious among the elderly. Often, the symptoms are not recognized until the affected person becomes truly alcohol dependent.

Suicide Attempts

A suicide *attempt* occurs when a patient has a genuine desire to die. Often, the person has planned the event. A suicidal *gesture* is something done by a person to ask for help rather than to die. The patient performs the act in a potentially reversible way, such as taking a few aspirin or a small handful of pills. Unfortunately, small amounts of certain medications can be very poisonous. These days, it is possible for patients to obtain large quantities of certain medications over the Internet. This possibility can increase the potential for a lethal overdose if there are many pills on hand. The EMS provider needs to treat suicidal gesture patients as poisoning patients and to pay careful attention to the behavioral emergency. Sometimes, people who intend to kill themselves take pills and then change their mind. Whether the event is an actual suicide attempt or only a suicide gesture, do not discount the patient's emotional state in any way. Do not be afraid to directly ask the patient, "Were you trying to kill yourself?" or "Did you want to die?" Many people are not aware of the resources available to them for help. A suicide gesture is the patient's way of seeking help. Always clearly document your findings on the prehospital care report and make sure you tell the emergency department physician that the patient said he was trying to harm himself.

Pleas for Help or Attention

Some behavioral calls are related to a patient's cry for attention, such as a suicide gesture or repeated calls by a hypochondriac or a lonely person who has no apparent medical problem but just wants to talk or visit. The patient with acute anxiety who is hyperventilating is often regarded as another example of a cry for help. Of course, hyperventilation is a diagnosis of exclusion, and it is essential that you consider all medical causes of the situation before concluding that it is emotional or behavioral. The patient with a medical cause for hyperventilating can appear identical to someone with only a simple anxiety attack. If these complaints are not taken seriously, a complete assessment may not be performed. This scenario can result in serious complications, as there are many serious and life-threatening medical illnesses that can cause hyperventilation. The safest approach is to assume something is seriously wrong until proved otherwise.

Often, people who want help are not aware of the resources available to them, but they do know that EMS and the people at the hospital are available, so they will call 911 for help. This call may come in the form of a suicide gesture or an alcoholic asking for detox or rehab. In addition to providing supportive psychological care for

the obvious complaint, the EMS provider must always be aware of the physical needs, so complete a physical assessment as well.

Assisting a Transportation

In some areas, EMS is called to transport a person for a mental health evaluation ordered by the county mental health officer. Police should have the order and be on the scene to assist with the transport. This person is usually not willing to cooperate with EMS or the police.

It is not uncommon for incarcerated people to feign unconsciousness or illness to get out of an arrest or just to get out of jail for a short time. These patients must still be evaluated very carefully. There have been cases in which a real medical problem was missed and the patient suffered or died. Another situation in which a patient must be transported against his will would be one in which the patient is a danger to himself or others.

The EMS provider may not be able to assess or interview the patient, and physical or chemical restraint may be necessary. The use of physical or chemical restraint on a patient is serious and carries a high risk of serious patient injury or death from inappropriate restraint techniques. The use of restraint should be based on local protocols in combination with medical control. However, many EMS agencies still have no formal protocol or training for the use of physical restraints. The major concerns are safety for the EMS provider and patient, including injury from excessive force and injury or death from hypoxia and positional asphyxia. Assessment includes the use of continuous pulse oximetry and end-tidal carbon dioxide ($EtCO_2$) and ECG monitoring.

Medical Conditions That Mimic Behavioral Disorders

Consider that conditions such as stroke, tumors, or trauma can affect speech, causing aphasia, dysphasia, or dysarthria. It is very important to consider other factors in addition to a psychiatric disorder. Look for clues that may confuse the presenting condition for something it is not. Medications, severe infections, hypoxia, and hypo- or hyperglycemia are just a few examples of conditions that can cause an altered mental status, depression, or psychosis.

A history of alcohol or substance abuse is a red flag for behavioral disorders because of the high use of addictive medications (Figure 16-2). A history of alcohol abuse and drug addiction is not uncommon in the behavioral patient and can worsen the underlying problem. Many psychotropic medications have powerful side effects and severe interactions with other medications.

STRESS AND THE EMS PROVIDER

EMS providers, as well as all emergency responders, are subjected to positive and negative stress as part of the job. This group is exposed to more negative stress than the average person (Figure 16-3), and they are not immune to the effects of stress and their coping mechanisms do occasionally fail. Stress disorders may be acute and then develop into chronic conditions if not recognized and managed. Some EMS providers "burn out" and leave the profession because of unmanaged stress. By being watchful and recognizing the emotional signs and symptoms of stress in yourself and your coworkers, you may help to intervene and possibly help to keep EMS providers healthy in the workplace.

Signs and symptoms of ineffective or failing coping mechanisms that may be seen in coworkers include increased absenteeism, withdrawal, depression, hyperactivity, irritability, increased smoking or alcohol consumption, sleep disturbances, headaches, poor concentration and decision making, and any of the abnormal behaviors described elsewhere in this chapter. The specific effects of stress on the body are shown in Table 16-7.

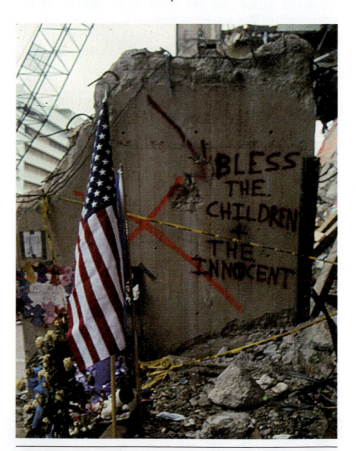

FIGURE 16-3 Some of the most stressful calls for EMS providers involve multiple casualties and the death or serious injury of children, as was the case in the bombing of the Alfred E. Murrah Federal Building in Oklahoma City. Learn how to access your regional critical incident stress management team before an incident like this occurs in your community. **(Courtesy of John O'Connell)**

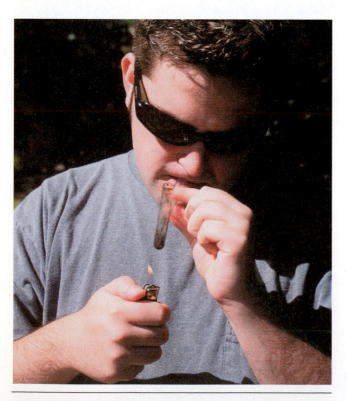

FIGURE 16-2 Substance abuse often leads to behavioral problems and depression.

TABLE 16-7
Effects of Stress on the Body

Organ Affected	Response	Organ Affected	Response
Eyes		Gallbladder and ducts	Relaxation
Radial muscle of the iris	Pupillary contraction	Urinary bladder	
Ciliary muscle	Relaxation for far vision	Detrusor	Relaxation
		Trigone and sphincter	Contraction
Heart			
SA node	Increased heart rate	Ureters	
Atria	Increased contractility and conduction velocity	Motility and tone	Increase
AV node	Increased conduction velocity	Uterus	Contraction (pregnant) Relaxation (pregnant and nonpregnant)
His-Purkinje system	Increased conduction velocity		
Ventricles	Increased contracility	Male sex organs	Ejaculation
Arterioles		Skin	
Coronary	Constriction, dilation	Pilomotor muscles	Contraction
Skin and mucosa	Constriction	Sweat glands	Slight, localized secretion
Skeletal muscle	Constriction, dilation		
Cerebral	Constriction	Spleen capsule	Contraction, relaxation
Pulmonary	Constriction, dilation		
Abdominal viscera	Constriction, dilation	Liver	Glycogenolysis (sugar breakdown)
Salivary glands	Constriction		
Renal	Constriction, dilation		
Systemic veins	Constriction, dilation	Pancreas	
		Acini	Decreased secretion
		Islets	Decreased insulin and glucagon secretion
Lungs			Increased insulin and glucagon secretion
Bronchial muscle	Relaxation		
Bronchial glands	Inhibition, stimulation		
		Salivary glands	Thick, viscous secretion Amylase secretion
Stomach			
Motility and tone	Decrease		
Sphincters	Contraction	Lacrimal glands	Secretion
Secretion	Inhibition		
Intestine		Adipose tissue (fat)	Lipolysis (fat breakdown)
Motility and tone	Decrease		
Sphincters	Contraction	Juxtaglomerular cells	Increased renin secretion
Secretion	Inhibition		

Exploring the Web

● Search the Web for information on coping with stress. What techniques can EMS providers use when they are feeling excessive work-related stress? What resources are available to EMS providers to combat work-related stress? What resources can you direct coworkers to when you see they are suffering from stress that is affecting the way they work?

CONCLUSION

Responses to a crisis vary from person to person. When stress becomes overwhelming and a person is unable to cope or feels he is losing control, stress reactions can cause impaired functioning. Some people become withdrawn or depressed, and others become overactive or even violent. Many factors can alter a patient's behavior, whether or not there is a history of mental illness. Whenever possible, obtain background information including concurrent disease processes, dystonic (muscle spasms) reactions to antipsychotic drugs, language problems, mutism, blindness, mental retardation, accidental or intentional overdose, injury, or mutilation. Never forget that personal safety comes first while taking an active role in controlling the situation and supporting the patient's emotional and physical needs.

REVIEW QUESTIONS

1. The highest priority when assessing a patient who may be having a behavioral emergency is:
  a. ruling out medical conditions.
  b. ruling out trauma.
  c. protecting yourself and your crew.
  d. determining the medications the patient is taking.

2. To assess a patient's intellectual function, the EMS provider considers orientation and:
  a. memory.
  b. concentration.
  c. judgment.
  d. all of the above.

3. Asking the patient his date of birth or Social Security number will help to assess his:
  a. long-term memory.
  b. short-term memory.
  c. recall.
  d. judgment.

4. Paying close attention to what the patient communicates concerning the current situation and his past medical history will help the EMS provider assess the patient's:
  a. orientation.
  b. judgment.
  c. recall.
  d. memory.

5. A false belief or idea that a person portrays as true is called a:
  a. memory block.
  b. recall disturbance.
  c. delusion.
  d. hallucination.

6. The expression of thoughts or emotions by means of gestures is known as:
  a. subliminal expression.
  b. hallucination.
  c. delusional behavior.
  d. body language.

7. Intonation, clarity, and pace should be considered when assessing a patient's:
  a. speech.
  b. perceptions.
  c. cognitive functions.
  d. affect.

8. Patients who are experiencing sleep disturbances and the inability to function should be evaluated for the possibility of:
  a. hypoglycemia.
  b. hyperventilation.
  c. depression.
  d. a cognitive disorder.

9. If the patient is hyperventilating, the EMS provider should:
  a. tell him to calm down.
  b. rule out any medical causes first.
  c. give the patient a paper bag to breath into.
  d. disregard this sign because it is emotional.

10. The signs and symptoms of ineffective coping with job stress seen in EMS providers often include:

    a. excessive alcohol consumption.

    b. sleep disturbances.

    c. headaches and poor concentration.

    d. all of the above.

CRITICAL THINKING QUESTIONS

1. You are called to a homeless shelter because one of the regulars is behaving erratically. Upon your arrival, you find a man in disheveled clothing. He is stumbling when he attempts to walk, is slurring his words, and is having difficulty concentrating. The woman working at the shelter said she hadn't seen him for several days. He keeps muttering weaten in several days. What could be the cause of this patient's problem? Is it a medical problem or a psychological problem? What additional information should you try to get from this patient?

2. You are called to a residence by the police who are on the scene of a domestic crisis. There is a female patient who has several self-inflicted knife wounds. Upon your arrival, the woman is sitting in a balled-up position on the floor and is visibly bleeding from wounds to the arms and legs. The police were able to secure the knife. She is rocking back and forth and has a vacant stare on her face. How would you approach this patient? What types of questions are pertinent to ask? What assistance can the police provide?

3. Lately, you notice a change in your partner. He has been very quiet and reserved and does not want to hang out socially with you or other coworkers. A couple of times, you have noticed the smell of alcohol on his breath during working hours. Attempts to talk to him about what is bothering him have gotten an angry response. What can you do to help your partner? What could be some causes of his behavior?

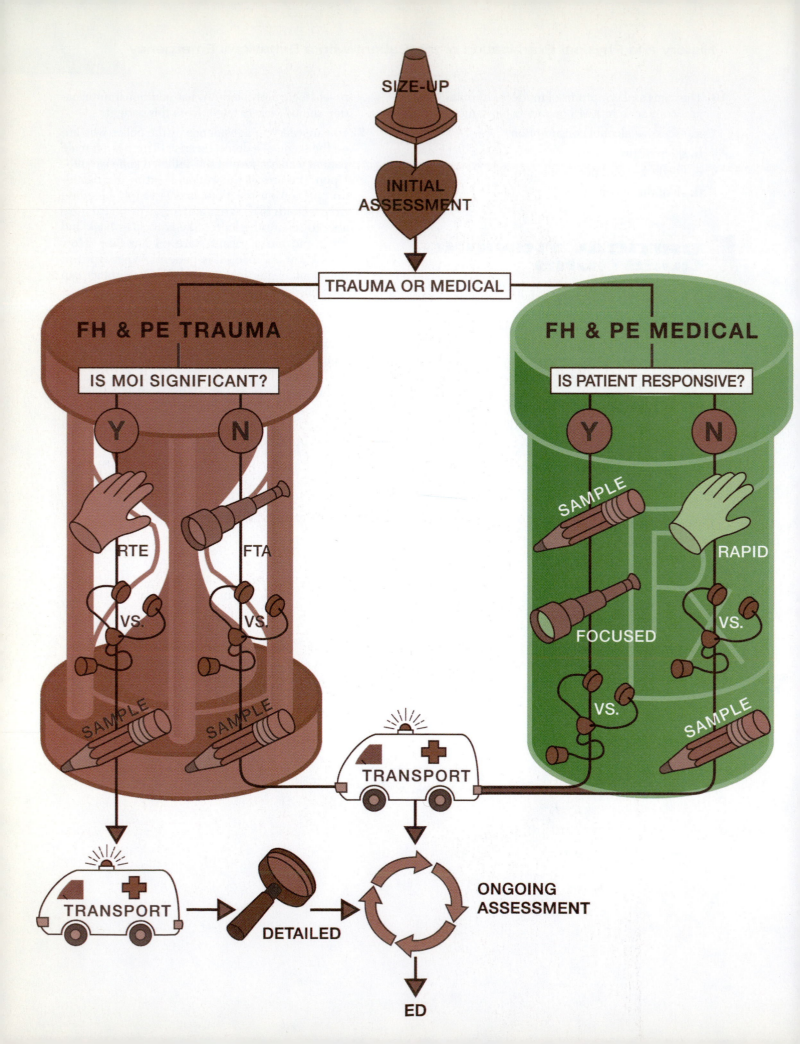

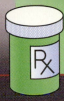

Chapter 17

The Assessment Approach for the Pediatric Patient

OBJECTIVES

Upon completion of this chapter, the reader should be able to:

- List and define the seven pediatric age groups.
- Define *emergency doctrine* and explain how it applies to the emergency care of a child.
- List the various references the EMS provider can use to find normal values for pediatric vital signs.
- Explain why temperature is such an important vital sign in the pediatric patient.
- Describe two characteristics of a normal pediatric heart rate.
- Describe two characteristics of normal respiratory muscle movement in children.
- Describe two ways an EMS provider can reduce a child's fear of having her blood pressure measured.
- Explain why capillary refill is usually a reliable indication of a child's circulatory status.
- Describe why a child's body weight is an important factor for the EMS provider and the emergency care of a child.
- Explain why the EMS provider's approach to the physical examination must incorporate the age of the patient as well as the emotional and psychological state of the patient and parents.
- Describe how the APGAR scoring system is used in the assessment of the newborn.
- Describe the differences between the airway anatomy of young and older infants and that of older children or adults.
- Explain why the physical examination is often performed from the toes to the head in toddlers and preschoolers.
- List some differences between the level of cognitive and social competency of the preschooler and that of a toddler or school-ager and how those differences are related to the EMS provider's interaction with a preschooler.

(continues)

OBJECTIVES *(continued)*

- Describe why the EMS provider should involve the child in the history-taking process and allow the child to make some choices during assessment and care.

- Describe the general assessment approach for the adolescent patient.

- List the most common causes of pediatric trauma death.

- List the risk factors that have been identified for pediatric suicide.

- List the warning signs that should alert the EMS provider to potential suicidal intentions that may be discovered during a focused history.

- List the risk factors found to be a common denominator in abuse situations.

- List the common causes of respiratory distress associated with specific age groups.

- Explain why dehydration is a significant problem in pediatric patients.

- List some of the equipment and devices the EMS provider may be called to assist with for special needs and technology-assisted children.

- List the complications that may arise with these devices.

KEY TERMS

acute life-threatening event (ALTE)

APGAR scoring system

asthma

ataxia

bronchiolitis

croup

diabetic ketoacidosis (DKA)

emergency doctrine

emergency information form (EIF)

epiglottitis

neonatal sepsis

pneumonia

rotavirus

sinus arrhythmia

sudden infant death syndrome (SIDS)

INTRODUCTION

This chapter focuses on the assessment approach to the various age groups of children, including children with special health care needs. It provides tips on taking vital signs, obtaining the focused history, and performing the physical examination. The signs and symptoms of the most common medical emergencies and the most common mechanisms of injury (MOIs) for traumatic injuries are also covered.

The key to assessing children is to understand and be able to integrate the physiological, psychological, and sociological changes that occur throughout human development. The EMS provider must be able to modify the examination to fit the age of the patient and to adjust the assessment approach in cases in which the child's chronological age does not match the emotional age. Pediatric age groups are classified as follows:

- Newborn: birth to first few hours of life

- Neonate: birth to 1 month
- Infant: birth to 1 year
- Toddler: 1 to 3 years
- Preschooler: 3 to 5 years
- School-ager: 6 to 10 years
- Adolescent (teenager): 11 to 18 years

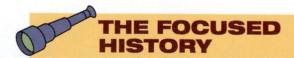

THE FOCUSED HISTORY

The younger the patient, the more the EMS provider will need to rely on the parent or caregiver for information. However, children as young as 2 years old may be able to answer simple questions about the current event. Fortunately, most children do not have an extensive medical history. Obtain the OPQRST and SAMPLE information just as you would for an adult patient.

Pediatric Pearl

● Injury is responsible for more childhood deaths than all other causes combined (Peters, Kochanek, & Murphy, 1998).

Schools, day care facilities, camps, and the like should have on file a record of the child's health history as well as a permission-to-treat form. When called to a medical or traumatic emergency that occurs away from a child's home, be sure to ask for them. When a parent or legal guardian is not present and there is no signed permission-to-treat form, the EMS provider may do what is necessary to sustain life under the concept of "implied consent," also referred to as the **emergency doctrine**. In the absence of a life-threatening emergency, the parent or legal guardian must be contacted to authorize treatment.

The OPQRST History

Anticipate the need to spend more time obtaining a focused history for a child than you would for an adult, especially for children with special medical needs or with technology-assistive devices. Using OPQRST, Table 17-1 highlights specific information pertaining to the focused history.

 ## The SAMPLE History

Use the SAMPLE acronym to obtain specific information pertaining to the focused history of a child, as outlined in Table 17-2.

TABLE 17-1
OPQRST for the Pediatric Patient

Information	Questions	Remarks
Onset	Is this a new problem? Is this a preexisting condition that has worsened?	Determine how the problem began. Many times, the worsening of a condition will initiate a call to EMS.
Provocation	What brought about the current condition? What was the child doing?	Obtain the details of the present episode. Determine what the patient was doing at the time of onset and try to differentiate trauma as a cause. Remember, trauma is the leading cause of pediatric death in the United States.
Quality	Can you show me where it hurts? Can you describe what it feels like?	Try to find out what the pain feels like and where the child is having the pain. Using some adjectives the child may understand to describe the pain may help.
Region, **R**adiation, **R**elief, **R**ecurrence	Does the pain feel like it is moving to anywhere else? Have you given the child anything to help alleviate the pain or other symptoms?	It is important to determine whether the parents have taken any actions to help relieve the pain and symptoms the child is feeling.

(continues)

TABLE 17-1 *(continued)*

Information	Questions	Remarks
Severity	What has the child's activity level been? Is the child behaving normally or behaving in an unusual manner?	Use a pain scale adapted for a child to determine the severity of the pain. Obtain a baseline assessment followed by serial assessments in order to determine whether the condition is improving or deteriorating. Parents can tell a lot about what a child is feeling on the basis of their knowledge of the child's patterns of behavior.
Time	When did the symptoms begin?	Determine when the problem first began and whether any time passed before EMS was called.

TABLE 17-2
SAMPLE for the Pediatric Patient

Information	Questions	Remarks
Signs and **S**ymptoms	What prompted you to call EMS? What is the child feeling? Has the child ever seen a doctor for this condition? Have you noticed changes in the child's behavior? Has the child vomited or had diarrhea? Is the child's urine output normal? Is the child producing tears when crying?	Determine how severe the problem is. If the child is under a doctor's care for the condition, more information may be obtained by calling the doctor. Behavioral changes, even subtle changes, may indicate a medical illness in children. Be alert to signs of dehydration such as reduced urine output, vomiting, diarrhea, or lack of tears when crying.
Allergies	Does the child have any allergies to medications or foods? Are there any procedures that should be avoided in the care of the child?	Determine whether the child has an allergic reaction to any medications that could be used in treatment. Also determine whether the child could be having an allergic reaction now. Parents would know best whether there is anything that should not be done to treat the child because they would know about past adverse reactions or experiences.

(continues)

TABLE 17-2 *(continued)*

Information	Questions	Remarks
Medications	What medications is the child taking? When did the child last take a medication? Did you give the child any aspirin or over-the-counter products to relieve the symptoms? Is there a possibility that the child accidentally ingested medications?	It is very important to get an accurate list of medications and doses. Determine when they were given last and whether any over-the-counter (OTC) or home remedies were tried. Determine whether it is possible that the child took an adult's medications by accident.
Pertinent past medical history	Is the child under a doctor's care for this condition? Does the child have any preexisting medical conditions? Has the child been injured recently?	Ask the parent or caregiver for detailed information about the child's disability or chronic illness and include all diagnoses, past procedures, baseline neurological status, baseline vital signs, baseline physical findings, prostheses, appliances, and the use of technology-assistive devices. Ask the parent or caregiver the child's weight and whether there are any other specific medical issues. Get the name of the patient's physicians, including the primary care pediatrician and current specialty physicians.
Last oral intake	When did the child last eat? When did the child last have anything to drink? Has the child been eating and drinking normally?	Determine the last time the child ate in the event any surgical interventions may be needed. Include feedings via a feeding tube. Find out the last time the parents performed pertinent procedures such as suctioning, flushing, lavage, cleaning or changing of tubes, and so on.
Events leading up to this incident	What prompted you to call EMS? Did the problem occur very suddenly, or has it been gradually getting worse? Is this a new occurrence, or is it an exacerbation of an ongoing condition?	Ask about the events leading up to the call for EMS. Circumstances relevant to the chronic illness or disability are not always the primary reason emergency care is required. The child may have fallen or had a seizure that resulted in an isolated extremity injury or a laceration, making the underlying disability or chronic illness secondary to splinting or wound care.

Taking Pediatric Vital Signs

It is important that pediatric assessment equipment such as electrodes, stethoscope, and blood pressure cuff be age appropriate to prevent false readings. Vital sign values vary with age, and, though it is not necessary to memorize the values for each age group, the EMS provider should be well practiced at reading pediatric reference charts. There are numerous pediatric references available in the form of pocket guides, charts, and weight- or length-based tapes (Figure 17-1). These small, handy resources allow the health care provider to quickly identify the proper size of equipment, medication doses, age-appropriate vital signs, and estimated weight. Keep a pocket reference or a weight- or length-based chart such as a Broselow tape handy or with the pediatric equipment. If pediatric calls do not occur frequently in your service area, refer to the guide now and again to maintain proficiency in using it. Children over the age of 12 have vital sign values similar to those of normal adults.

Temperature

Temperature is an important vital sign in children and should be taken routinely in the prehospital setting in cases in which an infectious disease or hypo- or hyperthermia is suspected. During the first 3 months of life, a fever is a serious sign and any temperature over 38°C (101°F) warrants a hospital visit and a complete workup. An infection from a virus or bacterium is the most common cause of fever in neonates. Assume that a fever in the neonate represents **neonatal sepsis** (severe overwhelming infection) until proved otherwise.

Wide fluctuations in body temperature can occur in small children because of their immature thermal control mechanism. Infants and small children do not have the ability to shiver to create body heat when they are cold. They are especially vulnerable to rapid changes in temperature (which may cause febrile seizure), and many pediatric illnesses are accompanied by a fever. Skin color is a good indicator of the child's condition. Red and flushed indicates hyperthermia, and pale, bluish, or mottled indicates hypothermia.

Rectal temperatures are the preferred method for infants and children younger than 5 years of age because of the difficulty in obtaining an accurate oral temperature. To obtain a rectal temperature, place the patient on her side or in a prone position. You can lay a small infant prone on your lap. While you separate the buttock with the thumb and forefinger of one hand, with the other hand gently insert a well-lubricated rectal thermometer through the anal sphincter: ½ inch for newborns, ¾ inch for infants, and 1 inch for preschoolers and older patients. Hold the thermometer firmly between your fingers to avoid accidentally inserting it too far. There is a potential for accidentally perforating the rectum, so tell the child to hold very still and ask the parent to help you hold the child still.

For the older child, temperature may be obtained by other methods as well as rectally. Tympanic and axillary temperatures are quick and painless; however, they are often less reliable than oral or rectal temperatures. When a thermometer is not available, the EMS provider can estimate a child's temperature by feeling the forehead and extremities with the back of his hand.

Heart Rate

The heart rate in infants may be observed by: auscultating the apical heart, or the pulsations of the anterior fontanel. To count the pulse, the brachial artery is palpated. Owing to the small chest size, heart tones can be heard easily with a stethoscope. The rhythm is usually **sinus arrhythmia** (a rhythm typical in children and healthy adults with a rate that increases and decreases rhythmically with breathing), and the rate can fluctuate significantly with activity (e.g., sleeping or crying). In an older child, palpate the radial artery at the wrist just as you would in an adult. As the child grows, the heart rhythm remains sinus arrhythmia, but the heart rate begins to slow with age (Table 17-3).

Respiratory Rate

The respiratory rate can easily be observed by watching the abdomen rather than the chest of infants and small children. The immature muscles of an infant's abdomen allow for the abdomen to protrude, making respiratory movement visible in the belly. The abdomen of older children protrudes (potbelly) when they are standing but flattens when they lie down. As the child gets older, diaphragmatic breathing becomes minimal, and chest excursion is more prominent. Respiratory muscle move-

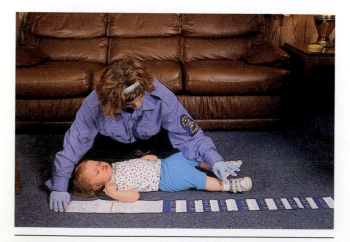

FIGURE 17-1 Using a Broselow tape.

TABLE 17-3
Resting Pediatric Heart Rates

Patient Age (yr)	Range (beats/ minute)	Average (beats/ minute)
Newborn	120–160	140
Infant (birth–1)	90–140	120
Toddler (1–3)	80–130	110
Preschooler (3–5)	80–120	100
School-ager (6–10)	70–110	90
Adolescent (11–14)	60–105	80–90

TABLE 17-4
Resting Pediatric Respiratory Rates

Patient Age (yr)	Range (breaths/ minute)	Average (breaths/ minute)
Newborn	30–50	40
Infant (birth–1)	25–40	30
Toddler (1–3)	20–30	25
Preschooler (3–5)	20–30	22
School-ager (6–10)	16–30	20
Adolescent (11–14)	12–20	18

ment can be observed or palpated in a child's chest as it is in an adult's. Normal values for the respiratory rates in pediatric age groups are listed in Table 17-4.

Blood Pressure

It is not always easy to take toddlers' and preschoolers' blood pressure (BP) because of their fear or uncooperativeness. Fortunately, taking the blood pressure on a child is not necessary to determine the circulatory status. Because children have such good circulation, the skin color, temperature, and condition (CTC) is a very reliable sign of circulation. If a child looks sick, she probably is sick! The skin should be warm and dry and should have a good color. Signs of poor circulation in a child would be mottled or blotchy skin on the extremities and, worse, on the body; delayed capillary refill; and cool, cold, pale, or cyanotic skin.

To reduce a small child's fear or anxiety about having a blood pressure taken, the EMS provider can demonstrate the skill on a doll, a parent, or himself before taking the child's blood pressure. The demonstration will show the child that having her blood pressure taken will not hurt. Another approach is to tell the child that it feels like a hug around the arm, while you take her upper arm in your hand and gently squeeze it as a demonstration. A proper-sized cuff should be centered on and cover about two-thirds of the upper arm. To estimate a normal systolic blood pressure, multiply the child's age by 2 and add 80: (child's age × 2) + 80 = systolic BP. Normal values for blood pressure by pediatric age group are listed in Table 17-5.

TABLE 17-5
Pediatric Blood Pressure Values

Patient Age (yr)	Systolic Range (mm Hg)	Diastolic Range (mm Hg)
Infants and toddlers (birth–3)	80 + (2 × age in years)	2/3 systolic
Preschooler (3–5)	78–116	48–64
School-ager (6–10)	80–122	46–68
Adolescent (11–14)	88–140	50–70

Capillary Refill

Because most children have good circulation, uncomplicated by heart disease, smoking, cholesterol, and so on, capillary refill is a reliable indicator of a child's circulatory condition. A refill time greater than 2 seconds is considered delayed (Figure 17-2). To assess capillary refill on the infant, press your thumb on the bottom of the foot. Even before a blood pressure is obtained, a combination of delayed capillary refill and poor skin

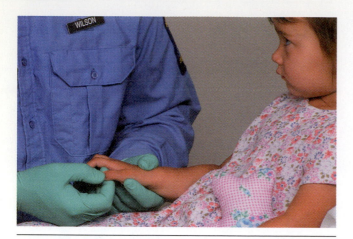

FIGURE 17-2 Assessing capillary refill on a young child.

CTC is considered a reliable indicator that the child's circulatory status is ailing.

Body Weight

The body weight of a child is an important factor, especially when emergency care involves the use of medications and fluid administration. When parents or caregivers are present, ask about the child's weight; most of the time they will know. When the weight of a child is not known, refer to a pediatric guide or use the following simple formula to estimate a child's weight in kilograms. Multiply the child's age by 2 and add 8: (child's age × 2) + 8 = weight (in kg).

THE PHYSICAL EXAMINATION

The EMS provider's approach to the physical examination is geared to the age of the patient as well as to the emotional and psychological state of the patient and parents. Children are very dependent on the quality of their home environment and familiar surroundings (e.g., day care, school) and their interactions with family members. EMS providers are in a unique position to observe the child in her own environment during an EMS call; therefore, the EMS provider should include an assessment of the child's environment and interactions with family or guardians as part of the general assessment. The following discussion on the pediatric physical examination includes anatomical, cognitive, and emotional differences by various age groups.

The Approach for the Newborn

The assessment of the newborn is performed immediately after birth. Respiratory effort, heart rate, and skin color (for perfusion) are evaluated by using the **APGAR scoring system** (Table 17-6) at 1 minute and 5 minutes after birth. The APGAR score is a well-accepted assessment score chart that assigns a rating of 0, 1, or 2 to each of five signs (appearance, pulse, grimace, activity, and respirations). Ten is the highest score; a good to excellent score is 7 to 10; 4 to 6 is fair; and less than 4 at 1 minute is poor and indicates the need to begin aggressive assisted ventilations. At 5 minutes an APGAR score of less than 7 indicates the baby is at high risk for central nervous system (CNS) impairment.

Once the baby is delivered, clear the airway of any remaining secretions, then quickly dry the baby and begin the assessment. Stimulate the baby as necessary and keep the baby warm. It is easier to manage and assess the baby once the cord is cut, so clamp and cut the cord and examine both ends for bleeding and tighten the clamps tighter if necessary.

Note the infant's skin color, activity, and muscle tone and assign the corresponding number from the APGAR scoring system. Listen to the chest with your stethoscope for breath sounds and heart rate. Because the chest is very small and the wall is very thin, it is nearly impossible to differentiate the two sides separately. The breathing and heart rate should be easy to hear; count the heart rate and respiratory rate while listening and then assign those a number and complete the scoring.

Weight, length, and other physical dimensions such as circumference of the head and chest are measured in the clinical setting. In the clinical setting, a newborn is initially classified by weight and gestational age. In the prehospital setting, it is rare to find an appropriate scale for weighing a newborn; therefore, the classification of gestational age is used in this setting. The baby is classified as preterm, term, or postterm:

- Preterm: <38 weeks' gestation
- Term: 38 to 42 weeks' gestation
- Postterm: >42 weeks' gestation

The Approach for the Neonate and Infant

Completing a physical examination on the infant can be done while the child is lying down or being held by a parent. Keeping the child and the parents calm is important both for getting an accurate assessment and for preventing the child from agitating the current condition or injury. If the child sees that the parent is upset, the situation will often become more difficult. The key with this age group is to distract the child, and the parent can help you do it. Infants usually give attention to only one thing at a time, and the EMS provider or the parent can use distraction with a flashlight or a toy or by playing peek-a-boo.

TABLE 17-6
APGAR Score (Maximum Score of 10)

	0	1	2
Appearance (skin color)	Blue or pale	Pink body, blue extremities	Completely pink all over
Pulse	Absent	Slow, <100 bpm	>100 bpm
Grimace (irritability)	No response	Grimaces	Cries
Activity (muscle tone)	Limp	Some flexion of extremities	Active extremity motion
Respirations	Absent	Slow, irregular	Good, crying

Infants and toddlers rely a great deal on facial expressions and the tone of voice for communication. They will look to a parent for reassurance, so distraught and frightened parents need reassurance and explanation. The EMS provider should pay close attention to his body language and keep a reassuring smile on his face while attending the patient and the family.

The infant's head is proportionately large (Figure 17-3) in relation to the body and remains so through the preschool years. The **fontanels** (sometimes spelled fontanelles) are the membrane-covered spaces between the incompletely ossified cranial bones of an infant's head. The posterior fontanel normally closes at 4 to 6 months of age, and the anterior fontanel closes by 12 to 18 months (Figure 17-4). The fontanels are normally soft and flat, but they can bulge during crying. The fontanels can be used as a diagnostic aid when assessing for dehydration, shock, or head injury with rising intracranial pressure (ICP) by observing whether they are sunken (dehydration and shock) or swollen (rising ICP).

The airway anatomy in young and older infants has distinct differences from that of older children and adults. The infant's tongue is very large in proportion to the size of the mouth. The small trachea is more anterior than an adult's airway, increasing the possibility for obstruction either by foreign bodies or when the head is hyperextended. The smallest diameter of the airway is the cricoid ring. Infants are obligate nose breathers until 6 months of age, and they might not open their mouth to breathe even when their nose becomes obstructed from a cold, so a stuffy nose is a problem and may create periods of apnea.

The potbelly appearance and belly breathing are normal. The infant's respiratory muscles are immature

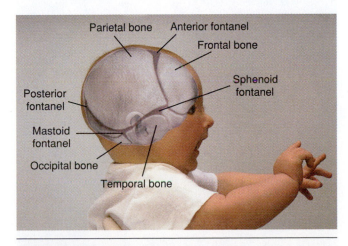

FIGURE 17-3 Proportionately large infant head.

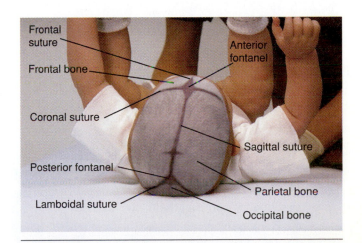

FIGURE 17-4 Fontanels.

and unable to sustain a rapid respiratory rate for long periods of time. In cases of severe respiratory distress, the infant will compensate with sternal retractions and a pronounced "see-saw" motion of the chest and abdomen.

The Approach for the Toddler

The toddler can be a bit more challenging to examine than the infant, but the primary concerns for this age group are similar to those for infants. Establish a rapport with the parents or caregivers while getting the information about the current emergency. Involve them as much as possible and observe the interaction between the parents and child. Upon approaching the scene, note the general appearance of the child. The child's appearance is a very reliable indicator of how ill the child is, and getting an impression upon approaching the scene may provide information before the fear, crying, and physical struggle that often results when the EMS provider begins a hands-on examination.

The physical examination for the toddler is often performed in a toe-to-head fashion in an effort to reduce fear and anxiety. This age group does not like the head or ears to be touched by strangers. Start the physical exam by getting on the same level as the child in an effort to make eye contact and watch facial expressions. The EMS provider should remember to warm his hands and equipment before touching the child's body. Smile and talk gently in simple terms to the child while holding her hand. Distract the child by counting her fingers while touching each one. If is often helpful to demonstrate the steps of many procedures on a toy, on the parent, or on yourself beforehand to help the child understand and to lessen her fears. Save the unpleasant procedures such as taking a blood pressure or rectal temperature or examining the head for last.

The Approach for the Preschooler

The preschooler has mastered the basics of language and will tell the EMS provider what hurts. Because the child's level of cognitive and social competency is directly related to the home environment, depending on the level of distress, the child may be very dependent and cling to the parent for comfort or she may be comfortably independent. This age group has developed imagination and can have fantasies (Figure 17-5). If they see blood or a distracting injury, they may think they are going to die. Use a Band-Aid or dressing to cover such injuries. Preschoolers can take the things an EMS provider says very literally, so be careful of the phrases used. For example, if you say, "I am going to take your pulse," the child may wonder where you are taking it and whether you will give it back. Gaining a child's trust is just as important as it is for an adult for getting cooperation and providing care. Do not lie to a child; rather, explain things in a way that is appropriate to her cognitive capability.

The approach for the physical examination of the preschooler is the same as that for the toddler. Use a firm but gentle tone with precise instructions when performing an act pertaining to the examination. Tell the child what to do rather than asking the child to do it. For example, say, "Open your mouth and stick out your tongue" rather than "Will you open your mouth for me?" The preschooler will often find comfort in holding a toy and having a parent near. Demonstrating procedures on a doll or on yourself is very effective.

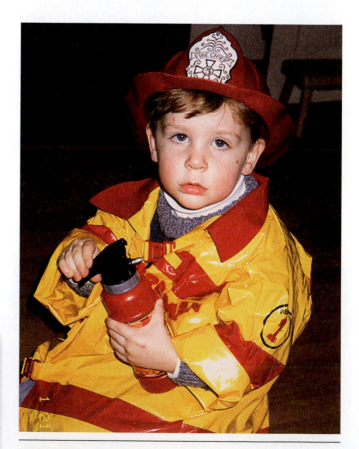

FIGURE 17-5 The preschooler.

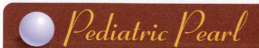

Pediatric Pearl

● Preschoolers can take the things an EMS provider says very literally, so be careful of the phrases used.

The Approach for the School-ager

Aside from modesty, school-agers become easier to assess than the younger age groups. It is very important that a child in this age group (Figure 17-6) not feel different from other children. In this age group, independence and self-esteem are developing rapidly. The EMS provider should involve the child in the history-taking process because she can provide reliable information. When information from this patient does not appear to fit with the circumstances, consider interviewing her when the parent is out of sight. Allow the child to make minor choices in order to increase her sense of control.

The Approach for the Adolescent

Approach the adolescent patient in the same manner as you would an adult. Preserve her modesty and, if possible, interview and examine her without the parent nearby. Teens often withhold information they do not want their parents to know. Take them seriously because they may be dangerous to themselves or others (e.g., suicidal or in a gang).

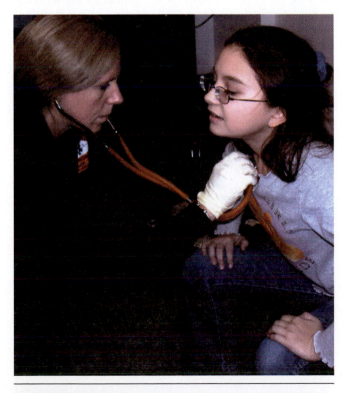

FIGURE 17-6 When assessing the school-ager, consider her modesty and need for privacy.

TRAUMA

The leading cause of death among children in the United States is trauma, and the most common causes of trauma in pediatrics are motor vehicle crashes (MVCs), abuse, auto–pedestrian accidents, bicycle injuries, falls, burns, drowning, and firearms. Many of the injuries from these causes can be prevented through education and diligence in using safe practices such as teaching children to always wear a seat belt, or putting small children in the proper car seat while in a motor vehicle, and making sure children wear a helmet while riding a bicycle. Prevention works, and EMS providers have contributed significantly by offering programs to educate the public, setting an example by wearing seat belts and helmets, and following safety guidelines and procedures themselves.

Suicide is a major cause of death among adolescents, and it is not uncommon among preteens. The incidence of pediatric suicide continues to rise each year. Recent statistics show suicide as the third leading cause of death among males age 15 to 24. Unfortunately, the number of suicide deaths among younger children is growing too. During the focused history, warning signs that should alert the EMS provider to suicidal intentions include dramatic changes in personality as reported by family or caregivers; self-destructive behavior; withdrawal from family and friends; lack of interest in favorite activities; expressing signs of depression, hopelessness, or excessive guilt; and obvious talk of suicide. There are certain risk factors that have been identified for pediatric suicide, and these are listed in Table 17-7.

TABLE 17-7
Risk Factors for Pediatric Suicide

- Access to lethal weapons
- Access to drugs and alcohol
- Access to motor vehicles
- Inadequate support system
- Family history of depression or alcoholism
- Exposure to domestic violence
- Abuse or neglect
- Divorced parents
- Loss of loved one (death in the family)
- Breakup of a romantic relationship

Another category of trauma is child neglect and abuse, which can be physical, sexual, or emotional and occurs when a child is injured or is allowed to be injured by someone who was entrusted with her care. The U.S. Department of Health and Human Services published data from the National Study of Child Abuse and Neglect that estimates that as many as 2.8 million children were actually abused or neglected in the United States in 1993. There are certain risk factors (Table 17-8) found to be a common denominator in abuse situations. The clues that should alert an EMS provider to the possibility of abuse are listed in Table 17-9. However, the

TABLE 17-8
Risk Factors for Abuse

- Lack of financial support
- Lack of emotional support
- Misunderstandings of the normal child developmental stages leading the parent or caregiver to have unrealistic expectations of the child's behavior
- A colicky child
- A chronically ill or developmentally delayed child
- A sibling of an abused child
- A parent who was abused as a child

TABLE 17-9
Clues Suggestive of Child Abuse

- Multiple bruises of various ages
- Unusual burn injuries such as skin burns (e.g., stocking or glove distribution, burns on genitalia from dunking in hot water)
- Central nervous system injuries
- Mouth injuries
- Injuries to the eyes, ears, or nose
- Inappropriate interaction with the parent or caregiver
- A child who is not comforted by a parent or caregiver

Exploring the Web

- Search the Web for the leading causes of trauma-related injuries in children. What are the top five traumatic injuries in children? What puts children at risk for these types of injuries? What patterns should you be alert for in these types of injuries? What preventive actions can be taken to reduce the risks of these injuries in children? What role can you play as an EMS provider in injury prevention?

presence or absence of these clues does not positively prove or disprove an abusive situation; they should serve to encourage the EMS provider to perform a detailed physical examination and obtain a detailed history that will aid in treating the patient.

Pediatric suicide risk factors and child abuse and neglect are two areas in which prevention can come only through recognition of certain signs and risk factors. EMS providers may be the child's first opportunity for recognition of such findings because they are the ones who see the child in her home environment and are able to directly observe key family interactions. Examples of environmental conditions suggesting the possibility of child abuse or neglect include evidence of alcohol or substance use, a report of a mechanism of injury (MOI) that does not fit the scene (e.g., a child with a severe head injury from "falling off the couch"), or family members giving different accounts of the incident.

MEDICAL EMERGENCIES

Respiratory distress is the leading medical complaint among children. Causes of respiratory distress in children are asthma, bronchiolitis, croup, epiglottitis, pneumonia, and foreign body airway obstructions (FBAOs). Table 17-10 lists the common causes of respiratory distress as they occur by age group.

Indications that a child is experiencing respiratory distress include altered mental status (AMS), poor skin CTC, and changes in respiratory effort and respiratory sounds. Always suspect a child with an altered mental status to be experiencing respiratory difficulties until proved otherwise. The appearance of cyanotic or mottled skin is a result of poor oxygenation and decreased perfusion. Nasal flaring and the use of accessory muscles to breathe (e.g., inspiratory sternal retractions in the intercostal, subcostal, and supracostal areas), and stridor

TABLE 17-10
Causes of Pediatric Respiratory Emergencies by Age Group

Patient Age (yr)	Causes
Infant (birth–1)	Asthma, croup, bronchiolitis, foreign body
Toddler, preschooler (1–5)	Asthma, croup, pneumonia, foreign body, epiglottitis
School-ager (6–10)	Asthma, pneumonia, foreign body, epiglottitis
Adolescent (11–18)	Asthma

with grunting on expiration are all abnormal findings and indicate distress (Figure 17-7).

Asthma can occur at any age but is prominent in the 3- to 12-year age group. The onset can vary from slow to sudden, but a history of allergies is what differentiates this disorder from croup, epiglottitis, and FBAO. Early symptoms of an asthma attack include wheezing and dyspnea characterized by the child's being able to inhale but having great difficulty exhaling. The child will attempt to compensate by increasing the respiratory rate (tachypnea) and effort to breath. The movement of the respiratory muscles will be exaggerated (sternal retractions) and there may be nasal flaring. Late symptoms occur as the child becomes physically exhausted and experiences respiratory failure. A major warning sign is a quiet-sounding chest in a patient who is obviously tachypneic and short of breath. A child with a low heart rate and a sharp decrease in mental status in the face of any acute asthma attack is in imminent danger of respiratory arrest.

Bronchiolitis is a viral infection of the bronchioles that causes swelling of the lower airways. Signs and symptoms are very similar to those of an asthma attack and include tachypnea, sternal retractions, and cyanosis. However, bronchiolitis is often consistent with a recent or current history of respiratory infections. Ask about nasal congestion, cough, and a low-grade fever.

Croup is caused by viral respiratory infections or other infections such as an ear infection. This infection settles in the upper airway tissues and causes swelling of the vocal cords, the trachea, and the tissue directly under the epiglottis, creating a partial airway obstruction. The patient will have a mild or severe seal-like barking cough, and there will be noticeable drooling. Croup is common in the 3-month to 3-year age group and is associated with a history of recent or current upper respiratory infection.

Epiglottitis is a relatively rare, but potentially life-threatening, infection that causes severe inflammation and swelling of the epiglottis and is associated with a history of mild flulike symptoms. The swollen epiglottis has the potential to completely obstruct the airway. Infection can occur at any age (including adult), but 3 to 6 years is the most common age. The condition develops into respiratory distress within 1 to 2 hours. There is pain and difficulty swallowing, profound drooling, a sore throat, little or no cough, and difficulty breathing.

Pneumonia may be caused by viral or bacterial infections and is associated with recent upper respiratory infections. Signs and symptoms include fever, tachypnea, crackles, consolidations in one or more lobes, and cough.

Foreign bodies are easily trapped in the narrow airway passages and should be suspected when respiratory distress is sudden or wheezing or stridor is present, especially in children 1 to 3 years of age.

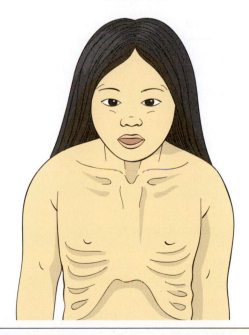

FIGURE 17-7 Inspiratory retractions indicate respiratory distress.

Additional Medical Emergencies

After respiratory distress, the other common medical emergencies seen in children are seizures, dehydration, nausea and vomiting, diarrhea, rotavirus infection, hypothermia, hyperthermia, hypoglycemia, hyperglycemia, shock, ataxia, delirium or coma, congenital heart defects, apnea, and problems associated with special needs children.

The most common cause of seizures in children is a rapid increase in body temperature (febrile seizure). Other causes of seizures in children include infection, epilepsy, poison ingestion, ICP, electrolyte disturbances (e.g., loss of sodium or calcium), and tumors. Often the cause is unknown.

Dehydration is a significant problem for pediatric patients, especially for young children because their fluid maintenance requirements are much higher than are those of adults. Diarrhea is the leading cause of dehydration in children. Other causes are fever, loss of appetite when a child is sick, **diabetic ketoacidosis (DKA)**, and extensive burns. Diabetic ketoacidosis is an inability to metabolize fats. Severe dehydration can cause death and is a common cause of hospitalization for children. Table 17-11 lists signs of moderate and severe dehydration.

Nausea and vomiting are symptoms of an illness or injury. Diarrhea may be caused by viral or bacterial infection and is very common in infants and children. Persistence of vomiting and diarrhea can lead to dehydration.

Rotavirus is a virus that infects nearly all children by age 2. Symptoms of rotavirus infection include vomiting and watery diarrhea, lasting from 24 hours to several days. The primary concern is dehydration, especially in infants. Signs include extreme sleepiness, decreased urine output, sunken eyes, poor skin turgor, and dry mucous membranes.

Hypothermia in children may be caused by exposure to extreme cold, ingestion of drugs or alcohol,

TABLE 17-11
Signs of Moderate and Severe Dehydration

	Moderate	Severe
Mental status	Irritable	Sleepy to comatose
Respiratory rate	Increased	Increased
Heart rate	Increased Decreased peripheral pulses	Increased, >130 bpm No peripheral pulses
Blood pressure	Normal	Systolic, <80 mm Hg
Skin color, temperature, and condition	Delayed capillary refill, 2–3 seconds Decreased skin turgor Mucous membranes dry Cool, pale skin Some tears with crying Sunken, darkened eyes	Delayed capillary refill, >3 seconds Significantly poor skin turgor Mucous membranes parched Cold, clammy, cyanotic skin No tears with crying Sunken, soft eyes
Urine output	Decreased	Decreased

metabolic disorders (e.g., hypoglycemia), prolonged infection (e.g., sepsis), or brain disorders affecting the thermoregulatory center. Hyperthermia may be caused by exposure to extreme heat or toxic doses of certain medications (e.g., aspirin, antihistamines) but more often is caused by a viral or bacterial infection with a resulting fever.

Hypoglycemia may be caused by too much insulin without adequate food intake or increased physical stress (e.g., exercise or fever). Hyperglycemia can occur with too little or missed insulin dosing and undiagnosed new onset of diabetes mellitus. In older children, abdominal pain is a common complaint associated with diabetic ketoacidosis (DKA).

Common causes of shock in children are dehydration, sepsis, burns, poison ingestion, anaphylaxis, DKA, adrenal insufficiency, and meningococcemia. **Ataxia** may be caused by poison ingestion, infection, or tumor. Delirium or coma can be caused by infection (e.g., meningitis, encephalitis), Reye's syndrome, DKA, hypoglycemia, hepatic failure, substance abuse, or head trauma.

Congenital heart defects are defects of the structures of the heart or diseases of the heart itself that occur while the fetus is developing and are present at birth. There are more than 35 types of heart defects and the causes are unknown. Depending on the defect, signs and symptoms may not appear for days after birth or even until adulthood. Signs and symptoms associated with congenital heart defects can range from cyanosis, with cold hands and feet, to congestive heart failure (CHF), tachycardia, weak pulses, poor feeding, failure to thrive, weakness, shortness of breath, and syncope.

Apnea in children may be caused by congestion due to a cold; a seizure disorder; cardiac arrhythmia; **sudden infant death syndrome (SIDS)**; or an **acute life-threatening event (ALTE)**, an event that is a combination of apnea, choking, gagging, and change in skin color and muscle tone and is not a sleep disorder. Sudden infant death syndrome is the sudden, unexplained death of an infant in the first year of life.

SPECIAL NEEDS AND TECHNOLOGY-ASSISTED CHILDREN

Significant improvements in medical procedures and technology have produced a steadily growing population of children with special health care needs living at home and attending schools. These children may be on life support equipment such as oxygen devices, ventilators, and apnea monitors (Figure 17-8). The prehospital provider now has to have a basic knowledge of such technology and the special medical needs of this growing population.

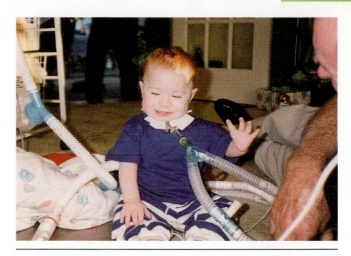

FIGURE 17-8 This child is on a mechanical ventilator.

Special needs children may have chronic illness, physical disabilities, cognitive or mental disabilities, or forms of technology used to assist the child. Special needs children may have prosthetics, tracheostomies or other ostomies, vascular access devices (VADs), or feeding tubes and may use suction, feeding pumps, and medication pumps. The family and caregivers are often very familiar with the equipment and very knowledgeable about the patient. They often call for transport or additional assistance after performing their own interventions. Examples of emergency complications seen in the home-care patient that can result in hospitalization include infections and sepsis, respiratory and cardiac failure, and emergencies with defective or inoperative equipment and access devices (e.g., plugged catheters, dislocated or accidentally removed tubes).

Obtaining a history in this population can be challenging because of communication difficulties, developmental delays, and the potentially lengthy list of prior treatments, medications, and surgeries. Utilize the parents or caregivers fully for getting the information about these children because they most often know the child's special needs best and are, in this case, the experts. They most likely performed some intervention before EMS arrived and often are able to assist the EMS provider.

The American College of Emergency Physicians (ACEP) in conjunction with the American Academy of Pediatrics (AAP) developed an **emergency information form (EIF)** containing standardized information that would be helpful to emergency personnel inside and outside of the hospital setting (see Appendix E). Be prepared to spend time with the family and the patient to obtain a history and perform a physical examination on these children. If there is any confusion regarding resuscitation of the child, make every effort to identify the parent or legal guardian responsible for making the decision and, if in doubt, begin resuscitation!

Airway Devices

Problems that can occur with airway devices found in the patient's home (Table 17-12) arise when they are improperly placed or become obstructed or when oxygen tubing becomes blocked or the oxygen runs out. Problems that arise with ventilation devices at home are due to power failures and pressures that are either too high or too low. Assessment findings associated with problems occurring with airway devices include dyspnea, decreased breath sounds, decreased tidal volume, decreased peak flow, decreased oxygen saturation, or respiratory failure or arrest.

Vascular Access Devices

Problems that may occur with vascular access devices (VADs) or shunts and medication ports (Table 17-13) are common in the home-care setting and often are due to infections, clotting, dislodgement, extravasation, hemorrhage, embolism, obstruction, equipment failure, or an infusion being given too rapidly. Assessment findings associated with problems occurring with these devices include signs of infection at the site (e.g., redness and swelling), hemorrhage, hemodyamic compromise, or signs of an embolus (pain or dyspnea or both).

Ostomies and Feeding Tubes

Problems that can occur with gastrointestinal or genitourinary devices (Table 17-14) result from improper patient positioning and feeding or emptying problems such as urinary tract infections, urinary retention, and urosepsis, which are often the same reasons that these devices were put in place initially. Assessment findings associated with complications of these devices include signs of aspiration, abdominal pain, abdominal distension, decreased or absent bowel sounds, distended bladder, dysuria, or change in urine output.

TABLE 17-12
Airway Devices Found in the Home-Care Setting

- Nasal cannulas
- Face masks
- Tracheostomies
- Suctioning devices
- Ventilators
- Pulmonary function meters
- Apnea monitors

TABLE 17-13
Vascular Access Devices and Medication Ports

Central venous catheters
- Port-A-Cath
- Hickman
- Groshong

Dialysis shunts

Peripheral vascular catheters
- Peripherally Inserted Central Catheter (PICC)
- Intracath

TABLE 17-14
Gastrointestinal and Genitourinary Devices Used in the Home-Care Setting

- External urinary catheters
- Indwelling urinary catheters
- Surgical urinary catheters
- Nasogastric tubes
- Feeding tubes
- PEG tubes
- J-tubes
- G-tubes
- Colostomy appliance

CONCLUSION

The key elements to assessing children are to modify the approach of the examination to fit the child's developmental age and to be willing to include the parent or caregiver when appropriate. Using age-appropriate pediatric assessment equipment (e.g., electrodes, stethoscope, blood pressure cuff) is very important to prevent inaccurate readings. Include the child's weight and body temperature routinely as part of the assessment. Be prepared to spend time obtaining a focused history on children, especially those with special medical needs or with technology-assistive devices. Take the time to become familiar with and obtain a basic knowledge of such devices and the special medical needs of this growing population.

REVIEW QUESTIONS

1. The pediatric age group that includes children from age 3 to 5 is called:
   a. infant.
   b. toddler.
   c. preschooler.
   d. school-ager.

2. The leading cause of pediatric deaths in the United States is:
   a. infectious diseases.
   b. trauma.
   c. cancer.
   d. heart disease.

3. Infants who have a fever should be:
   a. left at home with their parent.
   b. wiped down with rubbing alcohol.
   c. given baby aspirin.
   d. examined and taken to the hospital.

4. An ECG rhythm that is fairly common in children is:
   a. ventricular tachycardia.
   b. sinus arrhythmia.
   c. sinus bradycardia.
   d. atrial tachycardia.

5. Capillary refill is described as delayed if it takes longer than _____ second(s) for the color to return to the fingertip.
   a. 1
   b. 2
   c. 3
   d. 4

6. At _____ minutes, an APGAR score of less than _____ indicates the baby is at high risk for central nervous system impairment.
   a. 2; 10
   b. 2; 6
   c. 5; 7
   d. 5; 10

7. A full-term gestation is considered to be between _____ and _____ weeks.
   a. 32; 36
   b. 36; 38
   c. 38; 42
   d. 42; 44

8. An example of a difference between the adult and child airway would be that:
   a. the infant's tongue is very large in proportion to the size of the mouth.
   b. the small trachea is more anterior than an adult's.
   c. the smallest diameter of the child's airway is the cricoid ring.
   d. all of the above.

9. The age group that has a very well-developed imagination and fantasies is the:
   a. newborn.
   b. infant.
   c. toddler.
   d. preschooler.

10. A major warning sign of an asthmatic child in severe distress would be:
    a. nasal flaring.
    b. sternal retractions.
    c. a quiet chest.
    d. tachypnea.

CRITICAL THINKING QUESTIONS

1. You are called to the scene of an auto–pedestrian accident. Upon arrival, you discover that a 5-year-old boy was hit after he chased a ball out into the street. What types of injuries can you expect to see? What priority would this patient most likely be? What is the mortality rate in these types of injuries?

2. You are called to the elementary school for a child with breathing difficulties. Upon arrival, you are directed to the nurse's office. An 8-year-old girl is sitting in the tripod position and working very hard to breathe. The nurse tells you the child was out on the playground and began wheezing. She has a history of asthma and has used her inhaler, but it does not seem to be offering any relief. What assessment findings might you expect in this case? If the school does not have a consent-to-treat form on hand, is implied consent applicable in this case? Why or why not? What priority is this patient?

3. You are called to a residence for an unresponsive infant. Upon your arrival, you find a frantic mother attempting resuscitation on her 6-month-old. She tells you she went to check on the child while the infant was napping and found her not breathing. What could be the cause of this infant's emergency? What actions should you take? What is the priority of this infant?

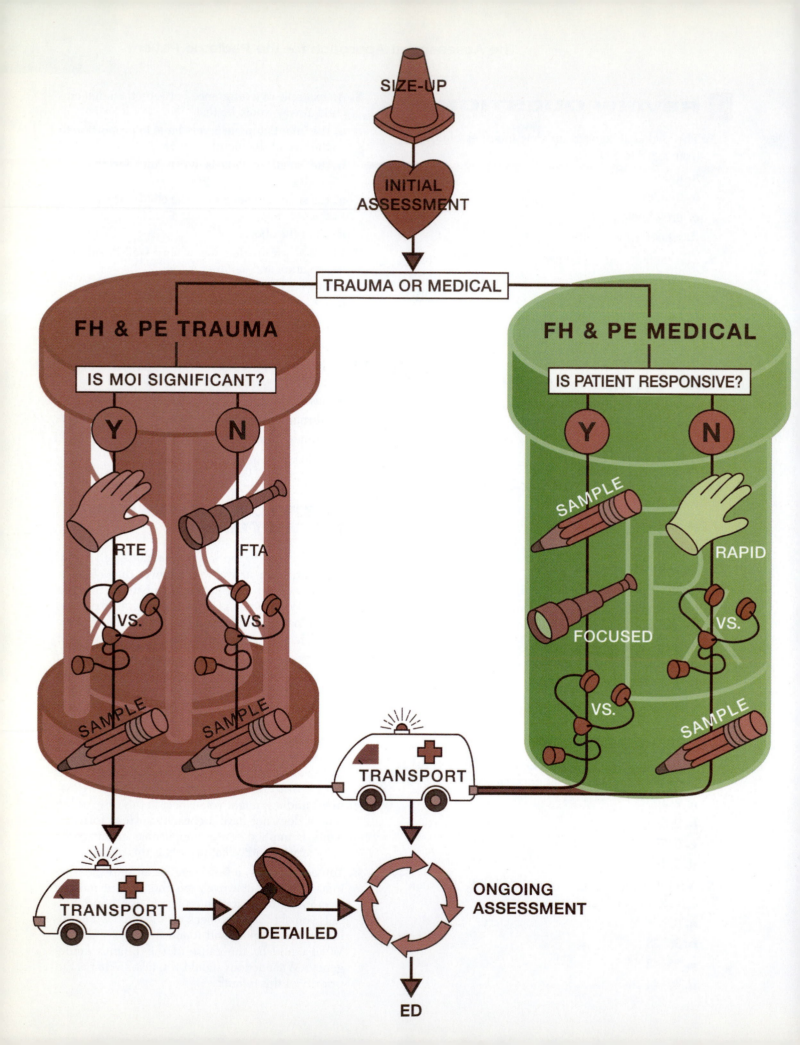

Chapter 18

The Assessment Approach for the Pregnant Patient

OBJECTIVES

Upon completion of this chapter, the reader should be able to:

- Describe the normal anatomical and physiological changes that occur during the first, second, and third trimesters of pregnancy.
- Explain why the pregnant woman is at increased risk for vomiting and aspiration.
- Describe the condition anemia of pregnancy and its significance in a patient who is hemorrhaging.
- Explain the importance of prenatal care and list some of the potential problems that can develop with inadequate or no prenatal care.
- Discuss the OPQRST history specific to the pregnant patient.
- Discuss the SAMPLE history specific to the pregnant patient.
- List additional information to obtain specific to the current pregnancy as well as to any prior pregnancies.
- Explain why positioning becomes an important consideration for the woman in late second trimester and third trimester pregnancy.
- Explain the condition of supine hypotension and describe how to correct the condition.
- List the gestational ages at which fetal movement can be felt by the mother and by the examiner.
- Describe fetal assessment, including measurement of the fundus, fetal heart rate, and palpation of uterine contractions.
- List the possible causes of fetal distress.
- List six complications associated with pregnancy and describe the characteristics of each.
- Differentiate signs of active labor from imminent delivery.

KEY TERMS

anemia of pregnancy

Braxton Hicks

chloasoma

fetal heart rate (FHR)

fetal heart tones (FHTs)

fundus

gravida

hemoglobin and hematocrit (H&H)

linea nigra

multiparous

nulliparous

parity

preterm labor

supine hypotension

trimester

true labor

INTRODUCTION

Assessing the pregnant patient is similar to assessing the nonpregnant female in that the extent of the physical examination is focused on the patient's chief complaint. The EMS provider must have an understanding of the normal anatomical and physiological changes to organ systems during pregnancy, and these changes need to be taken into account during the assessment process. Depending on the gestational age and number of fetuses, assessment may involve two or more patients (i.e., the mother and the fetuses). In the event the baby is born in the prehospital setting, the newborn assessment that will need to be performed is described in Chapter 17. This chapter focuses on the changes of pregnancy and how they are related to obtaining a focused history and physical examination of the pregnant patient.

NORMAL ANATOMICAL AND PHYSIOLOGICAL CHANGES OF PREGNANCY

The normal duration of pregnancy is 38 to 42 weeks. Pregnancy is broken down into three segments approximately 3 months each called **trimesters** (Figure 18-1). At 12 weeks' gestation, the top of the uterus (the **fundus**) is large enough to be considered an abdominal organ because it can be palpated above the symphysis pubis. This change also displaces the urinary bladder anteriorly and superiorly, leaving the bladder unprotected from the pelvis.

Excessive fatigue is a common complaint during early pregnancy, and the mother can become easily fatigued and short of breath with exertion throughout the pregnancy. Release of the hormone progesterone during pregnancy causes relaxation of the gastrointestinal (GI) tract and other smooth muscles. This slows normal peristalsis, and the patient often has nausea (morning sickness) and vomiting.

Clinical Carat

● Always consider the pregnant female to be at increased risk of vomiting and aspiration, especially during periods of altered mental status (AMS) or traumatic injury.

A significant change that occurs in the circulating blood volume during pregnancy is that the total volume has increased by nearly 50% by the end of the pregnancy. However, the hemoglobin does not increase proportionately to the blood volume, and there is a dilution effect. During the last trimester, **hemoglobin and hematocrit (H&H)** values are at their lowest. Maternal oxygen consumption increases by nearly 40%; this increase, together with the mismatch of hemoglobin to blood volume, creates a condition called **anemia of pregnancy**. This is a significant factor to consider when there is a possibility of injury or internal bleeding. With the increased blood volume and decreased H&H, internal bleeding will not become apparent with the normal signs of shock (e.g., tachycardia and changes in blood pressure) until a significant amount (30% to 35%) of blood is lost. The fetus can quickly become critically stressed because of hypoxia before signs of shock are apparent in the mother.

Clinical Carat

● With a nearly 50% increase in blood volume and diluted hemoglobin and hematocrit, internal bleeding will not be apparent with the normal signs of shock until a significant amount of blood (30% to 35%) is lost.

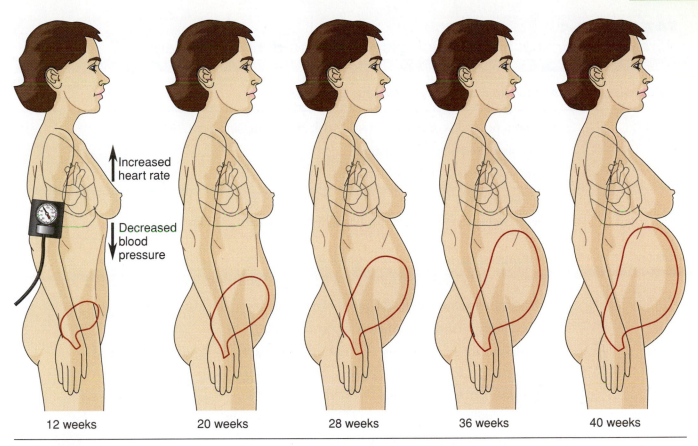

↑ Increased heart rate

↓ Decreased blood pressure

| 12 weeks | 20 weeks | 28 weeks | 36 weeks | 40 weeks |

FIGURE 18-1 Development of the mother through 40 weeks of pregnancy. Pregnancy is broken down into three trimesters of approximately 3 months each.

As the uterus enlarges, the fetus will displace and shift many internal organs. By the third trimester, the uterus displaces the diaphragm upward nearly 4 cm (1.5 inches), decreasing functional residual capacity by nearly 25%. To compensate for the decreased vertical diameter of the thoracic cage, an increase in estrogen levels helps to relax chest cage ligaments, thereby increasing the horizontal diameter. The enlarging uterus may also displace the lower esophageal sphincter into the thorax; this displacement, together with the upward stomach displacement, may result in gastroesophageal reflux.

Most changes that occur in the peripheral vascular system are apparent in the third trimester. Pressure from the fetus may impair venous return, causing hemorrhoids to show around the anus and varicose veins to be visible in the labia or legs. Low back pain is a common complaint in late pregnancy because of the increased lordosis (a forward curvature of the lumbar spine) and weakened ligament and joint support (Figure 18-2). Table 18-1 shows the normal anatomical and physiological changes occurring throughout the three trimesters of pregnancy.

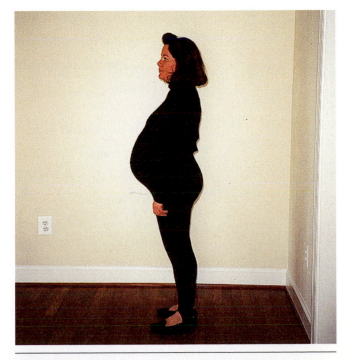

FIGURE 18-2 Lordosis of pregnancy.

TABLE 18-1
Normal Anatomical and Physiological Changes during Pregnancy

Trimester	Anatomical and Physiological Changes
First	• Slowed peristalsis, nausea, increased risk of vomiting and aspiration • Increased frequency of urination • Breasts increase in fullness, tenderness • Mother is easily fatigued • Tenth week, cardiac output increases by 1 to 1.5 liters per minute
Second	• Movements from the fetus can be felt by the mother • Over 12 weeks' gestation, fundus can be palpated above the symphysis pubis • Heart rate increases 10 to 15 bpm above resting rate • Blood pressure decreases slightly (10 to 15 mm Hg) • Fetal heart tones can be heard by 12 to 14 weeks with the handheld ultrasound or Doppler • 20 weeks' gestation fundus at the level of umbilicus • Mother easily fatigued and short of breath with exertion • Nausea and vomiting subside for many women • Constipation common due to reduced gastric tone and reduced motility • Breasts may secrete thick yellow colostrum
Third	• Fetus large enough for movement to be felt by the examiner • 36 weeks' gestation fundus at the costal margin • Tidal volume and minute ventilation increase by 30% to 40% • Blood pressure returns to normal but varies more with positioning (supine hypotension) • Respiratory rate usually remains normal or just slightly increased • Heart rate increases 15 to 20 bpm above resting rate • Cardiac output increases by 6 to 7 liters per minute by term • Total blood volume increases by nearly 50% by term • Uterus displaces the diaphragm upward nearly 4 cm (1.5 inches), causing the apex of the heart to be shifted up and slightly left, and rotated forward • ECG may show left axis deviation • Premature beats more frequent • Progressive lordosis, kyphosis, and the characteristic protruding abdomen commonly cause back pain • Mother easily fatigued and short of breath with exertion • Increased frequency of urination and nocturia (increased urination at night)

Exploring the Web

- Search the Web to learn more about the normal changes that occur during pregnancy. Create a list of all normal findings. If a woman is expecting twins, what additional changes might occur? What are some of the additional things to consider during assessment of the woman expecting multiple births?

THE FOCUSED HISTORY

Some of the most common reasons the EMS provider is called to care for a pregnant patient are traumatic injury, pain, and vaginal hemorrhage. However, it is important to remember that the pregnant patient is not immune to any of the causes of abdominal pain (e.g., appendicitis, gallbladder problems, or kidney stones) that the non-pregnant female may have. Obtain a complete history as well as specific information about the current pregnancy and any previous pregnancies. Ask about prenatal care. Prenatal care is essential to identify and manage potential complications of pregnancy and risk factors associated with premature birth and low-birth-weight infants (Table 18-2) or any preexisting medical condition. When prenatal care is noted, the information obtained from the

TABLE 18-2
Risk Factors Associated with Premature Birth and Low Birth Weight

- Gestational diabetes
- Hypertension syndromes
- Inadequate or no prenatal care
- Maternal hormonal imbalance
- Maternal use of drugs, alcohol, or cigarettes
- Mother is under age 16 or over age 35
- Multiple fetuses
- Premature labor
- Structural abnormality of the uterus
- Third-trimester hemorrhage
- Preexisting medical and neurological conditions

patient is usually considered reliable. When no prenatal care exists, be especially thorough during history taking and look for the possible risk factors listed in Table 18-2. In addition to gathering the OPQRST and SAMPLE information, obtain the information listed in Table 18-3.

The OPQRST History

Using OPQRST, Table 18-4 highlights specific information pertaining to the focused history of the female patient of childbearing age.

The SAMPLE History

Use SAMPLE to obtain specific information pertaining to the focused history of the female patient of childbearing age. Table 18-5 outlines the SAMPLE history and Table 18-6 lists substances that present dangers during pregnancy.

TABLE 18-3
The Obstetric History

- Date of last menstrual period (LMP)
- Weeks of gestation (38 to 42 is full term)
- Estimated due date (EDD)
- Number of fetuses (If more than one, was there use of fertility drugs?)
- Position of fetus
- Preterm labor or false labor (**Braxton Hicks**)
- Previous obstetric history
- Previous medical and surgical history
- Prior pregnancies
- **Gravida** (total number of pregnancies)
- **Parity** (total number of births)
- Duration of each prior gestation
- Number of preterm pregnancies
- Any abortions or miscarriages (how many and were they spontaneous or elective)
- Type of delivery: vaginal (spontaneous or induced) or cesarean section (use of forceps or vacuum extraction, episiotomy or laceration)
- Complications during pregnancy (hypertension, gestational diabetes)
- Length of labor(s), precipitous delivery (labor and delivery in less than 3 hours)

TABLE 18-4
OPQRST for the Pregnant Patient

Information	Questions	Remarks
Onset	When did you begin feeling this way?	Determine when the complaint began. Common complaints of the pregnant patient are pain, bleeding, labor, and traumatic injury.
Provocation	Can you describe what you are experiencing? What were you doing when the symptoms began? Are you having any other symptoms that may be related to the reason you called EMS? Have you recently had any injuries or illnesses?	Obtain the details of the present episode. Determine what the patient was doing at the time of onset, and try to differentiate trauma as a cause. Ask about any associated symptoms, and be alert for signs and symptoms of complications of pregnancy such as ectopic pregnancy, spontaneous abortion, hypertension, hemorrhage, infections (e.g., pelvic inflammatory disease), and gastrointestinal conditions.
Quality	What does the pain feel like? Will you show me where the pain is located? Are you having any discharge or vaginal bleeding? Have you been having a normal urinary and bowel output? Have you experienced this at any other time during your pregnancy? Have you experienced this during other pregnancies?	Determine whether the patient is experiencing contractions. If vaginal bleeding or discharge is present, determine the duration and quantity of discharge. Ask about associated pain and urinary and bowel symptoms. Determine whether the patient is guarding or is able to move without further provoking the pain.
Region, **R**adiation, **R**elief, **R**ecurrence	Is the pain in one spot, or does it seem to move to other areas? Have you done anything or taken anything to help relieve the symptoms? Has this been an ongoing occurrence during the pregnancy?	It is important to determine whether the patient has taken any actions to relieve the symptoms. Is it also significant to note whether this is a problem that has happened throughout the pregnancy.
Severity	On a scale of 1 to 10, with 1 being no pain and 10 being the worst pain ever, how would you rate the pain?	Obtain a baseline assessment followed by serial assessments in order to determine whether the condition is improving.

(continues)

TABLE 18-4 *(continued)*

Information	Questions	Remarks
Time	When did the symptoms begin?	Time is paramount when life-threatening conditions exist. Rapidly identify life-threatening conditions (e.g., toxemia), acute surgical conditions (e.g., ectopic pregnancy), and imminent delivery.

TABLE 18-5
SAMPLE History for the Pregnant Patient

Information	Questions	Remarks
Signs and **S**ymptoms	What are you feeling? Can you describe your symptoms?	Some of the signs and symptoms of pregnancy include amenorrhea, nausea, vomiting, breast tenderness, back pain, abdominal pain or cramping, vaginal discharge, urinary or bowel problems, dizziness, and syncope. Abnormal weight gain, generalized edema, severe continuous headaches, vision disturbances, and seizures are especially significant and require prompt evaluation at the emergency department.
Allergies	Are you allergic to any foods? Are you allergic to any medications? Do you have environmental allergies?	Increased sensitivity to environmental allergens is common.
Medications	Are you currently taking any medications? What form of birth control do you use? Are you using prenatal vitamins? Have you taken any over-the-counter or herbal remedies to attempt to relieve the symptoms?	Determine the patient's method of birth control and compliance, use of prenatal vitamins, recent changes in medications, use of over-the-counter (OTC) and herbal medications, and drug or alcohol use during pregnancy. The absence of prenatal vitamins from the list is a clue that the patient may not be getting prenatal care. During pregnancy, drugs, alcohol, and other agents can easily pass the placental barrier and are dangerous to the developing fetus. Table 18-6 lists substances that are dangerous if taken during pregnancy.

(continues)

TABLE 18-5 *(continued)*

Information	Questions	Remarks
Pertinent past medical history	Are you currently under a doctor's care for any illness or chronic condition? Have you had any recent injuries? Is this your first pregnancy?	Preexisting medical conditions can create complications during pregnancy. Be alert for a history of hypertension, diabetes, cardiac problems, and asthma. Ask about prior pregnancies and surgeries (e.g., partial or full hysterectomy, uterine surgery, cesarean section). Abdominal surgeries may have caused scarring or adhesions, leading to complications. Ask about any past ectopic pregnancies because a past ectopic pregnancy increases the risk for having one in this pregnancy.
Last oral intake, **L**ast menstrual period	When did you last eat or have anything to drink? When did you last have your menstrual period?	Determine the patient's menstrual history (regularity and length of cycles). Consider that dehydration can preceed labor pains.
Events leading up to this incident	What were you doing when the symptoms began?	Determine the reason why EMS was called (e.g., trauma, pain, hemorrhage, ruptured waters, labor).

TABLE 18-6
Substances That Are Dangerous during Pregnancy

Alcohol	Lithium
Androgen and testosterone derivatives	Organic mercury
Angiotensin-converting enzyme (ACE) inhibitors	Phenytoin
	Streptomycin and kanamycin
Carbamazepine	Tetracycline
Coumadin derivatives	Trimethadione and paramethadione
Diethystilbestrol (DES)	Valprioc acid
Folic acid antagonists	Vitamin A and its derivatives
Lead	

THE PHYSICAL EXAMINATION

Perform the initial assessment of the mental status and ABCs as with any other patient. The depth of the physical examination is focused on the patient's chief complaint. For the woman in late second trimester and third trimester pregnancy, positioning becomes important for patient comfort and for circulation. Let the patient assume a position of comfort and offer a pillow for the low back. When a patient needs to be immobilized to a longboard because of a traumatic injury, after securing

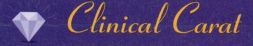

Clinical Carat

- To avoid the possibility of supine hypotension, do not lay the pregnant patient in a supine position.

the patient to the board be sure to tilt the board 15 degrees to the patient's left to avoid the possibility of supine hypotension, which is caused by the fetus's lying on the inferior cava (Figure 18-3). Do not lay the patient in a supine position.

Vital Signs and Skin Color and Condition

Obtain vital signs, keeping in mind the changes in heart rate and blood pressure during the three trimesters of pregnancy. Assess the respiration, pulse, and blood pressure. The respiratory rate is usually normal or slightly increased, although the tidal volume and minute ventilation may increase by 30% to 40% in late pregnancy. The resting heart rate increases 15 to 20 beats per minute (bpm) throughout the pregnancy. This normal increase can distort the evaluation of tachycardia. A decrease in peripheral vascular resistance causes blood pressure to be slightly lower (10 to 15 mm Hg) during the second trimester. Blood pressure returns to normal values during the third trimester, but it will vary more with positioning, especially when the mother is supine. When the mother is supine, the weight of the fetus lies on the inferior vena cava and can restrict blood return from the lower extremities, causing a drop in pressure (**supine hypotension**) with the associated symptoms of dizziness, light-headedness, and even syncope. This condition is easily and quickly reversed with repositioning, ideally to a left lateral position. Pregnancy-associated hypertension—a new onset of hypertension (≥140/90 mm Hg) during pregnancy—is an indication of possible toxemia (preeclampsia and eclampsia).

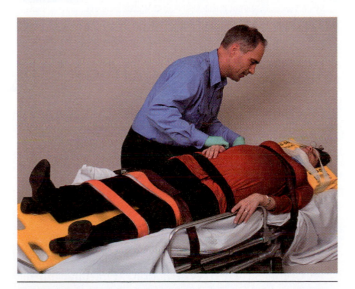

FIGURE 18-3 Tilting the backboard as little as 15 degrees can prevent supine hypotensive syndrome.

Clinical Carat

● Be alert for orthostatic changes in any pregnant female, and suspect supine hypotension in third-trimester patients.

Assess skin color and condition, and note the presence of generalized edema. Changes in skin color are common because of increased levels of estrogen. Typically, the pigmentation around the nipples (areola) will darken, and the pale line that runs midline from the umbilicus down to the pubic bone also darkens (**linea nigra**). Some women develop mild darkening on the face (**chloasoma**), which is commonly called the mask of pregnancy. Other areas of the skin that may darken during pregnancy are the perineum, armpits, and inner thighs.

The presence of edema in the patient with no history of edema is an indicator of hypertensive disorders specific to pregnancy (preeclampsia and eclampsia). Assess the hands, face, and feet for generalized edema.

Changes Assessed during Visualization

Postural changes include progressive lordosis, kyphosis, and the characteristic protruding abdomen. The rib cage may look wider, with flare of the lower ribs. When vaginal bleeding or discharge is reported or imminent delivery is suspected, the EMS provider should examine the external genitalia for the presence of a prolapsed cord, crowning, or the progression of labor.

Changes Assessed during Palpation

While palpating the neck, the EMS provider may note an enlarged thyroid gland, a normal change due to increased vascularity and hyperplasia of the tissue. During palpation of the thorax, the costal angle may feel wider than normal (Figure 18-4). Assess the abdomen for tenderness, guarding, and fundal height. By 12 weeks' gestation, the top of the uterus (the fundus) is large enough to be palpated above the symphysis pubis. In cases of retroversion, or a tipped uterus, the fundus may not be palpable until 16 weeks' gestation. By 20 weeks, it is at the level of the umbilicus, and by 36 weeks it has reached the ribs, or costal margin (Figure 18-5). By the third trimester, the fetus is large enough for the examiner to feel movement.

When contractions are reported, measure the duration of each contraction and the time between contractions.

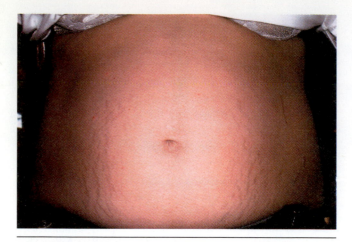

FIGURE 18-4 Widening of the costal margin.

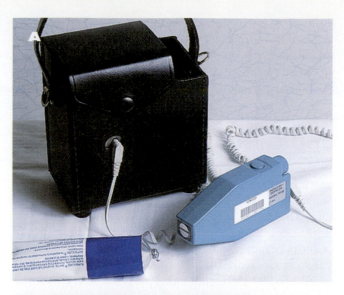

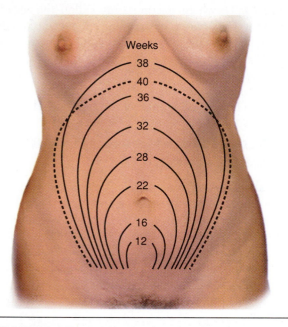

FIGURE 18-5 Uterine and abdominal enlargement of pregnancy.

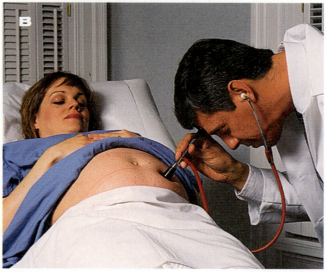

FIGURE 18-6 (**A**) Doppler. (**B**) Fetoscope.

Perform a fetal assessment, including measuring the fundal height, the fetal heart rate, and the fetal movement.

Changes Assessed during Auscultation

The mother's heart sounds may change because of the increased blood volume and workload. The S1 sound is often louder than normal, and an S3 sound is easily heard. In a high percentage of patients, a systolic murmur (an abnormal heart sound that occurs at systole) develops, but it disappears soon after delivery. Fetal heart tones can be heard by 12 to 14 weeks with the handheld ultrasound or Doppler and can be heard with the Fetoscope (Figure 18-6) by 18 to 20 weeks.

FETAL ASSESSMENT

Fetal assessment includes measuring fundal height and fetal heart rate, palpating uterine contractions, and checking for fetal movement. The EMS provider performs fetal assessment during active labor to check the cardiac status of the fetus. Possible causes of fetal distress include:

- Trauma
- Hypoxia
- Eclampsia
- Umbilical cord obstruction (typically during strong uterine contractions)
- Prolapsed cord
- Placental insufficiency

- Drug effects
- Bacterial sepsis
- Postterm gestation (>42 weeks)

Fundal Height

The height of the fundus is measured to estimate gestational age: by 12 weeks the fundus is at the symphysis pubis and is considered an abdominal organ. At 16 weeks the uterus is between the symphysis pubis and the umbilicus; by 20 weeks, it is at the umbilicus; and at 36 weeks, it is at the costal margin. Greater than 24 weeks is the gestational age at which the fetus may survive outside the womb. Uterine size that is smaller or larger than expected is an abnormal finding.

For the height of the fundus to be measured, the patient should be supine (be watchful for supine hypotension). With a measuring tape, place the zero centimeter mark at the symphysis pubis and measure in the midline up and over the abdomen to the top of the fundus and note the centimeter mark (Figure 18-7). Each centimeter equals approximately 1-week gestational age.

Fetal Heart Rate

Fetal heart tones (FHTs) may be heard at 12 to 14 weeks with the handheld ultrasound or Doppler or with the Fetoscope by 20 weeks' gestation. The normal **fetal heart rate (FHR)** is 110 to 160 bpm. A rate below 110 bpm is an abnormal finding and considered bradycardia, a sign of fetal distress or drug use. A rate above 160 bpm is also abnormal and is considered tachycardia. Periodic changes in the FHR are normal during fetal movement, sleep, and uterine contractions. The absence of FHTs is abnormal; however, the inexperience of the evaluator may be a factor in difficulty locating FHTs.

To measure the FHR, place the patient in the supine position (be watchful for supine hypotension). Place the microphone of the Doppler probe or Fetoscope on the abdomen and slowly move it around in circles until FHTs are heard and count the rate for a minute. During early pregnancy, the FHR is most often identified in the midline between the symphysis pubis and the umbilicus. As the fetus gets larger listen for FHTs in the right lower or left lower quadrant of the abdomen. Fetal heart tones are best heard through the back of the fetus. Ideally, the FHR should be measured as often as maternal vital signs.

Listening for FHTs with a stethoscope is difficult and time consuming. More often in the prehospital setting, the EMS provider's time is limited to performing other tasks such as completing the maternal assessment and treatment plans.

Fetal Movement and Uterine Contractions

The mother can feel fetal movement in the second trimester, and the examiner may feel fetal movement during auscultation of FHTs in the third trimester. Ask the patient when the last fetal movement was felt. The EMS provider assesses for contractions or fetal movement by placing her hand on the abdomen at the fundus (Figure 18-8). When the patient reports the contraction is beginning, the movement of the contraction is felt as a firming or rigidness, followed by a loosening of tension.

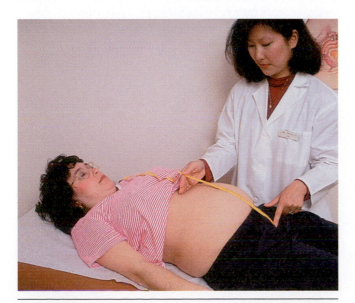

FIGURE 18-7 Measuring fundal height.

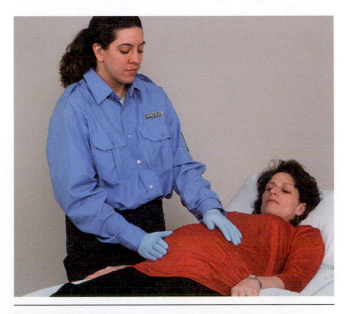

FIGURE 18-8 Hand placement on the fundus. Feel for point tenderness as well as for fetal movement.

Measure the duration of the contraction as well as the time from onset of one contraction to onset of the next contraction to get the time between two contractions.

True labor is recognized with persistent regular contractions. When contractions are irregular and inconsistent, then false labor (Braxton Hicks contractions) is most likely occurring. **Preterm labor** is true labor that occurs before 38 weeks' gestation. Patients experiencing any contractions should be transported for evaluation.

COMPLICATIONS ASSOCIATED WITH PREGNANCY

As it is for the nonpregnant patient, the physical examination is focused on the patient's chief complaint. Complications of pregnancy are not common, but when they do occur the object of the prehospital assessment is to rapidly identify life-threatening conditions (e.g., metabolic disturbances such as eclampsia), acute surgical conditions (e.g., ectopic pregnancy), and imminent delivery.

Ectopic Pregnancy

When pregnancy is unknown or is in the first trimester, suspect that the female patient of childbearing age who is complaining of lower abdominal pain, with or without vaginal bleed, has an ectopic pregnancy. During the first trimester of pregnancy, ectopic pregnancy and spontaneous abortion, or miscarriage, may be life-threatening conditions when not quickly recognized and managed appropriately. During the first weeks of pregnancy, the woman may not realize she is pregnant or may choose to deny the pregnancy. These factors may contribute to the late recognition of a life-threatening condition.

The chief complaint is usually abdominal pain or vaginal bleeding or both. Uncontrolled vaginal bleeding can lead to hypovolemia, shock, or death of both the fetus and the mother. Therefore, regardless of the history, for any female of childbearing age (12 to 50) with a complaint of lower abdominal pain or vaginal bleeding, the presumption is that she is pregnant until pregnancy is ruled out at the emergency department.

Ectopic pregnancy is a pregnancy that occurs in a location other than the uterine cavity (Figure 18-9), most often the fallopian tubes. The catastrophic problem is significant intra-abdominal bleeding, often unrecognized or recognized too late, making ectopic pregnancy a major cause of maternal death. The chief complaint is abdominal pain. Vaginal bleeding may be light or absent.

Spontaneous abortion, or miscarriage, is a loss of a fetus of less than 20 weeks' gestation. Miscarriage is the layperson's term for spontaneous abortion, which occurs in 20% to 30% of all pregnancies. In some instances, the woman may not even have known that she was pregnant. The chief complaint is vaginal bleeding with or without abdominal pain. Bleeding may be heavy, and often there is a passing of fetal tissue, which the patient may describe as clotting.

Other symptoms associated with either ectopic pregnancy or miscarriage include normal symptoms of pregnancy—amenorrhea, nausea, and breast tenderness—and orthostatic symptoms such as dizziness, syncope, and shock.

Diabetes

Hormones that are released during the second trimester of pregnancy cause an increased insulin release from the pancreas; for the insulin-dependent diabetic, insulin requirements increase dramatically. New-onset diabetes or gestational diabetes typically begins in the second or

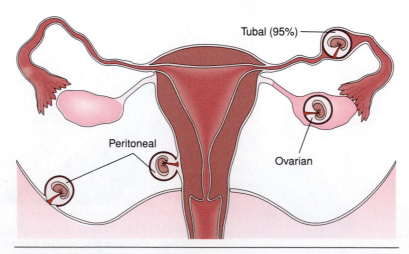

FIGURE 18-9 Locations of ectopic pregnancy.

third trimester and usually subsides after delivery. Diabetes must be monitored very carefully during pregnancy to decrease the high risk of birth defects and pregnancy complications such as hypertension and eclampsia.

Blood Pressure Disorders and Other Third-Trimester Complications

Hypertension, supine hypotension, abruptio placentae, and placenta previa are the complications seen in third-trimester pregnancy. Blood pressure (higher than 140/90) is abnormal and dangerous during pregnancy. Pregnancy-induced hypertension not only leads to stroke, acute pulmonary embolism, and renal failure but also can progress to preeclampsia, eclampsia, and death.

Signs and symptoms of pregnancy-induced hypertension include an increase of 30 mm Hg systolic and 15 mm Hg diastolic above the baseline, abnormal weight gain, headaches, visual disturbances, and the clinical analysis of protein in the urine. More severe signs and symptoms include abdominal pain, generalized edema, and decreased urine output (oliguria).

Preeclampsia and Eclampsia

Preeclampsia is the leading cause of maternal and fetal morbidity and death. Signs and symptoms of preeclampsia are the same as those of pregnancy-induced hypertension. More severe signs and symptoms include severe headaches, blurred vision, diplopia (double vision), nausea, vomiting, right upper quadrant or epigastric pain and tenderness, anuria, hematuria, oliguria, dizziness, confusion, fetal distress, and abruptio placentae. Without rapid interventions, the condition of preeclampsia progresses to eclampsia, the most serious complication of pregnancy-induced hypertension. This condition is recognized by seizures, coma, and death

Abruptio Placentae

Abruptio placentae is a sudden separation of the placenta from the uterine site (Figure 18-10A). Signs and symptoms of abruptio placentae vary with the extent of detachment and bleeding and include severe abdominal pain. There may be little or no vaginal bleeding with orthostatic symptoms (e.g., dizziness, syncope, and shock).

Placenta Previa

Placenta previa is an abnormal condition in which the placenta has implanted in a lower uterine site (Figure 18-10B). Signs and symptoms of placenta previa include symptoms of shock and vaginal bleeding *without* abdominal pain.

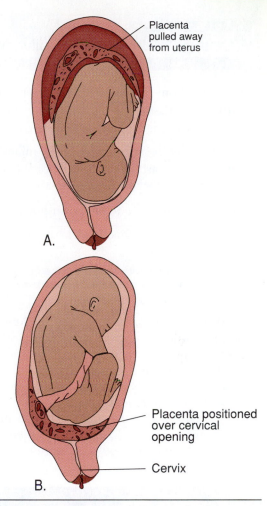

FIGURE 18-10 (**A**) Abruptio placentae, separation of the placenta from the uterine site. (**B**) Placenta previa, placenta implanted in lower uterine site.

Prehospital Delivery

Active labor typically progresses slowly in the woman who has never given birth (**nulliparous**) and rapidly in the women who has (**multiparous**). To assess active labor:

- Palpate the fundus during contractions.
  Measure the duration of each contraction.
  Measure the time of onset of one contraction to the onset of the next contraction to get the time between the two.
  Measure the height of the fundus (to estimate gestational age).
- Inspect the external genitalia for the presenting fetus.
- Ask the patient about leaking fluid (amniotic fluid or blood) from ruptured membranes.

TABLE 18-7
Warnings of Imminent Delivery

- Contractions that are strong and very close in time (1- to 2-minute intervals between contractions lasting 45 to 60 seconds)

- Crowning: the appearance of the infant's presenting part (normally the head) in the birth canal

- The mother's urge to move her bowels

- A multiparous woman's declaration that she is going to deliver

Exploring the Web

- Search the Web for additional information on each of the complications of pregnancy discussed in this chapter. Create index cards that list the signs and symptoms of each complication, assessment findings that will present with each complication, and techniques that can be used to assess and manage patients presenting with these complications.

Warnings that alert the EMS provider to prepare for imminent delivery are often declared by the patient, but contractions and crowning also give warning (Table 18-7). The woman may report an urge to bear down or to move her bowels or may just tell you she is going to deliver. Signs of imminent delivery include regular contractions lasting 45 to 60 seconds at 1- to 2-minute intervals, crowning (Figure 18-11), and, sometimes, loss of the mucous plug or a bloody discharge.

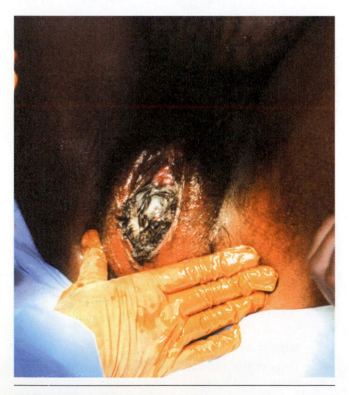

FIGURE 18-11 Crowning.

CONCLUSION

The approach to the pregnant patient is directed by the chief complaint, which is typically pain or bleeding or both, and obtaining accurate details in the focused history. Information obtained in the focused history is key for directing both the order and the content of the physical examination. When pregnancy is unknown or is in the first trimester, suspect the female patient of childbearing age who is complaining of lower abdominal pain with or without vaginal bleed to have an ectopic pregnancy and manage it as a life-threatening condition. During assessment, the EMS provider should take into consideration any preexisting conditions such as diabetes and hypertension, include the patient's priorities, and remember to consider other causes of abdominal pain such as appendicitis and gastric reflux.

REVIEW QUESTIONS

1. The normal duration of pregnancy is approximately _____ weeks.
   a. 34
   b. 36
   c. 40
   d. 42

2. Another name for the top of the uterus is the:
   a. apex.
   b. fundus.
   c. placenta.
   d. pubis.

3. The hormone progesterone causes _____ of the gastrointestinal tract and _____ muscles.

a. relaxation; smooth

b. relaxation; cardiac

c. contraction; skeletal

d. contraction; smooth

4. The mismatch of hemoglobin to blood volume in the _____ trimester can lead to _____ in the mother.

a. first; anemia

b. second; gestational diabetes

c. third; anemia

d. third: hypoxemia

5. The mismatch of hemoglobin to blood volume in the _____ trimester can lead to _____ in the fetus.

a. first; anemia

b. second; gestational diabetes

c. third; anemia

d. second: hypoxia

6. If taken during pregnancy, which drugs can be harmful to the developing fetus?

a. alcohol and coumadin

b. lead and lithium

c. ACE inhibitors

d. all of the above

7. Fetal bradycardia is considered to be present when the fetus has a heart rate below:

a. 180 bpm.

b. 150 bpm.

c. 120 bpm.

d. 100 bpm.

8. A pregnant woman who is full term is having contractions that are irregular and inconsistent may be having:

a. a prolapsed cord.

b. Braxton Hicks contractions.

c. an ectopic pregnancy.

d. placenta previa.

9. Close to _____ percent of all pregnancies end in _____ .

a. 15%; eclampsia

b. 30%; a spontaneous abortion

c. 45%; a premature birth

d. 60%; a cesarean section

10. A condition in which the placenta implants on the lower uterine wall is called:

a. prolapsed cord.

b. placenta previa.

c. vena cava syndrome.

d. placental abruption.

CRITICAL THINKING QUESTIONS

1. You are called to a residence for a pregnant woman who has fallen down a flight of stairs. She is having pain in her leg and ankle but otherwise feels fine. What complications related to the pregnancy could occur? What should you be watchful for? What is the priority of this patient?

2. You are called to a residence where a woman is in active labor. She tells you this is her third child, labor came on fast and furious, and she is ready to start pushing. What should you expect to find with this patient? What will you need to do? What priority is this patient?

3. You are called to a residence for a 15-year-old girl who is having severe abdominal pain. She is unwilling to discuss her sexual activity. What can you do to further your assessment of this patient? How should you handle her reluctance to provide information? What do you suspect might be the cause of her pain? What priority is this patient?

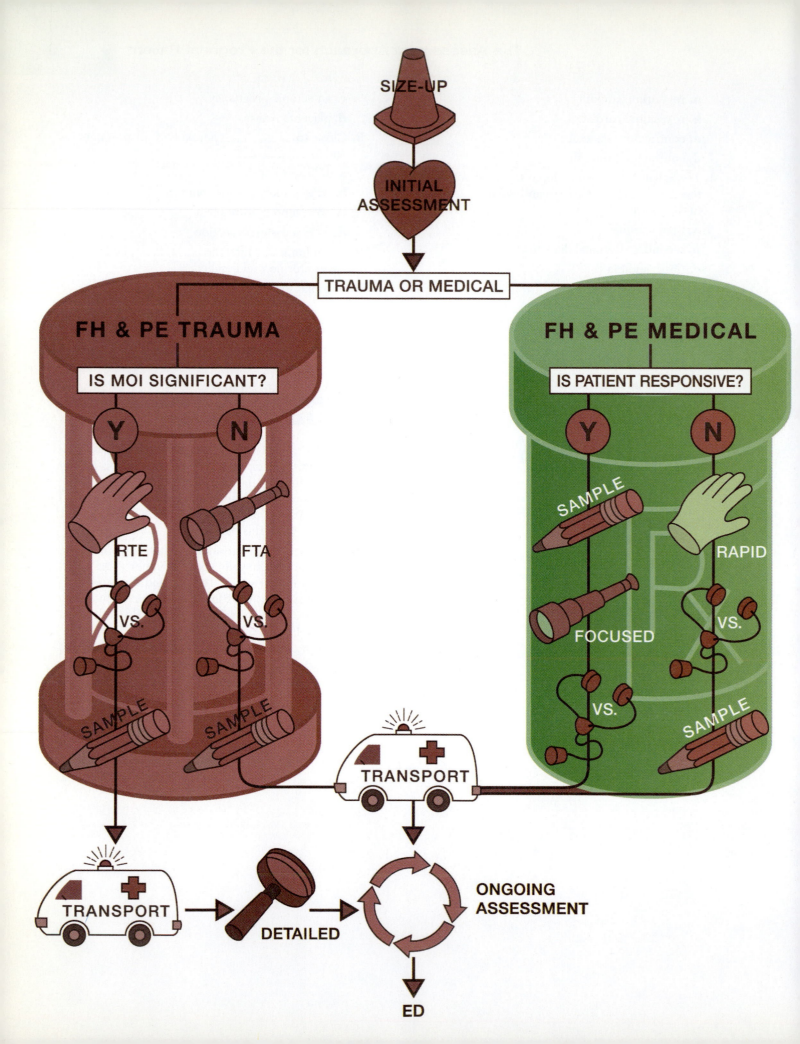

Chapter 19

The Assessment Approach for the Elderly Patient

OBJECTIVES

Upon completion of this chapter, the reader should be able to:

- Describe the physiological changes of aging that are related to the body senses, including changes in vision, hearing, taste, smell, and pain response.
- Describe the physiological changes of aging that are related to specific body systems, including the immune, endocrine, gastrointestinal, genitourinary, renal, cardiovascular, respiratory, nervous, integumentary, and musculoskeletal systems.
- Discuss the effects of aging as they are related to vital signs.
- Explain why body temperature is an important vital sign in the elderly.
- List the factors related to aging that lead to concern about the patient's psychological status.
- Discuss how anticipating the potential for deficits and modifying the approach for the patient will ease the assessment process for both patient and provider.
- Describe how the approach for obtaining a focused history from the elderly patient is different from that for a younger adult.
- Describe how the approach to performing the physical examination on the elderly is different from that for a younger adult.
- Describe why the assessment and management of the elderly patient includes evaluation of mental status, physical functional status, emotional functional status, and social functional status.
- List the common diseases found in the elderly and discuss specific factors and the signs and symptoms associated with each.
- Discuss specific types of trauma that are prevalent among elderly populations and explain why traumatic injury is so devastating to the elderly.

KEY TERMS

cardiomegaly

carotid artery disease (CAD)

kinesthetic

opacification

polypharmacy

presbycusis

INTRODUCTION

The fundamental aspects of the assessment approach for the elderly patient are to care for emergent and life-threatening problems first, then to continue with the symptom-based assessment as would be done for any other patient. After the initial assessment, some additional components are important to consider for the overall health of the often-complex and frail aging patient. In addition to the medical aspect of patient assessment, psychosocial and functional problems and capability components should be considered whenever time and personnel permit. This chapter discusses many of the normal physiological changes that occur with the aging process and how they are related to the focused history and physical examination. Also included is information on some of the most common diseases among the elderly and the emergencies associated with them as well as findings associated with traumatic injury.

PHYSIOLOGICAL CHANGES OF AGING

Before beginning the focused history and physical examination on the elderly patient, the EMS provider should consider the physiological changes that occur with the aging process. Everyone ages at a different pace, but ultimately the aging process affects all body organs and systems.

The Senses

The hearing loss that occurs with aging (**presbycusis**) makes it difficult to hear whispered words and to hear consonants during speech. Speak in a normal tone, and never shout at a hearing-impaired patient. Be sure to look at the patient's face when speaking because the patient may be a lip reader. Ask whether the patient uses a hearing aid, and ask the patient to adjust it so she can hear you.

Kinesthetic (body position) sense is decreased, which results in a loss of balance. This decrease is a contributing factor to falls among the elderly, often with devastating consequences (e.g., hip fracture).

Visual acuity and accommodation are diminished,

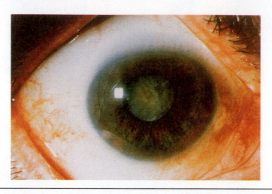

FIGURE 19-1 Cataract opacification. (Courtesy of the National Eye Institute, National Institutes of Health, Bethesda, MD)

and loss of vision is commonly due to cataract **opacification** (Figure 19-1). Opacification is the loss of transparency caused by the cloudiness of cataracts. Vision loss, together with a decreased kinesthetic sense, leads to increased risk of falls. If the patient needs glasses to see, let the patient wear them or bring them to the hospital. When a patient's vision is poor, take care to explain what you are doing before proceeding.

A decrease in the pain response is one of the reasons the elderly often have vague complaints such as atypical chest pain. Sometimes the elderly patient may simply state, "I just feel weak." A person's diminished perception of pain increases the risk of injury, especially from cold and heat. Note the ambient temperature in her environment and incorporate that into your assessment findings. A decreased pain perception may result in development of a serious condition such as appendicitis with severe symptoms.

Taste and smell sensations are decreased and may lead to a loss of appetite. A decreased sense of thirst is a common finding in the elderly. The result is that the person is in a persistent state of dehydration that may be mild, moderate, or severe and could be a contributing factor to an acute medical complaint (e.g., syncope or dysrhythmias). In taking the history, the EMS provider should routinely ask about daily fluid intake and recent changes in oral intake, both liquid and solid, especially when the patient is taking water pills (diuretics). Electrolyte imbalances resulting from the use of diuretics and a baseline state of dehydration cause many medical problems.

The Immune System

The inflammatory response is affected with the loss of T-cell function, making the healing process longer. The overall decrease in the immune system makes the elderly population highly susceptible to infection. EMS providers need to be aware of the increased risk of infection from cross-contamination (e.g., from patient to patient) and to be diligent about handwashing and routine cleaning and decontaminating of high-use equipment such as stethoscopes, blood pressure cuffs, and stretchers.

The Endocrine System

Cortisol is a steroid produced by the adrenal glands that has anti-inflammatory and other immunity effects. Because cortisol production diminishes by nearly 25%, the elderly do not handle bodily stresses such as severe infection well. Insulin production also decreases, leading to abnormalities in glucose metabolism. A decrease in thyroid hormone (T3) production predisposes the elderly to hypothyroidism. Reproductive organs stop or slow down hormone production in both sexes, though changes are more obvious in women. The pituitary, or "master gland," which is responsible for regulating the entire endocrine system, can become nearly 20% less effective. The result is a generalized decrease in all endocrine function.

The Gastrointestinal and Genitourinary Systems

The mouth, teeth, saliva, digestion, and excretion are all affected by aging. The teeth will weaken and may be missing. Salivary enzymes decrease in volume and potency, leading to digestive difficulty. Secretion of stomach acids decreases, leading to poor absorption of nutrients and making vitamin and mineral deficiencies common problems. Peristalsis decreases in the gastrointestinal tract, causing bowel slowdown (ileus) and blockage (obstruction). Muscular sphincters (e.g., esophageal, rectal) become less effective, resulting in acid reflux, increased incontinence, and increased risk of urinary tract infections (UTIs). Urinary tract infections are a common source of fever in the elderly and a frequent cause of sepsis, especially in hospital and nursing home environments.

The Renal System

Decreased blood flow and decreased elimination of waste are the effects of aging on the renal system. Nearly 50% of functioning nephrons are lost. As a result, excretion of fluid, salts, and waste products (e.g., urea and creatinine) may decrease. Changes in renal functions have a major effect on the metabolism of many drugs.

Medication dosages are often decreased in the elderly to keep the patient from reaching toxic levels due to poor elimination of waste.

The Cardiovascular System

Major changes in cardiovascular function affect blood cells, blood vessels, and the heart. Coronary artery disease is prominent among the elderly. Cardiac output decreases with age as a decreased catecholamine response affects the heart's ability to increase its rate in response to stress and exercise.

There is a decrease in blood volume as well as a decrease in bone marrow production of red blood cells and platelets. Decreased iron levels from poor nutrition or malabsorption further decrease the levels of red blood cells, making low-grade anemia relatively common (although not normal) in the elderly.

The walls of blood vessels thicken, often because of arteriosclerosis; this thickening causes an increase in peripheral vascular resistance with variable reductions in blood flow to the organs. By approximately 80 years of age, there is a 50% decrease in blood vessel elasticity. Baroreceptors (pressure sensors) within blood vessels lose their sensitivity. As a result, the elderly are highly sensitive to orthostatic (positional) changes. Postural hypotension becomes common because of inadequate compensatory mechanisms.

The heart muscle (myocardium) becomes less elastic and less able to respond to exercise and stress. This reduction leads to an increased workload on the aging heart. Cardiac reserves become limited, and stress such as tachycardia is not well tolerated. The heart can increase in size (**cardiomegaly**) for many reasons, including mitral or atrial valve disease. Cardiomegaly further increases the workload of the heart. The conduction system develops fibrous (scar) tissue, particularly in the sinoatrial node, and loss of normal cardiac pacemaker cells makes arrhythmias common in the elderly.

The Respiratory System

Changes occur in the mouth, nose, and lungs. Tissues atrophy and there is a loss of normal mucous membrane linings; as a result, inhaled air is not well humidified. Decreased muscle mass leads to relative chest wall weakness, and the chest wall becomes still and rigid, making the ribs vulnerable to fracture. Ventilation and gas exchange are affected as lung compliance diminishes with the loss of elasticity. Older persons have an ineffective cough reflex as a result of the weakened diaphragm muscle and chest wall structure (ribs, vertebrae, and sternum). A decrease in cilia and diminished cough and gag reflexes increase the risk of infectious pulmonary diseases.

The Nervous System

Normal aging results in a loss of neurons and neuro-transmitters. The clinical effects are variable. Reflexes and reaction times become slower, and memory impairment may develop. Often the sleep-wake cycle is disturbed. The brain shrinks (atrophies) with age, increasing the risk for injury. The sharp bone edges within the skull can cause bleeding as a result of rapid acceleration or deceleration forces.

The Integumentary System

With aging, the skin thins, and subcutaneous fat diminishes from the extremities and redistributes to the hips and abdomen. The loss of sebaceous glands and vascularity in the skin affects thermoregulation, increasing the risk of hypothermia. Dry skin is common, and elasticity decreases. The loss of the elastic fiber causes sagging and wrinkles.

The Musculoskeletal System

Changes in weight and height are progressive as muscle and bone mass decrease. After 70 years of age, body weight decreases because of muscle atrophy, and the extremities become disproportionately longer than the trunk owing to shrinking of the spinal column; the long bones remain the same length and postural kyphosis becomes apparent (Figure 19-2).

Abdominal muscles become thinner, making abdominal organs easy to palpate. Changes in the head and neck impair or limit physical mobility. Swallowing

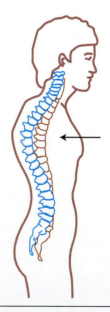

FIGURE 19-2 Kyphosis, an excessive convexity of the thoracic spine, occurs in the elderly.

becomes impaired (dysphagia). The EMS provider should not routinely palpate the carotid arteries of the elderly patient because plaque can be dislodged, leading to stroke. Visually inspect the neck for jugular venous distension (JVD), and note the presence of any scars related to **carotid artery disease (CAD)**, which is any breakdown or blockage in the carotid artery.

Vital Signs

The heart rate, respiratory rate, and blood pressure will depend on the patient's physical and health status. Distal pulses in the lower extremities become difficult to palpate because of changes associated with arterial insufficiency. Ectopic beats that create an irregular pulse are common among the elderly. Orthostatic changes occur easily with change of position, such as from sitting to standing or from lying down to sitting up.

Pulmonary function gradually deteriorates with age. Therefore, even mild dyspnea is a significant finding in the elderly. The normal ranges for respiratory rate are the same as for the younger adult; the respiratory effort is of more concern. In addition to visually observing and listening, the EMS provider should ask the patient about ease or effort of breathing.

A gradual rise in systolic pressure over the years is a normal finding owing to thickening of the walls of blood vessels and the development of cardiovascular disease. Many elderly adults have a high blood pressure when it is taken by blood pressure cuff, but it is relatively normal when direct intra-arterial measurements are taken. This difference is due to their stiffer vessels. Arterial hypertension (hypertension caused by thickening of the arteries) is considered currently the greatest health problem in the United States. According to the American Heart Association, one in five Americans has high blood pressure. One of the major problems associated with hypertension is that it is often asymptomatic until severe complications (e.g., stroke or transient ischemic attack) occur. It is estimated that more than 50% of all Americans will have hypertension by age 60. Women and African American men have an even higher prevalence.

The normal temperature remains 37°C (98.6°F) for most elderly people. However, slightly lower, but not dangerous, temperatures of 36.2°C (97.2°F) can be noted owing to impaired control mechanisms. Temperature is an important sign in the elderly because of the age-related decline in function of the thermoregulatory system and the body's impaired ability to maintain homeostasis. Except as noted, even modest elevations or decreases in temperature are indications for concern, especially when they are associated with confusion, loss of appetite, or other behavioral changes. Slight changes in temperature are consistent with pneumonias, UTIs, and sepsis.

Exploring the Web

- Search the Web for additional information on the effects of aging on the body systems. For each body system, create index cards for review that highlight the changes you may encounter and how to effectively make assessments based on those changes.

PSYCHOLOGICAL STATUS

Aging leads to numerous concerns about psychological status due to the decline in well-being as health problems arise. Decrease in self-worth may develop, as previously productive persons are no longer able to work. Financial burdens often come with retirement and a fixed income. Increased medical costs and poor or no insurance coverage pose a real concern to all patients, especially in late adulthood. The death or dying of friends and companions brings home the reality of our limited life span. The loss of a close friend or spouse further solidifies the fact that we are not immortal.

The loss of a support system (family and friends), a decreased quality of life, disfigurement, reduction or loss of mobility, lowered self-esteem, and decreased independence are all contributing factors to depression, alcohol or substance abuse, and suicide in the elderly population.

Depression is common among the elderly, and the rate of suicide in the elder population is higher than in the general population. The causes can be physiological and psychological. Always remember to ask the depressed patient about suicidal thoughts. Alcoholism is particularly insidious among the elderly and can lead to a number of illnesses, including hypoglycemia, chronic gastritis, pancreatitis, cirrhosis, heart and brain damage, impotence in men, and enlarged blood vessels in the skin. Symptoms are not easily recognized until the affected person becomes truly alcohol dependent.

THE FOCUSED HISTORY

The dimishment or loss of hearing and vision can make the assessment process difficult for both the patient and the EMS provider. Anticipating the potential for deficits and modifying the approach to the patient will ease the assessment process for both patient and provider. The elderly patient can easily become overwhelmed, confused, or fatigued when too many people ask too many questions too fast or if there is a lot of noise on the scene. The EMS provider can get frustrated when he does not get answers quickly. Be careful not to rush, and be prepared to give the patient a break as needed. If the patient appears to be getting flustered or overwhelmed, the EMS provider can slow down and give the patient a little breathing space by getting a history from the family or caregivers. When necessary, control the crowd, including other responders and family or caregivers.

Be prepared to give the patient a little extra time for responses to questions. The elderly patient tends to describe her history more slowly than a younger patient. For many reasons, elderly patients may not report what their symptoms are. They may be poor historians because of dementia or Alzheimer's disease or the presenting problem, or the patient may feel that the symptoms she is experiencing are just part of aging and not worth reporting. The patient may be afraid of a diagnosis that may not permit her to stay at home. Patients may be embarrassed, or too tired to face the discomfort of a trip to the hospital, or reluctant to impose the inconveniences they perceive they are creating. Avoiding the expenses of a hospital stay is a major concern for many people and a reason they may downplay symptoms. In addition to the patient's unreliability, concomitant disease processes can distort symptoms, making symptom-based assessment confusing.

When appropriate, attempt to determine what the patient's daily living activities consist of and how well the patient functions at home. Have there been any changes recently? The patient may now need temporary or permanent help with daily living activities, such as preparing meals, grooming, or dressing.

The OPQRST History

Using OPQRST, Table 19-1 highlights specific information pertaining to the focused history of the elderly patient.

The SAMPLE History

Use SAMPLE to obtain specific information pertaining to the focused history of the elderly patient (Table 19-2). When time and available personnel permit, take into consideration physical functional status, emotional status, and social functional status.

Clinical Carat

- If an elderly patient is on a medication, assume that it could be contributing to just about any health problem.

TABLE 19-1
OPQRST for the Elderly Patient

Information	Questions	Remarks
Onset	Is this a new problem? Have you ever experienced this before?	Determine whether this is a new problem or a preexisting condition suddenly worsened. Whenever possible, determine what the patient's baseline status is. This can be a very difficult and often impossible task. Seek out a spouse, family member, caregiver, or neighbor, or call the patient's physician when necessary to verify patient information.
Provocation	What were you doing when the problem began? Do you have a medical condition that could be contributing to the problem? Have you recently been injured?	Obtain the details of the present episode. Determine what the patient was doing at the time of onset, and try to differentiate trauma as a cause.
Quality	What are you feeling? Can you describe your symptoms? Are you having any pain? Can you describe the pain?	Determine what the pain feels like and where it is located. Be alert to subtle clues, and remember that mild dyspnea is often the only indication of a cardiac emergency.
Region, **R**adiation, **R**elief, **R**ecurrence	Is the pain located in only one spot? Does the pain appear to move around to other areas? Are you under a doctor's care for any medical conditions? Have you tried anything or taken anything in an attempt to relieve the symptoms?	Determine whether the pain or symptoms radiate from a point of origin. Concomitant disease processes often present with complicated findings. It is important to determine whether the patient attempted any interventions to improve the condition (e.g., taking nitroglycerin or just waiting to see whether the condition would get better).
Severity	On a scale of 1 to 10 with 1 being no pain and 10 being the worst pain ever felt, how would you rate the pain?	Obtain a baseline assessment followed by serial assessments in order to determine whether the condition is improving.
Time	When did the symptoms begin?	It is important to determine whether the current episode occurred suddenly or has progressively worsened over time. It is also critical to determine how long the patient waited before calling EMS.

TABLE 19-2
SAMPLE for the Elderly Patient

Information	Questions	Remarks
Signs and **S**ymptoms	What are you feeling? Can you describe the symptoms you have?	Determine what problem the patient is having and whether this is a medical or a trauma-related event.
Allergies	Are you allergic to any foods or medications?	Ask about allergies to medication and other substances (e.g., sulfa drugs, penicillin, lidocaine, latex products) and sensitivities to medications such as aspirin.
Medications	Are you currently taking any prescription medications? Has your medication changed or your dosage changed recently? Have you taken any over-the-counter medications in an attempt to relieve the symptoms?	Get an accurate list of medications and doses. Determine when they were taken last and how good the patient's compliance is. The elderly patient may be taking multiple medications (**polypharmacy**) for multiple medical problems. These medications can interact with other medications, potentiating side effects (e.g., taking a beta-blocker to control blood pressure and starting a new water pill that also lowers blood pressure can drop the pressure too much), or neutralizing each other (certain antibiotic medications can neutralize other medications). A poor response to drug therapy due to a decline in liver and kidney functions can present as an acute medical problem. Many medications are a predisposing factor for hypothermia, especially with a depressed thermoregulatory system.
Pertinent past medical history	Are you currently under a doctor's care for any medical illnesses? Have you had any injuries recently? Have you ever experienced anything like this in the past?	When the history is unreliable, seek out a family member, caregiver, or the patient's physician to verify detailed information about the disability or chronic illness, and include all diagnoses, past procedures, baseline neurological status, baseline vital signs, baseline physical findings, and any other specific medical issues. Get the name of the patient's physicians, including the primary care physician and current specialty physicians.

(continues)

TABLE 19-2 (continued)

Information	Questions	Remarks
Last oral intake	When did you last eat or have anything to drink? When did you last take your medication?	Ask about changes in appetite and any problems with eating, drinking, bowel movements, and urination.
Events leading up to this incident	What prompted you to call EMS? Did this problem occur suddenly, or is it a condition that has worsened over time? Is this the first time you have ever experienced this type of condition?	Be alert for clues such as subtle recent changes in mental status; changes in mobility; inability to perform daily living activities; and signs of depression, alcohol or substance abuse, and abuse or neglect.

THE PHYSICAL EXAMINATION

The physical examination of the elderly patient in the prehospital setting can present many challenges. Many of the normal physiological changes that occur with the aging process, such as loss of sensation, can obscure findings during the physical examination, and often there are concurrent illnesses involved that can present confusing signs and symptoms. Elderly patients are often cold and wear many layers of clothing year-round, or they wear supportive clothing (e.g., a full body girdle or support stockings). Just gaining access to the patient's body for the physical examination or to apply ECG electrodes can be a challenge. The older patient must be handled gently so as not to cause any additional injury.

It is important to respect the patient's modesty and to explain the steps being taken. All these things can take extra time, so be prepared to spend time with these patients. Serious problems are often underestimated because the complaint is vague. Picking up on vague clues and using them to guide the examination is a key component in the assessment of the elderly patient.

Medical Assessment

The EMS provider should introduce himself, begin the initial assessment, determine the patient's mental status (MS), and manage the patient's airway, breathing, and circulation (ABCs). Be respectful and courteous and ask permission to assess before touching the patient; also explain the steps being taken. Perform the physical examination on the basis of the patient's chief complaint and findings from the initial assessment. Treat life threats as they are discovered during the initial assessment.

Psychological Assessment

Consider the patient's MS and affect while obtaining a focused history. Are there signs of a healthy well-being, of loneliness or depression? Many times, EMS is called because the patient is simply lonely. This is a call for help and should not be quickly dismissed. Consider helping the patient get support services from the county or town.

Social Assessment

Ask about the patient's support system. Do family members live nearby? Does anyone (e.g., family, friends, support services, or clergy) come to visit if the patient is unable to get out?

Assessment of Functional or Physical Limitations

Inspect the patient's surroundings. Does the patient appear to be able to perform activities of daily living such as eating, bathing, dressing, and toileting? Did the patient call EMS because she fell and could not get up? Perhaps the home needs some improvements to make the daily routine a little easier (e.g., more lighting in the hallways, railings, handholds in the tub, removal of throw rugs to prevent tripping). The EMS provider may be able to get the patient support services to make the difference.

Use of Diagnostic Tools

Obtain an ECG on any patient with an irregular pulse, orthostatic changes (e.g., dizziness or weakness), shortness of breath (often the only symptom of a cardiac problem in the elderly), altered mental status (AMS), and both typical and atypical chest pains.

Obtain a glucose reading and temperature on any patient with a suspected AMS. Even a modest drop or elevation in temperature is an indication for concern, especially when combined with symptoms such as confusion, loss of appetite, or behavioral changes. The home should feel warm. If it is not warm, the patient may be on a limited fixed income and trying to save money on heat to be able to eat. When the environment is not the apparent cause of the hypo- or hyperthermia, assume that the elderly patient has developed a severe infection until proved otherwise.

COMMON DISEASES AMONG THE ELDERLY

The most common diseases in the U.S. population aged 65 and older include heart disease as the leading cause of death, followed by cancer, stroke, chronic obstructive pulmonary disease (COPD), pneumonia and influenza, and diabetes (Centers for Disease Control and Prevention, 1999). The most prevalent chronic diseases are arthritis, hypertension, heart disease, cancer, diabetes, and stroke. Additional common medical conditions that may result in a call for EMS include thyroid, Alzheimer's, and Parkinson's disease and nonacute states of confusion. Trauma is a significant problem in the elderly population. Abuse, head injury, hip or femur fracture, and burns are especially troublesome, leading to devastating life changes and morbidity.

Heart Disease

The pathology of cardiovascular emergencies in the elderly differs from that in younger adults in that the elderly tend to die from heart failure (HF) more often than from an acute myocardial infarction (AMI). The elderly do not have the reserves that younger adults have, so when they experience conditions such as fever, infection, hypertension, dysrhythmias, anemia, aneurysm, or MI, heart failure can easily develop.

Signs and symptoms of cardiac emergencies in the elderly can be very vague, and this vagueness often results in misdiagnosis and undertreatment. Subtle findings associated with cardiac emergencies include:

- Fever
- Weakness or fatigue
- Mild shortness of breath (SOB), especially with exertion
- AMS, including confusion or new-onset dementia
- Irregular heartbeat
- Epigastric, back, or neck pain
- Dysrhythmias

The more obvious assessment findings associated with cardiac emergencies include:

- Severe SOB
- Nausea or vomiting
- Dizziness
- Syncope
- Heartburn or indigestion
- Diaphoresis
- Tingling and numbness

Hypertension

Arterial hypertension, defined as consistent elevations of systolic or diastolic blood pressure >140/90, affects nearly 40 million people in the United States (Cleveland Clinic, 2000). Research has shown that controlling hypertension helps to prevent cardiovascular disease, increasing longevity. However, one of the main problems associated with hypertension is that it often is asymptomatic until severe complications (e.g., stroke or heart attack) occur.

Pulmonary Disease

Respiratory emergencies among the elderly are usually associated with complications of COPD (e.g., chronic bronchitis, emphysema, asbestosis, black lung disease, or a combination). Persons with COPD are at an increased risk for developing pneumonia, influenza, and other respiratory infections. Pneumonia and influenza are the fifth leading cause of death by disease in the U.S. population aged 65 and older.

The chief complaint is usually dyspnea, exertional dyspnea, orthopnea, or tachypnea; the patient exhibits accessory respiratory muscle use and pursed-lip breathing. Lung sounds can vary throughout the chest, ranging from wheezing to coarse crackles in the upper airways to wet or absent (consolidation) sounds in the bases. Signs and symptoms associated with respiratory emergencies are often complicated by concurrent disease processes, such as congestive heart failure (CHF) or pneumonia.

Upper respiratory infections and pneumonia are common precipitants to acute exacerbations of asthma and COPD. This relation may make it difficult for the EMS provider to differentiate respiratory problems from acute pulmonary edema (APE). Associated findings include changes in mental status and cyanosis due to poor perfusion, chronic productive cough, and recent weight loss. Getting an accurate history is key to making a field impression. Additional findings may be associated with specific conditions:

- Chronic bronchitis. The patient has a history of respiratory infections, constant coughing, and cigarette smoking or high exposure to secondhand smoke.
- Emphysema. The patient has a history of cigarette smoking or high exposure to secondhand smoke. Classic physical findings associated with the emphysemic patient include clubbing of the fingers or toes, barrel chest, signs of right heart failure (peripheral edema and wheezing), persistent cough (usually in the morning), and possibly weight loss.
- Pneumonia. The patient often has a history of recent respiratory infection, coughing, fever, adventitious or diminished breath sounds (usually on one side but may be bilateral).
- Pulmonary embolism. The patient has a history of heart failure, recent surgery, immobilization, or estrogen use. The patient complains of dyspnea that has marked progressive worsening. There may be pleuritic chest pain, leg pain, and high anxiety but no cough or fever.

Diabetes

Nearly 20% of elderly patients are diabetic. The EMS provider must consider diabetes a significant cause of AMS. Approximately half of all diabetes cases occur in people older than 55 years of age (American Diabetes Association, 2002). Another special consideration is that the physical and cognitive impairments that come with the aging process can make diabetes very difficult to manage. Slower metabolism affects carbohydrate absorption, and declining senses of thirst and taste, declining appetite, and poor dental condition may contribute to the patient's not getting nutritious meals at the appropriate times. Neuropathy is prevalent in the elderly, and they have high susceptibility to infections and slow healing processes.

Thyroid Disease

Thyroid hormones tell the body how fast to work and use energy. When the thyroid begins to decline and fail, it may overproduce hormones (hyperthyroidism), causing the body to use energy faster than it should, or it may underproduce hormones (hypothyroidism), making the body use energy more slowly than it should and predisposing the person to risks such as hypothermia.

Signs and symptoms of a thyroid problem are very vague and simulate many different conditions. Most symptoms are nonspecific and may include nonacute confusion, muscle aches and pains, weakness and falling (which lead to decreased mobility), incontinence, changes in appetite, and weight loss or gain.

Alzheimer's Disease

Alzheimer's disease is a progressive neurological condition that robs memory and intellect. Emergencies associated with Alzheimer's patients tend to fall into one of three categories: behavioral, metabolic, and psychiatric or psychological. Behavioral problems include wandering around and combativeness. Metabolic problems fall along the lines of dehydration, complications with infection, and drug toxicity. Psychiatric and psychological problems include depression, acute anxiety, hostility, and paranoia.

Parkinson's Disease

Parkinson's disease damages nerve cells. The average age of onset for this disease is 57. Emergencies associated with Parkinson's usually result from falls, dementia, or dysphagia, and medication toxicity may result in exacerbation of symptoms.

Cancer

More than 60% of cancer patients are aged 65 and older (American Cancer Society, 2001). Assessment is symptom-based, and symptoms will vary greatly depending on the treatments and progression of the disease.

Nonacute Causes of Confusion

Dementia comes on gradually over months or years. The patient experiences impaired memory function and impairment of at least one other area of cognition: judgment, abstract thinking, ability to comprehend words (aphasia), or ability to recognize familiar objects (agnosia). Dementia may also involve apraxia (difficulty moving).

Delirium has a mildly acute onset of hours to days, and, in most cases, it is reversible. The patient experiences disorganized thinking and a decreased attention span.

Depression can cause inability to concentrate, impaired memory, and decreased cognitive functions.

TRAUMA

Any older person could become a victim of abuse or neglect. The most common abusers are family members; however, caregivers, landlords, neighbors, and so-called friends are not excluded. Abuse is often not reported because the patient is being abused by someone she relies on to meet her needs for living. The abused person may not tell because of the fear of a worse situation (e.g., increased abuse or being moved to a nursing facility), or she may not be able to tell because of a physical or mental disability.

Falls are the leading cause of death from injury among persons over 65 years of age in the United States. Common injuries from falls among the elderly include hip and upper-limb fractures and head injuries. Hip or femur injuries are associated with high mortality rates in the first year following the injury. The injuries reduce the quality of life significantly through the effects of reduction or loss of mobility, lowered self-esteem, and decreased independence. Complications from surgery and the lengthy period of immobilization often lead to blood clots or pneumonia. Head injury often results in a poor outcome because of the increased potential for bleeding and swelling. As do other organs, the brain atrophies with age. The shrinkage allows for the subdural space to enlarge, and veins become stretched. When the patient experiences a rapid acceleration or deceleration force, the brain and blood vessels tear on the sharp bony edges within the skull and subdural hematomas develop.

The elderly do not survive severe burns well because of changes in the skin, a decreased immune response, and preexisting illnesses. Their thin skin also makes them highly susceptible to burn injury, as shown in Figure 19-3.

CONCLUSION

Assessment and management of the elderly patient include evaluation of mental status, physical functional status, emotional functional status, and social functional status. EMS providers get a firsthand look at the patient's living environment and can transfer that information to the next clinician, thereby helping to complete an integral part of the total health assessment. However, the EMS provider rarely would have the time to complete a full evaluation of all four components of a health assessment. By taking just a little more time and modifying the assessment approach to the elderly, the EMS provider can make a significant difference in the quality of life during the "golden years" of the people they care for.

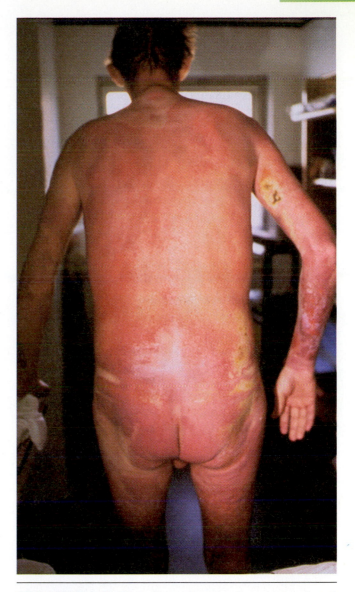

FIGURE 19-3 A first-degree burn received by an elderly patient who was unable to turn off the hot water from the shower in time to prevent being burned. (Courtesy of Ernest Grant, North Carolina Jaycee Burn Center, Chapel Hill, NC)

REVIEW QUESTIONS

1. If an elderly patient is awake yet does not seem to follow commands, the EMS provider should consider:

   a. that the patient has Alzheimer's disease.

   b. checking to see whether the patient has a hearing deficit.

   c. checking to see whether the patient is aphasic.

   d. none of the above.

2. Falls are common among the elderly because of vision loss and:

　a. decreased kinesthetic sense.

　b. increased sense of equilibrium.

　c. chronic dizziness.

　d. forgetfulness.

3. Effects of the aging endocrine system involve:

　a. decreased insulin production.

　b. decreased cortisol production.

　c. decreased reproductive hormones.

　d. all of the above.

4. Some elderly patients are prone to a persistent state of dehydration owing to:

　a. an increased sense of taste.

　b. chronic internal bleeding.

　c. a decreased sense of thirst.

　d. all of the above.

5. Effects of aging on the renal system can normally cause _____ of the nephrons to no longer function.

　a. 10%

　b. 25%

　c. 50%

　d. 80%

6. Patients in their seventies and eighties are very sensitive to _____ changes.

　a. meal

　b. orthostatic

　c. light

　d. color

7. The workload of the heart is increased in the elderly patient owing to:

　a. bradycardia.

　b. cardiomegaly.

　c. peristalsis.

　d. hypotension.

8. The carotid arteries of the elderly patient should rarely be palpated because:

　a. there is no pulse there anymore.

　b. elderly patients' strongest pulse is in their legs.

　c. palpation can cause plaque to become dislodged.

　d. none of the above.

9. Getting a SAMPLE history can help the EMS provider uncover problems that may be related to:

　a. polypharmacy.

　b. when the pain started.

　c. the type of pain the patient has.

　d. the degree of distress.

10. You note in your assessment of an elderly patient's living environment examples of home improvements that can help prevent injuries. They include:

　a. better lighting in the hallways.

　b. handrails and handholds in the tub.

　c. removal of throw rugs.

　d. all of the above.

CRITICAL THINKING QUESTIONS

1. You are called to a residence for an 80-year-old woman who has fallen in the bathroom. She is unable to get up. She tells you she has been diagnosed with osteoporosis. What do you suspect may be the problem? What additional information do you need to get from this woman? What can you do to prevent falls in the homes of the elderly in your community?

2. It is a very hot summer day, and you are called to the state park, where an elderly man was found wandering around aimlessly. The police are on the scene, and they tell you he is not able to tell them who he is or where he lives. He does not have any identification on him. What do you suspect is the problem? What can you do to adequately assess this patient? What additional factors must you consider?

3. What complications might you encounter when working with an elderly patient? How can you overcome these complications and improve your assessment of the elderly patient?

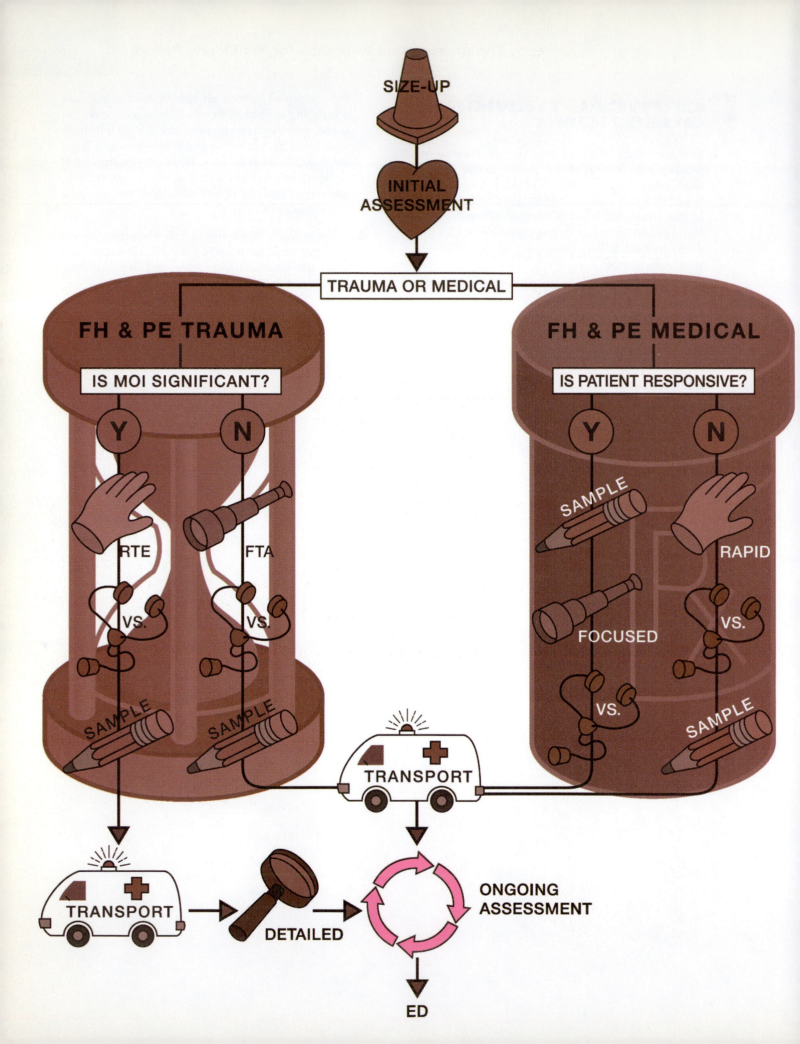

Chapter 20

The Ongoing Assessment

OBJECTIVES

Upon completion of this chapter, the reader should be able to:

- List the steps of the ongoing assessment.
- List three objectives of the ongoing assessment.
- Define trending and describe why trending is an important tool in patient care.
- Provide two examples of trending.
- Describe the typical information included in a radio report.
- Discuss the appropriate use of a patient assessment card.
- Explain why it is not appropriate to complete the prehospital care report en route to the hospital or facility.
- Explain how to document statements made by the patient while under your care.

KEY TERMS

assessment card

ongoing assessment (OA)

prehospital care report (PCR)

trending

INTRODUCTION

Recent U.S. Department of Transportation curricula have given a name to the phase of assessment and patient management that EMS providers have been doing since the "ambulance attendant" began riding in the patient compartment. This phase of care, provided to the patient while en route to a hospital or other medical facility, has come to be known as the **ongoing assessment (OA)**. Clearly, the title or phrase *ongoing assessment* may be new, but the steps involved are not! This chapter reviews the steps of the ongoing assessment and discusses them in detail.

The steps in the ongoing assessment are repeating the initial assessment and reevaluating the patient's priority, reassessing and recording the vital signs, repeating the focused assessment, and checking interventions.

BEGINNING THE ONGOING ASSESSMENT

Once the patient is in the ambulance, the EMS provider needs to ensure that the patient is properly belted to the stretcher and warm or cool enough, depending on the environmental conditions. Secure the IV, fasten down any loose equipment, and transfer the oxygen from the portable tank to the onboard tank. Make sure the ECG monitor, the pulse oximeter, and the capnograph are in a location where the EMS provider can easily observe dynamic changes. Once the patient is settled in, maintain a continuous concerned conversation with the patient, when appropriate, to help keep him informed of what is being done and to help deal with his anxiety about the trip to the hospital. It is also recommended that the EMS providers buckle themselves in to avoid being thrown about in the rear of the ambulance should a collision occur en route to the hospital.

Repeating the Initial Assessment

Once everyone is secure and the ambulance is ready to roll, repeat the initial assessment to deal with any potential life threats that may have developed and reevaluate the patient's priority. The initial assessment is described in detail in Chapter 4 and summarized in Figure 20-1. All steps of the ongoing assessment should be conducted with three objectives in mind:

1. To observe and note trends (changes over time of a symptom or condition)
2. To communicate with medical control or the receiving facility during transport

---

The initial assessment is the EMS provider's first assessment of the patient. It is designed to find and begin to deal with life threats as well as to prioritize the patient for care and transport. The general steps are:

- Body substance isolation (BSI) precautions
- Mental status evaluation
- Airway assessment
- Breathing assessment
- Circulation assessment
- Determining patient priority and the need for additional assistance (e.g., helicopter, critical care transport unit)

FIGURE 20-1 The initial assessment.

3. To document assessment findings and care of the patient

Reassessing and Recording Vital Signs

Trending is an important tool in patient care. **Trending** is the process of obtaining a baseline assessment, repeating the assessment a number of times, and using the information to determine whether the patient is getting better or worse or showing no change. Obtaining serial sets of vital signs is one example of trending. Another example of the use of trending is noting the subtle changes in mental status in the head-injured patient. By careful monitoring of the patient, the EMS provider can pick up subtle changes in the mental status, establishing a trend long before the obvious physical changes, such as a blown pupil on the injured side, occur. Examples of trends can be found in Table 20-1.

During the ongoing assessment, make some notes of the trends, serial vital signs, and patient findings. These notes will be necessary for documentation purposes as well as for helping to prepare for communications with the hospital or medical control. Traditionally, EMS providers provided a report over the radio to medical control or the receiving hospital to give them a good understanding of a patient's condition before arrival and

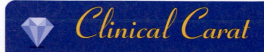

Clinical Carat

- **Trending is an important tool in patient care.**

TABLE 20-1
Acute Trends

Previous Check	Upon Reevaluation	Possible Indication
Tachycardia and pallor	Increased tachycardia, hypotension, and pallor	Shock
Normal pulse, hypertension, and altered mental status (AMS)	Bradycardia, hypertension, and AMS	Intracranial bleeding
Tachycardia and normal blood pressure (BP)	Increased tachycardia and hypotension	Shock Cardiac dysrhythmia
Pallor	Cyanosis	Hypoxia or shock
Normal respirations	Tachypnea	Respiratory distress Anxiety, overdose, or shock Head injury Hypoglycemia
Alert	Confused or unconscious	AMS and hypoglycemia Head injury Hypovolemia Overdose Any of AEIOUTIPS conditions (see Chapter 14)

the opportunity to prepare as necessary for critical patients. Although this advance information is also provided via more high-tech methods, such as a cellular phone, it is still referred to as the radio report. Depending on the extent of the prehospital protocols, the EMS providers may also need to communicate with medical control for consultation and permission to administer specific medications and treatment interventions. In some EMS systems, the EMT-Basics may need permission to assist or administer to the patient with one of the medications within the scope of their training such as nitroglycerin, an epinephrine self-injector, activated charcoal, glucose, or a single-dose bronchodilator inhaler.

Information obtained during the ongoing assessment will be a large part of the radio report given by the EMS provider en route to the hospital. Use of a template (see Table 20-2) helps new EMS providers give a complete, yet brief, transmission to medical control.

Documenting

It is important to document assessment findings as well as patient management. An **assessment card**, or patient profile (Figure 20-2), should be used to prompt the

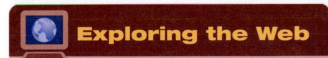

Exploring the Web

● Search the Web for information on the progressive deterioration of the following conditions: shock, respiratory distress, hypoglycemia, and overdose. Create an index card that lists the signs of deterioration for each, and use these cards to review.

TABLE 20-2
Radio Report Template

The typical radio report is given in the following format. There may be some local variations based on hospital needs and the medical director's wishes.

- Unit identification (ambulance number)
- Level of provider
- Estimated time of arrival (ETA)
- Patient's age and gender
- Chief complaint (CC)
- Brief, pertinent history of present illness or injury
- Major past illnesses
- Mental status
- Baseline vital signs
- Pertinent findings of the physical examination (PE)
- Emergency medical care given
- Response to emergency medical care
- Does medical control have any questions or orders?

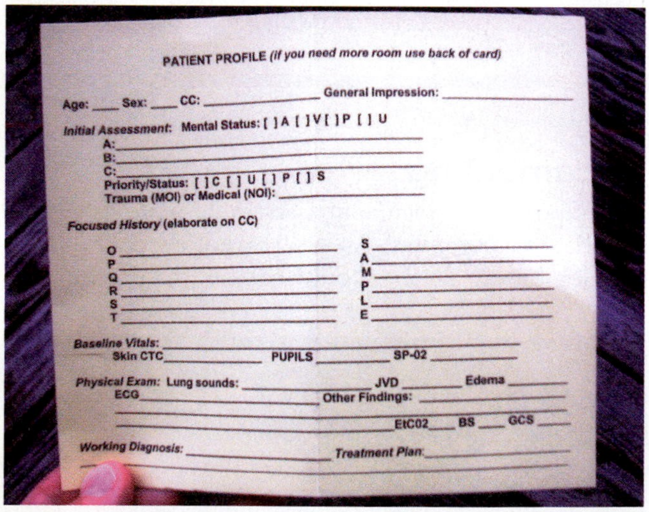
PATIENT PROFILE (if you need more room use back of card)
Age: ___ Sex: ___ CC: ___ General Impression: ___
Initial Assessment: Mental Status: [ ] A [ ] V [ ] P [ ] U
A:
B:
C:
Priority/Status: [ ] C [ ] U [ ] P [ ] S
Trauma (MOI) or Medical (NOI):
Focused History (elaborate on CC)
O S
P A
Q M
R P
S L
T E
Baseline Vitals:
Skin CTC ___ PUPILS ___ SP-02 ___
Physical Exam: Lung sounds: ___ JVD ___ Edema ___
ECG ___ Other Findings:
EtC02 ___ BS ___ GCS ___
Working Diagnosis: ___ Treatment Plan: ___

FIGURE 20-2 Consider using a patient profile or assessment card for information obtained on the scene (scene size-up, initial assessment, focused history and physical examination) and en route (ongoing assessment and detailed physical examination) to the hospital.

EMS provider regarding the appropriate questions to ask the patient for the focused history. It is also a place to jot down the vital signs and information obtained during the scene size-up, initial assessment, focused history and physical examination, and ongoing assessment. Some EMS providers use a personal digital assistant (PDA) or pocket reference to prompt them about the questions to ask and to provide useful information, such as normal pediatric vital signs, while doing their assessment. An assessment card can be a very helpful tool.

The **prehospital care report (PCR)**, on the other hand, was not designed to be completed in the back of a moving ambulance. This report needs to be neat, complete, and accurate as well as well thought out. It makes good sense that the EMS provider who was responsible for the patient assessment complete the PCR in a quiet corner of the emergency department. The PCR should be prepared after an oral report has been given to the emergency department staff and the patient has been carefully moved to the hospital stretcher. When documenting, always try to use objective language and not make any subjective judgments. Instead of writing "the patient's home was dirty and disorganized," write "There were cobwebs and piles of papers all over the bedroom." Rather than writing "The patient vomited a lot of times last night," be specific and write "The patient stated he vomited three or four times last night."

Be concrete by documenting exactly what is seen, heard, felt, or smelled. Avoid adding an interpretation of the reasons why the patient exhibited specific behavior. For example, do not write "The patient was crying from his depression"; instead, write "The patient was crying during the initial assessment." Be especially careful to document the pre- and postimmobilization (or splinting) assessments of pulse, motor, and sensory (PMS) function, the times vital signs were taken, and relevant pertinent negatives. If a patient makes a statement that is very important, document the statement in quotes such as, "I drank two six-packs," "I was trying to kill myself," or "I only shook the infant a little bit before he stopped crying."

Whenever using abbreviations on the PCR, be sure to use standard medical abbreviations that will be understood by health care providers who may read the form a day or even weeks later. The standard abbreviations commonly used by EMS providers appear in Table 20-3.

Repeating the Focused Assessment

Repeating the focused assessment is the next part of the ongoing assessment. For a responsive medical patient,

TABLE 20-3
Standardized Abbreviations

=	equal	L or l	liter
+	positive	mA	milliamps
−	negative	mg	milligram
>	greater than	mL or ml	milliliter
<	less than		
R	right	mm	millimeter
L	left	mm Hg	millimeters of mercury
×	times or multiply	n/a	not applicable
@	at	ohm	electrical resistance
ā	before		
AC	alternating current	PSI or psi	pounds per square inch
Bid	twice a day	oz	ounce
c̄	with	p̄	after
CC or c/c	chief complaint	prn	as needed
		q	every
cc	cubic centimeters	qd	every day
		qh	every hour
cm	centimeters	qid	four times a day
c/o	complained of		
D5W	5% dextrose in water	qod	every other day
		r/o	rule out
d/c	discontinue	s̄	without
DC	direct current	tid	three times a day
Dr.	doctor		
h	hour	w/	with
h/o	history of	WNL	within normal limits
Hz	hertz	w/o	without
kg	kilogram	y/o	year old

exams is discussed in detail in other chapters. For a trauma patient, a focused examination is done when there is no significant mechanism of injury (MOI). In this instance, as may be the case of a patient with a sprained ankle, the specific injured body part is examined, and distal pulse, motor, and sensory function are assessed. For a patient with a significant MOI, the rapid trauma examination is performed

Checking Interventions

Anything the EMS provider does to a patient that is expected to change the patient's condition should be reassessed to see whether the intervention had a positive effect (desired improvement), negative effect (undesired deterioration), or no observed effect. Vital signs should be reassessed every 5 minutes on the unstable patient and every 15 minutes on the stable patient (Figure 20-3). Examples of interventions and what should be reassessed during the ongoing assessment appear in Table 20-4.

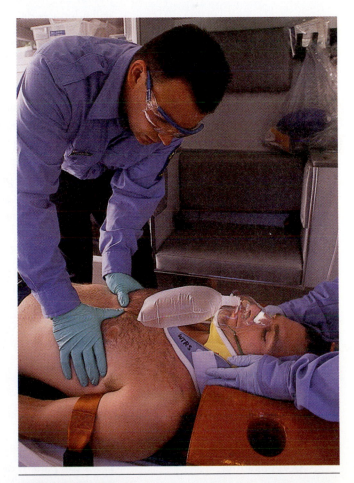

FIGURE 20-3 Reassessing the patient en route to the hospital.

this step will involve a focused examination of the respiratory, cardiac, neurological, abdominal, or psychological status of the patient, depending on the specific presenting medical problem. Each of these specific

TABLE 20-4
Interventions to Check

Patient Care Intervention	Reassessment
Oxygen administration	Check tank pressure. Make sure the non-rebreather valves are not covered and the bag is filling properly. Is the patient with chronic obstructive pulmonary disease (COPD) getting sleepy? What is the skin color?
Sugar administration	Recheck blood sugar, mental status, and patency of the IV.
Bronchodilator	Auscultate lung sounds, measure the peak flow, oxygen saturation (SpO_2), and end-tidal carbon dioxide ($EtCO_2$). Assess for physical signs of respiratory distress.
Nitroglycerin administration	Check for headache, pain relief, the need for an additional dose or paste or a stronger analgesic. Check the impact on the blood pressure (BP).
Splinting	Is the splint still effectively immobilizing the bone ends and adjacent joints? Is there still a distal pulse, or is the splint too tight? Is the traction still adequate?
Cold application	Is it effective? Is it still cold? Is another cold pack needed? Is it too cold on the skin?
Humane restraint	Is the restraint too tight? Check circulation. Is the restraint loosening up? Does the restriction affect the patient's breathing? Consider monitoring oxygen saturation with a pulse oximeter.
Spinal immobilization	How is the distal pulse, sensory, and motor (PMS) function? Assess the level of sensation and motor activity (check dermatomes). Observe for distal flushing from vasopooling in the extremities. Is the patient warm enough?
Antidysrhythmic medications	Is the ectopy diminished? Was there an impact on the underlying rhythm? Is there a need to rebolus or to set up a drip?
Pacing	Is there mechanical capture? Do you still have effective body surface interface? Are the batteries still charged?
Blood drawing and placing an IV	Label tubes and package and handle them carefully.
Fluid administration	Do you still have a patent line? Is the bag of fluid almost empty? Is the fluid too cold?
ECG application	Does the patient need to be shaved? Are the electrodes adhering? How are the monitor's batteries, paper, cables, and alarms?

(continues)

TABLE 20-4 *(continued)*

Patient Care Intervention	Reassessment
Patient positioning and comfort	Does the patient need repositioning, a pillow, or to have his head or legs raised? Is the patient warm enough?
Diagnostic equipment	Are the IV lines running? Are the ECG leads connected and electrodes adhering? Are the pulse oximeter and capnograph probes connected? Is the glucometer calibrated? Is the electronic BP cuff properly applied?
Temperature management	Does the patient's temperature need to be rechecked? Do blankets need to be added or removed? Is the air conditioning or heater in the ambulance working properly? Does wet clothing need to be removed?
Intubation	After all patient moves, periodically check the tube number at the teeth, the lung sounds, the pulse oximeter, the need for suctioning, and the capnograph.
Psychological support	Do you need to reorient the confused patient? Do you need to provide ongoing support, reassurance, and compassionate concerned conversation to the patient?
Suctioning	Is the patient becoming bradycardic? Are there signs of hypoxia? Is there gurgling from a partially obstructed airway? Is there a need for another catheter? Do the batteries on the suction unit need to be changed?
Body substance isolation (BSI)	Do you have the proper personal protective equipment (PPE) for yourself and the patient for this situation? Is there a need for a HEPA or N-95 mask or gown?
Pain management	Does the patient require positioning, icing, supportive conversation, or pharmacologic intervention?
Nausea	Will the patient require an emesis basin or vomit bag? Should an anti-emetic (e.g., Phenergan) be considered?
Bleeding control	Is a pressure bandage working? Will a pressure point be required to control the bleeding? Is cold or elevation needed?
Narcotic antagonist	When a drug such as Narcan is being administered, it is necessary to rebolus occasionally. What is the status of the airway and ventilations? Will the patient require restraint? Are withdrawal symptoms occurring?
Needle thorocostomy	Has the patient's breathing gotten better or worse? How is the patient's color? Is there a need for another needle? Is it necessary to remove one side of the occlusive bandage?

(continues)

TABLE 20-4 *(continued)*

Patient Care Intervention	Reassessment
PASG/MAST	Is the pressure being maintained in the pants? Reassess the BP and mental status. Is it necessary to add IV fluid to the patient before removing the pants?
Automated external defibrillator (AED)	Have the pulses returned? Is there a need to do CPR? Are the batteries still working? Is there still good electrode adherence?
Inducing vomiting by ipecac or charcoal administration	Are there any changes in the mental status? Do you need to collect the vomit for analysis?
Family support	Are you giving the family updates on the patient's condition? How can they help you help their loved one? Recognize the stages of grieving.
Recognition of death	When CPR is not appropriate, prepare the appropriate documentation and notify the police and medical examiner. Console the family.
Social or economic living condition adjustment	Notify social services resources of the need for assistance with daily living activities.
Mandatory reporting	Report child abuse, elder abuse, neglect, and so on (per state law).
Other	Additional interventions that are not directly patient care–oriented include: radio communications with dispatcher and medical control, scene safety, hazard control, rescue skills, emergency vehicle operations, and securing the patient's home, vehicle, and pets.

CONCLUSION

The ongoing assessment is done on every call when the patient is transported to the hospital or some other medical facility. Its steps involve reassessing the initial assessment, obtaining serial vital signs, and observing for trends in the patient's condition. For most calls, the ongoing assessment can easily be done as the EMS provider prepares to give the radio report. Remember to make some notes for documentation. There is often plenty of time to learn more about the patient, his family, his home and daily living activities, and his needs. In calls involving the critically ill or injured patient, there may not be enough time to perform an ongoing assessment.

REVIEW QUESTIONS

1. The ongoing assessment includes each of the following steps except:
   a. repeating the initial assessment.
   b. checking interventions.
   c. taking baseline vital signs.
   d. repeating the focused assessment.
2. Settling the patient into the ambulance includes:
   a. securing the IV bag.
   b. transferring the oxygen to the onboard.
   c. securing all loose equipment.
   d. all of the above.

3. Obtaining more than two sets of vital signs helps to establish:

  a. trends.

  b. convergence.

  c. priorities.

  d. reference points.

4. Examples of when an EMT-Basic might need to consult with medical control before treating a patient would include:

  a. an overdosed patient needing activated charcoal.

  b. a patient having a severe allergic reaction and needing epinephrine.

  c. a patient experiencing chest pain who has not yet taken his nitroglycerin.

  d. all of the above.

5. It is not uncommon for the EMS provider to give the emergency department a radio report while en route to the facility. Of the following items, which would not routinely be stated in this radio report?

  a. ETA

  b. the patient's name

  c. the treatment that was given

  d. the baseline vital signs

6. Documentation should be:

  a. neat.

  b. accurate.

  c. complete.

  d. all of the above.

7. Vital signs should be reassessed every _____ minutes for the stable patient.

  a. 5

  b. 10

  c. 15

  d. 20

8. If a patient made a dying statement, the EMS provider should:

  a. document the statement in quotes.

  b. not write it down.

  c. paraphrase it on the assessment card.

  d. report it to the police.

9. When reassessing a splint during the ongoing assessment, the EMS provider should check to see whether:

  a. the splint is still immobilizing the bone ends and adjacent joints.

  b. there is still a distal pulse.

  c. the traction is still adequate.

  d. all of the above.

10. Before and after a splint is applied, the _____ should be assessed and documented.

  a. bandage

  b. PMS

  c. level of consciousness

  d. SAMPLE history

CRITICAL THINKING QUESTIONS

1. Explain the importance of the ongoing assessment in terms of its usefulness in identifying deterioration of the patient while in your care. What are the possible legal consequences if you fail to complete the ongoing assessment? What are the moral or ethical consequences?

2. Explain your role in alerting the emergency department to the condition of the patient. How does appropriate communication help the patient? How does appropriate communication help you as a care provider? What might be the consequences of a lack of communication between EMS providers en route to the emergency department and the emergency department staff?

3. Explain the importance of making objective statements on the PCR and using direct quotes from the patient when documenting care. What are the legal considerations? What are the ethical and moral considerations?

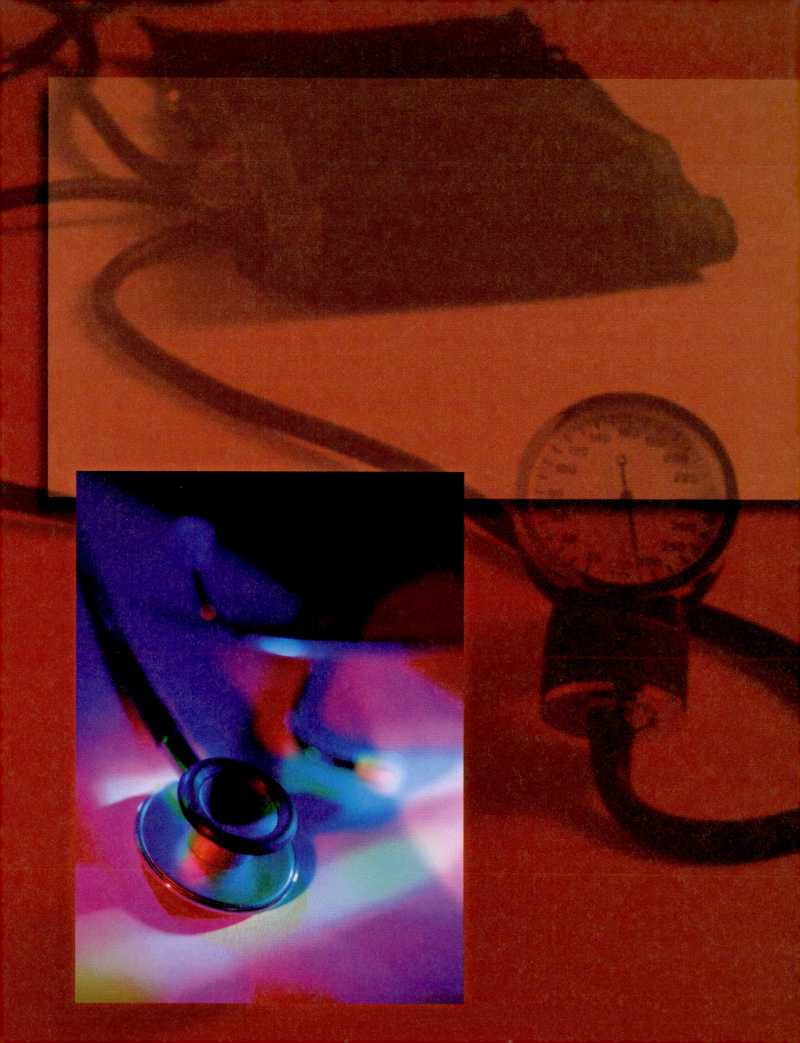

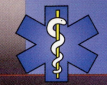

Chapter 21

Comprehensive Examination and Health Assessment

OBJECTIVES

Upon completion of this chapter, the reader should be able to:

- List the categories included in the comprehensive examination.
- Describe how the EMS provider uses the senses of vision, hearing, and touch to perform the comprehensive examination.
- Describe the possible findings associated with a patient's mental status, including AVPU, Glascow Coma Scale, behavior, appearance, speech, mood, thought content, perceptions, and memory.
- List the components incorporated into the general survey of a patient.
- Describe the technique used to examine the skin and the specific features to be assessed.
- Describe assessment features of the skin.
- Describe assessment features of the head, ears, eyes, nose, and throat.
- Describe assessment features of the chest.
- Describe assessment features of the cardiovascular system.
- Describe assessment features of the abdomen and genitalia.
- Describe assessment features of the upper and lower extremities.
- Describe assessment features of the spine.
- Describe assessment features of the peripheral vascular system.
- Describe assessment features of the nervous system.
- Describe the patient information obtained in the comprehensive patient history and health assessment.

KEY TERMS

bruit

comprehensive examination and health assessment

drowsiness

dysphonia

HEENT

hyphema

illusions

ophthalmoscope

otorrhea

otoscope

paralytic ileus

peritonitis

range of motion (ROM)

stupor

INTRODUCTION

The National Standard EMT-Paramedic curriculum describes a **comprehensive examination and health assessment**, which is an examination of the body as a whole. This is often completed on patients in the emergency department, a medical clinic, or a physician's office when the patient's condition is stable and time is not of the essence. The comprehensive examination and health assessment has not traditionally been a part of the responsibilities of EMS providers in the field. That is why it does not neatly fit into the assessment algorithm used throughout this book, which is primarily designed for the field assessment of a patient. With the expanding scope of practice in some areas, as well as remote areas where the transportation times may be quite lengthy, it makes sense to help the EMS provider understand the additional steps involved in a comprehensive assessment of the patient.

This chapter discusses both the comprehensive examination, with an emphasis on the areas that are new or different for the EMS provider, and the process of health assessment. Whether a particular EMS service area will be providing these assessments is clearly a function of training availability and of the decision of the service medical director.

USING THE SENSES

The comprehensive examination involves using the senses to inspect, auscultate, palpate, and percuss, as appropriate, each body part or region. Inspection, or looking at the patient, is used in conjunction with the skills of palpation and auscultation. Inspection, both visual and using the sense of smell, is used immediately as the EMS provider begins to form a general impression of the patient. Look for signs of distress and begin to differentiate normal from abnormal findings. Specific features to look at are discussed throughout this chapter.

Inspection

Upon forming a general impression of the patient, consider the location of the call and who else is present:

family, friends, caregivers, coworkers, or strangers. Observe the patient for signs and level of distress. Signs of distress can be obvious or quite subtle. The more practiced one becomes with physical examination and what normal findings are, the easier it becomes to recognize the less obvious signs of distress. Note the patient's age, gender, behavior, and skin: (CTC) color, temperature, and condition and whether the patient's dress is appropriate for the surroundings. Identify any unusual odors or visual clues that are pertinent to the patient's current condition.

Auscultation

Auscultation, or examining by listening to the body, may be performed using the ear alone or with the use of a stethoscope or Doppler (a special tool for listening to the body). Listening to the body is first employed in the initial assessment but may be a part of forming a general impression of the patient, as when the patient is presenting with wheezing audible from a few feet away. Listening skills become honed as the EMS provider learns how to auscultate lung sounds, heart sounds, bruits, bowel sounds, and blood pressures in places with loud ambient noises.

Palpation

Palpation is examination through touch or feel. Using light touch and deep touch and feeling for symmetry, compare one side of the body with the other. Before palpation, the EMS provider should warm his hands and equipment, such as the stethoscope. The EMS provider can reduce anxiety, fear, and muscle tensing by explaining where and how he is going to touch the patient.

Percussion

Percussion is a skill that is occasionally used in physical examination but not regularly in the field. This skill combines touching and tapping the fingertips on various body parts while listening to determine size, position, and consistency of underlying structures. Various areas of the body have what is called normal percussion tone. Think of this as the normal sound when that part is tapped. Diseases or illnesses that cause an accumulation of fluid in the lungs will have a flattened tone and sound dull (hyporesonant). Abnormal collections of air in the chest cavity, such as pneumothorax, make the percussion tone louder or hollow (hyperresonant).

THE COMPREHENSIVE EXAMINATION

The categories of a physical examination included in the comprehensive examination are mental status; a general impression; the vital signs; the integumentary system (skin, hair, and nails); the head, eyes, ears, nose, and throat (**HEENT**); the chest and cardiopulmonary system; the abdomen; the external genitalia; the extremities; the spine and posterior body; the peripheral vascular system; and the nervous system.

The head-to-toe method of performing the physical examination is a systematic approach used to keep the evaluator in sequence and to avoid overlooking any body parts during the exam. In the prehospital setting, a complete head-to-toe examination is primarily used for trauma patients so as not to overlook any injuries. However, this general rule does not preclude the EMS provider from completing a comprehensive examination on the medical patient when appropriate. After the initial assessment, in most cases, the EMS provider should focus the physical examination on the chief complaint and the source of the illness or injury as discovered in the initial assessment.

Mental Status

The mental status is evaluated by observing the patient's appearance and behavior. Initially, the EMS provider assesses the patient's level of consciousness, using AVPU (*a*lert, *v*erbally responsive, *p*ainful response, *u*nresponsive). This assessment determines whether the patient is alert, responsive to verbal stimuli, responsive to a touch or shake of the shoulder, and responsive to painful stimuli. Patients who do not respond at all are considered unresponsive. The range of possible findings when assessing a patient's mental status may include:

- Normal. The patient is aware of her surroundings and can state her name, where she is, and the day of the week (i.e., oriented to person, place, and day).

- Drowsiness. The patient is alert but sleepy; however, when questioned, the patient is oriented to person, place, and day.

- Obtundation. The patient is insensitive to unpleasant or painful stimuli owing to a reduced level of consciousness from an anesthetic or analgesic.

- Stupor. The patient is in a state of lethargy and unresponsiveness and appears to be unaware of her surroundings.

- Coma. The patient is in a state of profound unconsciousness, absent of spontaneous eye movements and exhibiting no response to verbal or painful stimuli.

Although terms such as *drowsiness*, *obtundation*, and *stupor* appear in the comprehensive examination, they are not commonly used because they are vague and very subjective and it is difficult to find multiple health care providers who have the same definition of these terms. Using the AVPU or the Glasgow Coma Score (GCS) is more exact. Be sure to take note of the patient's posture and motor behavior (e.g., purposeful withdrawal from pain or decorticate or decerebrate posturing), especially if it is necessary to apply painful stimuli.

Appearance

Observe the patient's dress, grooming, and personal hygiene, and note any signs of neglect. Facial expressions may provide a hint as to the affect and emotions such as anxiety, depression, elation, anger, and withdrawal. They may also indicate that the patient is responding to imaginary people or objects.

Behavior

Observe the patient for emotions and character of responses as well as for appropriateness of physical movements and **range of motion (ROM)**. The ROM is the span of movement of the joint. Consider whether the patient's behavior is appropriate for the current situation. Pay attention to the patient's manner, affect, and relation to persons and the surroundings. Does the patient get along, or is she short tempered? The variety of possible behavioral findings may include restlessness, agitation, excessive calmness, withdrawal, bizarre posture, immobility, and involuntary movements, or tics.

Pediatric Pearl

- After it has been ensured that the airway, breathing, and circulation (ABCs) are secure, the pediatric physical examination is often performed in the opposite direction, from toe-to-head. The order is reversed so as not to frighten the child. For infants and small children, the ears and throat are the most uncomfortable to have examined and that part of the exam may upset a child.

Pediatric Pearl

- If the EMS provider walks into the room to begin the assessment on a child and the child just does not seem to notice or care about his presence, the child is probably very sick!

Speech

Listen to the patient's speech and use of language. Pay close attention to the quality, rate, and loudness, and listen for any speech impairments. There are four general types of speech impairment: language disorders, articulation disorders, voice production disorders and fluency disorders. When a speech disorder is recognized, it is important to ascertain whether it is a new or existing condition. New-onset speech disorder is a critical finding and is associated with such conditions as stroke, brain tumor, and traumatic brain injury. The patient with a preexisting condition may need a little extra time to respond to questions and may become frustrated by the inability to communicate. Provide any aids as needed (e.g., writing tablet, pictures) and allow the patient time to respond. The following terms are associated with speech disorders:

- Aphasia: the loss of the ability to speak
- Dysphasia: abnormal speech due to lack of coordination and failure to arrange words in the proper order
- Dysarthria: imperfect articulation
- **Dysphonia:** a classical disorder of the voice involving discomfort when talking due to laryngeal disease.

Mood

Possible findings in mood assessment may include happiness, elation, depression, anxiety, or indifference. Some patients have diagnosed mood disorders and may exhibit changes with these disorders. Evaluate the following:

- What is the stability of the patient's mood? Is the patient on an even keel, or does she exhibit a range of moods?
- How intense is the patient or the feeling?
- What is the duration of the mood?
- Is the patient at risk for suicide (e.g., depressed)? If she is, ask her whether she was thinking about hurting herself or another.

Thought Content

The EMS provider listens to the patient's thought content and perceptions to assess whether they are logical and relevant and whether the thought processes are organized and coherent. Assess the patient's insight into her own illness and her judgment in making decisions or plans about her daily routine or care. The EMS provider may find that the patient's recognition or denial of mental causes of her symptoms is bizarre, impulsive, or unrealistic. Assess thought content by listening for unpleasant or unusual thoughts (e.g., threatening statements or talk of death or gore). Possible findings, including abnormality of thought content, may include:

- Phobias: intense fears of objects or situations (e.g., of spiders, snakes, heights, enclosed spaces)
- Hypochondriasis: feeling sick without any actual physical reason or pathology (hypochondriacs tend to abuse the EMS system)
- Obsession: feeling overwhelmed by persistent thoughts or impulses, such as a patient who is obsessed by the possibility of becoming infected or contracting a disease
- Compulsion: unwanted but irresistible need to repeat some purposeful act such as handwashing or checking and rechecking to be sure the oven is turned off.
- Delusions: false beliefs despite physical evidence to the contrary, such as "I am the Emperor"

Perceptions

Assess the patient's perceptions. Does the patient believe she hears things or sees things that are not actually there (e.g., "They told me to do it" or "I see dead people")? She may be experiencing **illusions** (misperceptions of actual existing stimuli by any sense) or hallucinations (a sensory perception of something that is not actually present). A hallucination may affect visual, auditory, tactile, olfactory, or gustatory senses. Possible findings about a patient's thoughts and perceptions may include:

- Blocking: a sudden interruption in train of thought such as a patient who says, "Oops, I forgot what I was going to say."
- Confabulation: fabricating events to cover memory gaps. Some people call this embellishing; others refer to it as pathological lying.
- Neologism: a new made-up word that has a meaning only for the person who made it up
- Circumlocution: substituting a phrase when unable to remember a word such as "the thing you shock the patient with" instead of "defibrillator"
- Circumstantiality: talking in excess with details unnecessary to answer the original question. For example, patients commonly elaborate on their medical history, jumping around from story to story and including lots of irrelevant details.

- Loosening associations: shifting from topic to topic without any clear connection. This is also called stream of consciousness.
- Flight of ideas: rapid skipping from topic to topic with recognizable associations between them
- Word salad: illogical mixture of words or phrases that are disconnected and incoherent
- Perseveration: continued repeating of verbal and motor responses. This is not the same as a confused patient with amnesia asking questions about the collision over and over.
- Echolalia: repeating others' words in a mumbling or mocking tone
- Clanging: choosing words on the basis of their sounds rather than their meaning as in nonsense rhymes

Memory

Memory and attention are assessed initially when the EMS provider determines whether the patient is alert to person, place, and day provided the patient is conscious. If the patient is disoriented, assess her attention span by using a simple test such as spelling a word backward or counting by sevens. Assess the patient's ability to access remote memory by asking the date of birth, as long as this can be verified. Access recent memory by quizzing the patient on the events of the day ("What did you eat today?" "When did you take your last medication dose?"). Assess new learning ability by telling the patient a phrase and asking her a few minutes later to repeat the phrase.

Blood Sugar Assessment

As a part of the comprehensive examination, it is helpful to assess the patient's blood sugar level if there is any reason there may be an altered mental status or the patient has a history of diabetes. There are two general methods for obtaining blood glucose in the field.

- Glucometers. Many brands are available. These are fast and easy to use and are reliable when calibrated to the manufacturer's specifications. The meters provide an LCD (liquid crystal display) readout very quickly after a drop of capillary or venous blood is placed on the test strip and the strip is inserted into the meter.
- Chemstrips, BGS, Dextrostix, and others are reagent strips and are not as accurate as glucometers but are still used in the field. Testing with these strips requires placing a drop of capillary or venous blood on a test strip and waiting a specific number of seconds for a color change and then comparing the color on the strip against a chart. Several variables can affect the reading, which is always more accurate when combined with a meter.

General Survey

The general survey in the comprehensive examination of a patient includes assessment of the following:

- Level of consciousness. Include whether the patient is awake, alert, and responsive to voice and painful stimuli.
- Signs of distress. Include signs that indicate cardio-respiratory insufficiency (e.g., labored breathing, wheezing, a cough), pain (e.g., sweating, guarding, wincing), and anxiety (e.g., furrowed brow, fidgety movements, cold moist palms).
- Apparent state of health. Does the patient appear acutely or chronically ill? Is the patient frail and feeble or robust and vigorous?
- Skin color and obvious lesions. Does the skin have an overall abnormal color such as pallor, cyanosis, or jaundice? Are there rashes, bruises, or scars? Pay particular attention to patients who have multiple bruises in different stages of healing in areas that are not commonly injured accidentally (e.g., upper arms, back, or buttocks) because these are possible indications of neglect or abuse.
- Height and build. Is the patient unusually tall or short for her age? Does the patient have a petite, slender, lanky, muscular, or stocky build?
- Sexual development. EMS providers do not unnecessarily disrobe anyone, especially children. However, in the assessment of the patient, the EMS provider may take note if the voice, hair (facial, axillary, and pubic), and breast size are age and gender appropriate. Malnourishment or developmental disorders may be a factor.
- Weight. Does the patient look emaciated, slender, average, obese, or morbidly obese? Emaciation is excessive leanness and a wasted condition of the body, which is associated with several causes (e.g., starvation, poor nutrition, or cancer). When obesity is noted, is the extra weight distributed in a normal or an abnormal pattern (e.g., a Cushing's syndrome patient would have centripetal obesity and wasting of the arms and legs)? Obesity is defined as 20% to 30% over normal body weight and results when a person's caloric intake exceeds the calories burned. There are numerous underlying and often related causes such as a low inherent metabolic rate. There is also a genetic predisposition to body type and the distribution of fat cells. Current thinking has shown that many obese people have an underlying metabolic defect involving excess insulin secretion. Many of these individuals gain weight even on a normal or moderately reduced-calorie diet. Several drugs, such as steroids, cause a temporary weight gain. Cessation of cigarette smoking also causes temporary weight

gain because nicotine normally stimulates a compound that breaks down fat in the body. In addition, many obese people have psychological problems related to their body image. *Morbidly obese* refers to the patient who has such a large amount of fat (adipose) tissue that it creates a significant negative impact on the rest of the body; for instance, a person who is 100 pounds over the ideal body weight would be considered morbidly obese. Obesity places the patient at risk for coronary artery disease (CAD), hyperlipidemia, hypercholesterolemia, diabetes, hypertension, sleep apnea, degradation of the knees and hips, vertebral disk degeneration, stroke, and chronic disorders.

- Posture, gait, and motor activity. What is the patient's preferred posture? Is it tripodal (e.g., respiratory distress) or paralytic (e.g., stroke)? Does the patient limp (e.g., old injury)? Can the patient walk easily? Look for balance, discomfort, fear of falling, and any abnormal motor patterns.

- Dress, grooming, and personal hygiene. Is the patient dressed appropriately for the temperature and weather conditions? Is the clothing clean and buttoned and zipped up properly? How does the clothing compare with that worn by people of similar age, lifestyle, occupation, and socioeconomic group? Are the shoes clean and laced, or are holes cut in the shoes or the soles completely worn? Does the patient wear any unusual jewelry such as a copper bracelet for arthritis or a medical identification bracelet or necklace? Do the hair, fingernails, and use of cosmetics reflect a specific lifestyle, mood, or personality, or are they basically traditional? Unkempt hair may indicate a decreased interest in appearance, or it can be a clue to the length of illness. Perhaps no one is available to assist the elderly patient with grooming, as would be indicated by long, hardened, and curling toenails.

- Odors. Breath odors may indicate underlying conditions. Does the patient smell of body odor (inability to bathe), alcohol, acetone (as in diabetic coma), infection, liver failure (urea), vomitus, gas (flatulence), bloody stool, or any other substance?

- Observe the facial expressions. Check the expressions when the patient is at rest, during conversation, during the examination, and when the patient does not know you are looking at her.

Vital Signs

Obtain a complete set of vital signs. This topic is discussed in detail in Chapter 6.

The Integumentary System

The examination of the integumentary system includes assessment of the skin, hair, and nails. The EMS provider should note the following characteristics:

- Color of skin. The colors (e.g., red of oxyhemoglobin, pallor) are best seen where the epidermis is thinnest. The fingernails, lips, and mucous membranes of the mouth and conjunctiva are good spots to observe the color changes in a patient's skin. For a dark-skinned patient, the palms and soles may also be useful areas to assess.

- Temperature and moisture of the skin. The skin can be assessed for moisture by feeling the forehead with the back of the hand. The temperature of the skin is also roughly assessed with the back of the hand on the forehead. If it seems too hot or too cold, the patient's temperature should be measured. The antiquated mercury glass thermometer found in a patient's home might be the only instrument available for some EMS providers to measure a temperature. However, the patient must be able to follow instructions. The two and a half minutes it takes to get a reading makes it untimely in emergent situations. The rectal route using the same device is utilized when other routes are not practical. There is also a hazard with accidental perforation of the rectum. Various types of electronic thermometers are available for use as an oral, rectal, or continuous monitoring device. The tympanic probe placed in the ear is safe and fast and uses a one-patient disposable probe cover. These methods are designed for a single patient use. These devices must be calibrated and charged on a regular basis. The temperature of a patient suspected of hypothermia should be measured with a special thermometer that covers temperatures lower than most normal thermometers do.

- Condition of the skin. Is it excessively dry, moist, scaly, or oily?

- Turgor of the skin. Assessing the elasticity of the skin, or turgor, can help to indicate the patient's state of hydration. To assess the skin turgor, gently pinch a small section of the patient's skin on the forearm, back of the hand, anterior chest, or abdomen. When the skin is released, it should return to its original shape quickly. Skin that remains pinched (tenting) or returns slowly to the natural contour indicates dehydration. It is possible to have increased skin turgor due to increased tension or connective tissue disease. Aging affects turgor, and it is common for geriatric patients to have poor skin turgor due to the loss of elasticity in connective tissue.

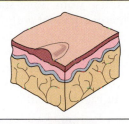

A **papule** is a small solid raised lesion that is less than 0.5 cm in diameter.

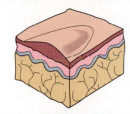

A **plaque** is a solid raised lesion that is greater than 0.5 cm in diameter.

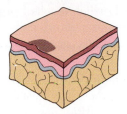

A **macule** is a flat discolored lesion that is less than 1 cm in diameter.

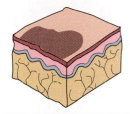

A **patch** is a flat discolored lesion that is greater than 1 cm in diameter.

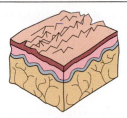

A **scale** is a flaking or dry patch made up of excess dead epidermal cells.

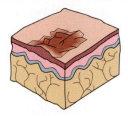

A **crust** is a collection of dried serum and cellular debris.

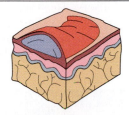

A **wheal** is a smooth, slightly elevated swollen area that is redder or paler than the surrounding skin. It is usually accompanied by itching.

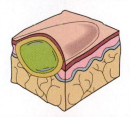

A **cyst** is a closed sack or pouch containing fluid or semisolid material.

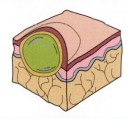

A **pustule** is a small circumscribed elevation of the skin containing pus.

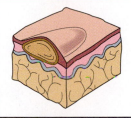

A **vesicle** is a circumscribed elevation of skin containing fluid that is less than 0.5 cm in diameter.

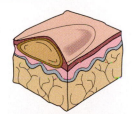

A **bulla** is a large vesicle that is more than 0.5 cm in diameter.

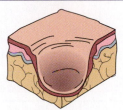

An **ulcer** is an open sore or erosion of the skin or mucous membrane resulting in tissue loss.

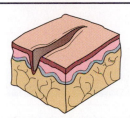

A **fissure** of the skin is a groove or cracklike sore.

FIGURE 21-1 Types of skin lesions.

- Lesions. Observe the skin for lesions that may be an indication of disease or injury. There are many types of skin lesions, as illustrated in Figure 21-1. Does the patient have psoriasis, a skin condition whose etiology is in part genetic and is thought to be aggravated by cold weather, infection, and trauma? Some medications, such as steroids, create abnormal skin conditions (e.g., dry skin or thin skin prone to tears).

- Hair. Inspect and palpate the hair, noting its quantity, distribution, texture, and the presence of lice or nits.

- Nails. Inspect and palpate the fingernails and toenails, noting the color and shape and whether any lesions are present. Findings in or near the nails may include any of the following:

  - Acrocyanosis. This is a disorder of the arterioles of the exposed parts of the hands and feet involving abnormal contraction of the arteriolar walls intensified by exposure to cold and resulting in bluish mottled skin.

  - Beau's lines. Transverse furrows on the fingernails are caused by a stopping in nail growth at the matrix (nail bed) (Figure 21-2A). Beau's lines are associated with acute infectious disease, anemia, and malnutrition.

- Clubbing. This results from long-standing hypoxia, as in the case of a patient with COPD or lung cancer. In early clubbing, the nail base may feel spongy and there will be a 180-degree angle or greater as between the nail base and the plane of the nail. Fully developed clubbing of the nails is shown in Figure 21-2B.

- Onycholysis. This is a loosening or separation of a nail from its bed, which results from hypo- and hyperthyroidism, repeated nail trauma, Raynaud's disease, syphilis, eczema, and acrocyanosis.

- Paronychia. This is an inflammation of the tissue folds surrounding the fingernails caused by *Candida albicans* (a parasitic fungus), bacteria, or repeated exposure of the nails to moisture (Figure 21-2C).

Head, Eyes, Ears, Nose, and Throat

The head, including the scalp, skull, face, and skin, should be closely examined. Observe the scalp by parting the hair in several places. Look for scaliness, lumps, and lesions. Observe the general size and contour of the patient's skull. Palpate and inspect for any tenderness,

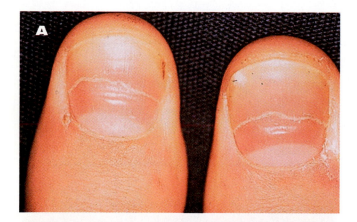
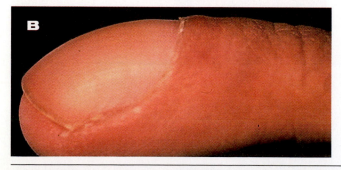
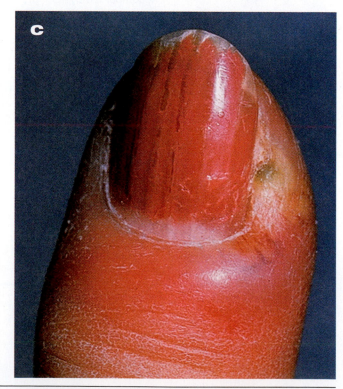

FIGURE 21-2 Abnormalities of the shape and configuration of the nail: (**A**) Beau's lines (**B**) clubbing (Courtesy of Robert A. Silverman, MD, Clinical Associate Professor, Department of Pediatrics, Georgetown University, Washington, DC), (**C**) paronychia.

lumps, and all the DCAP-BTLS items (*d*eformities, *c*ontusions, *a*brasions, *p*enetrations or *p*unctures, *b*urns, *t*enderness, *l*acerations, and *s*welling). The face should be observed, and the facial expressions and contours noted. Observe the face for asymmetry; involuntary movements, or tics; masses; and edema. Does the patient have a facial droop (e.g., some stroke patients)? Take a close look at the patient's skin about the head. Note the color, pigmentation, texture, thickness, hair distribution, and any lesions. Does the nose have spiderweb-like veins (spider nevus)? These are associated with liver disease but also are found on children and pregnant women.

The Eyes

The eyes should be assessed for visual acuity by asking the patient to read some printed material, to tell how many fingers you are holding up, and to distinguish between light and dark as in shades of white to black. First determine whether the patient wears glasses or contact lenses normally. The Snellen vision chart (Figure 21-3) can be used to test visual acuity. The chart is designed to be used at a distance of 20 feet from the patient. The

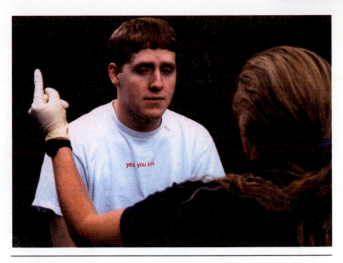

FIGURE 21-4 Assessing a patient's visual field.

provider assesses a patient's visual field by asking the patient to look directly at his face while he holds his own arms extended to the sides and his elbows at right angles (Figure 21-4). The EMS provider now wiggles both index fingers at the same time. The patient is asked which finger is moved, and, if the patient states both, the visual field is normal. This test should be performed in all four directions (left, right, up, and down). By positioning yourself in front of the patient, the EMS provider should also be able to survey the eyes for their position and alignment.

Inspect the eyebrows, and note the quantity and distribution and scaliness of the underlying skin. Note the position of the eyelids in relation to the eyeballs. Inspect for the following: width of the palpebral fissure (the space between the upper and lower eyelids) on each eye (Figure 21-5), edema and color of the eyelids, lesions, condition and direction of the eyelashes, adequacy with which the eyelids close, and the presence of any drainage. Look at the lacrimal apparatus and briefly inspect the regions of the lacrimal glands (Figure 21-5). Look for excessive tearing or dryness of the eyes.

Ask the patient to look up while gently depressing both lower lids with both thumbs, exposing the sclera and conjunctiva. Look at the sclera and palpebral conjunctiva for color and unusual vascular patterns. With oblique lighting, inspect the cornea of each eye for opacities. Also look at the iris to see whether the markings are clearly defined. Inspect the pupils for their size, shape, and symmetry. Does the patient have a cataract (opacity in the lens of the eye that gives the pupil a pearly gray appearance) (Figure 21-6)? Test the papillary reactions to light, and look for direct reaction and consensual reactions.

From about 2 feet in front of the patient, shine a light into the patient's eyes and ask the patient to look at it. To test for accommodation, ask the patient to focus on

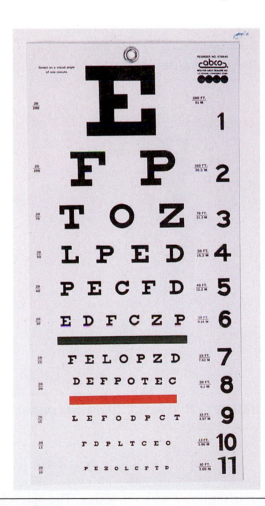

FIGURE 21-3 The Snellen vision chart.

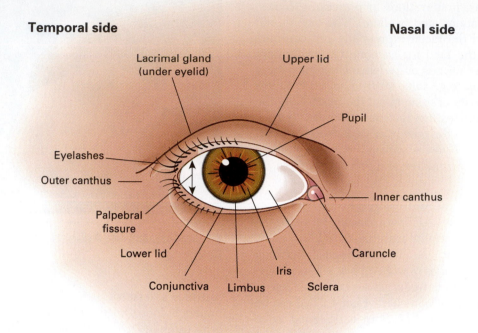

Temporal side

Nasal side

Lacrimal gland
(under eyelid)

Upper lid

Pupil

Eyelashes

Outer canthus

Inner canthus

Palpebral
fissure

Caruncle

Lower lid

Iris

Conjunctiva   Limbus   Sclera

RIGHT EYE

FIGURE 21-5 The lacrimal gland is on the underside of the eyelid.

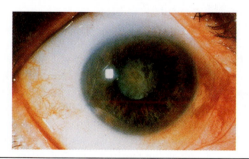

FIGURE 21-6 A cataract. (Courtesy of the National Eye Institute, National Institutes of Health, Bethesda, MD)

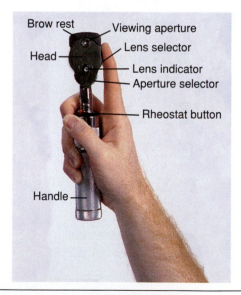

Brow rest

Viewing aperture

Lens selector

Head

Lens indicator

Aperture selector

Rheostat button

Handle

FIGURE 21-7 The ophthalmoscope is used to examine the eyes.

a distant object. Then ask the patient to shift her gaze to a near object. A normal pupil will constrict. Observe for convergence of the eyes as a finger is brought closer to the patient's face.

The **ophthalmoscope** is a tool used by health care personnel to perform a detailed examination of the eye (Figure 21-7). This skill requires practice. If this skill is used routinely by the EMS service, the EMS providers should ask the medical director to give additional training and supervision in the use of the device for proficiency in its use. An ophthalmoscope is a combination of

several lenses and a light source. The EMS provider looks through the ophthalmoscope, at the patient's eye, by focusing the scope with the lenses. The ophthalmoscope is used to visualize foreign bodies, lacerations,

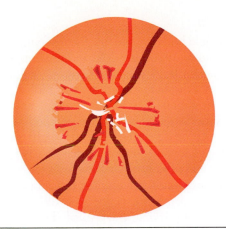

FIGURE 21-8 Retinal structure abnormalities such as papilledema.

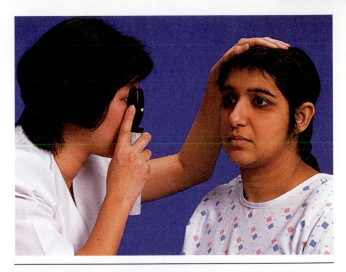

FIGURE 21-10 Eliciting the red reflex with an ophthalmoscope.

infection, some corneal abrasions and other external eye injuries, **hyphema** (blood in the anterior chamber), hypopyron (pus in the anterior chamber), as well as numerous conditions within the globe. These include:

- Papilledema: swelling of the optic disc due to increased intracranial pressure (Figure 21-8)
- Diabetic retinopathy: changes in the blood vessels due to diabetes (Figure 21-9)
- Hypertensive retinopathy: changes in the blood vessels due to high blood pressure
- Bleeding into the globe

The examination of the retinal structures should be conducted with the ophthalmoscope in a darkened room with the patient's glasses or contact lenses removed. The patient should be instructed to look at a distant object to help dilate the eyes. With the ophthalmoscope set on the 0 lens and held in front of the right

eye, from a distance of 8 to 12 inches away from the patient and 15 degrees to the side, shine the light into the patient's pupil. The light should elicit a light reflection from the patient's retina known as the red reflex (Figure 21-10). With a red reflex in view, slowly move closer to the patient, approximately 1 inch away, and change the diopter setting from 0 to the positive (+) or black numbers to focus on the anterior ocular structures. Next, move the diopter settings into the negative (–) or red numbers to focus on the posterior structures in the eye. Focus on the optic disc, which is on the nasal side of the retina, and follow retinal vessels centrally (Figure 21-11). If the disc is difficult to find, reverse direction on the vessel to attempt to find it.

Observe the retina for color and lesions, the vessels for configuration and characteristics of their

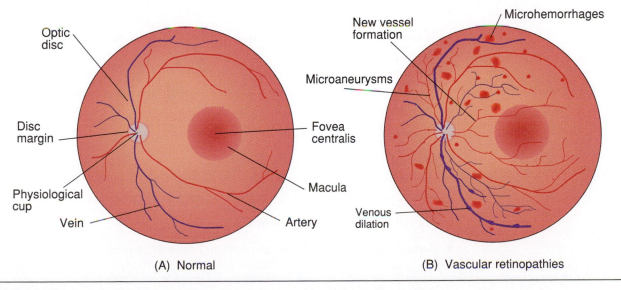

(A) Normal   (B) Vascular retinopathies

FIGURE 21-9 Vascular changes caused by diabetic retinopathy.

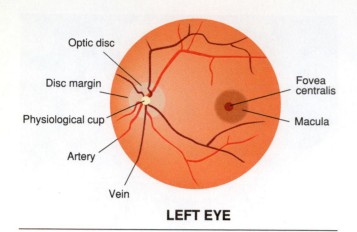

Optic disc

Disc margin

Physiological cup

Artery

Vein

Fovea centralis

Macula

LEFT EYE

FIGURE 21-11 The optic disc can be seen on examination with an ophthalmoscope.

crossing, and the optic disc for color, shape, size, margins, and cup-to-disc ratio. Describe the size, position, and location of any abnormality. The disc can be used as a clock face as a reference point to describe the location of the abnormality. The abnormality can be described in relation to the size of the optic disc. The optic disc is normally pinkish orange and has a yellow-white excavated center known as the cup. The ratio of the cup to the entire disc size should be 1:3. Examples of retinal color variations are shown in Table 21-1.

The Ears

The ears should be examined first by observing the auricle and surrounding tissue for deformities, lumps and skin lesions, drainage, tenderness, and redness (Figure 21-12). **Otorrhea** is a discharge from the ear and an indication of an ear infection. The **otoscope** is a tool used by health care personnel to perform a detailed examination of the ear. An otoscope consists of a light source projected through a cone-shaped device that is placed into an orifice, either the nose or the ear (Figure 21-13). It enables the examiner to visualize the inner structures, such as the eardrum, for redness, swelling, purulence, and foreign bodies. The portion of the device that is actually placed into the patient's nose or ear is usually disposable; if it is not, it must be disinfected properly before being used on a different patient.

The otoscope is used to evaluate for any discharges, foreign bodies, redness, and swelling in the eardrum. The eardrum can be visualized and observed for its color, contour, fluid or infection behind the drum, and perforation. The most common findings that may be helpful to observe with an otoscope include:

- Inflammation of the eardrum, suggestive of middle ear infection, or otitis media (Figure 21-14)

- Inflammation of the ear canal, as in an external ear infection (e.g., swimmer's ear)

TABLE 21-1
Retinal Color Variations

Findings	Characteristics
Fair-skinned individual	• Retina appears a light red-orange • Tessellated appearance of the fundi (pigment does not obscure the choroid vessels)
Dark-skinned individual	• Fundi appear darker grayish purple to brownish (from increased pigment in the choroid and retina) • No tessellated appearance • Choroidal vessels usually obscured
Aging individual	• Vessels are straighter and narrower compared to a younger person • Choroidal vessels are easily visualized • Retinal pigment epithelium atrophies and causes the retina to become paler

From Estes, M. E. Z. (2002). *Health assessment and physical examination* (2nd ed.). Clifton Park, NY: Delmar Learning.

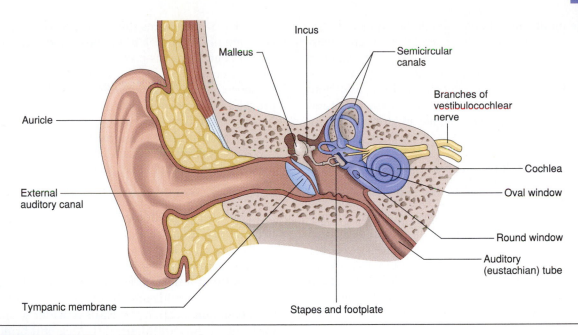

FIGURE 21-12 The ear.

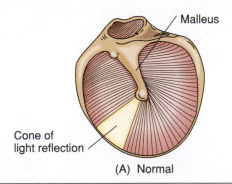

FIGURE 21-13 The otoscope can be used in the ear or the nose.

- Rupture of the eardrum (e.g., hyperbaric, or pressure injuries, and explosion injuries)
- Foreign bodies

An EMS provider who suspects that the patient has a foreign body in the ear should be very careful not to advance the tip of the otoscope blindly so as not to push the foreign body in farther. Acute changes in hearing are significant findings and should be evaluated. The patient's gross auditory acuity should be assessed by determining how well the patient can hear normal conversation and the sounds around her.

The Nose and Throat

Next evaluate the nose. Inspect the anterior and inferior surfaces of the nose for asymmetry, deformity, rhinorrhea (watery discharge), and DCAP-BTLS. The otoscope can be a useful tool in determining whether the patient has a foreign body obstructing the nares.

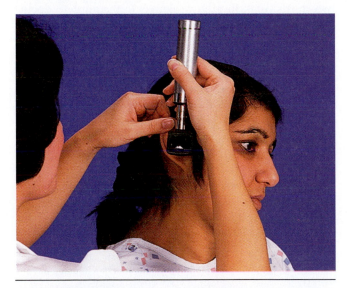
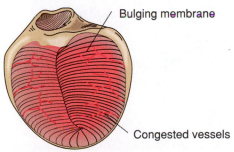

FIGURE 21-14 In the examination of the middle ear with an otoscope, a bulging tympanic membrane is indicative of otitis media.

The mouth and pharynx should be evaluated next. Inspect the patient's lips, observing for color and moisture and noting any lumps, ulcers, cracking, or scaliness. Use a penlight to look into the patient's mouth. A tongue blade can be helpful to inspect the oral mucosa. Note the color of the gums and teeth. Look at the color and structure of the hard palate, tongue, and tonsils.

The external throat (neck) should be inspected and the symmetry and any masses or scars on the neck noted. Note any swelling, redness, deviations, or abnormal structures (pierced body parts and jewelry are common sources of infection). Close inspection can reveal the tiny scars of carotid artery surgery present on a surprising number of people. Palpate the lymph nodes and inspect the trachea for any deviation to one side or the other. Inspect the anterior neck for the thyroid gland, noting enlargement. The EMS provider can inspect the thyroid gland by positioning himself behind or in front of the patient, as shown in Figure 21-15.

A

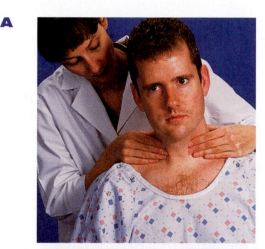

B

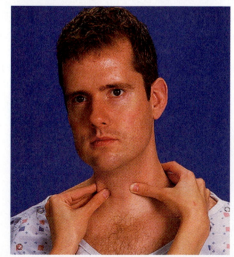

FIGURE 21-15 Examination of the thyroid gland from (**A**) the posterior approach and (**B**) the anterior approach.

The jugular veins should be assessed. The jugular veins are like a dipstick to the heart and give an estimation of central venous pressure (CVP). Distension indicates increased CVP. To accurately assess for the presence of jugular venous distension (JVD), the EMS provider must place the patient in a semi-Fowler's position, with the head raised at a 30-degree to 45-degree angle (Figure 21-16). The semi-Fowler's position is halfway between sitting up and lying supine. Position is important because JVD is a normal finding in a patient who is lying supine, whereas in a patient in a position of 45 degrees it is abnormal and JVD at 90 degrees may indicate serious pathology such as severe right heart failure, pericardial tamponade, or tension pneumothorax. Unilateral JVD is abnormal and may indicate a local vein blockage or restriction.

A **bruit** is a swishing turbulent sound heard over the arteries that indicates blockage of blood flow. The most common location the EMS provider would assess for bruits is the carotid arteries. A carotid bruit can be heard when the lumen becomes occluded by one-half to two-thirds (e.g., in atherosclerosis). A complete occlusion would result in no bruit or no sounds because no blood is flowing through the artery. To auscultate for carotid bruits, the EMS provider places the patient's neck in a neutral position and lightly places the bell of the stethoscope over the carotid artery. Listen first at the base of the neck, then halfway up the neck, and last at the angle of the jaw. Perform this procedure with extreme care so as not to compress the artery. Compression may dislodge plaque or stimulate a vagus nerve response.

The temporomandibular joint can be examined by asking the patient to open her mouth and jut out her jaw. The cervical spine can be inspected and palpated for tenderness and deformities. Range of motion should be

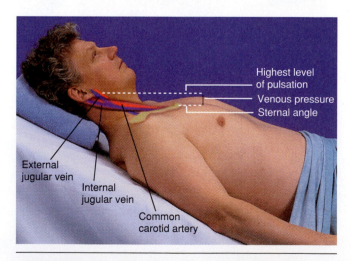

Highest level of pulsation
Venous pressure
Sternal angle
External jugular vein
Internal jugular vein
Common carotid artery

FIGURE 21-16 The proper position for inspection of the jugular vein for distension.

assessed, provided the patient does not have a suspected cervical spine injury. Have the patient first flex her neck, attempting to touch her chin to her chest. Next, test for rotation by looking to see whether the patient can touch her chin to each of her shoulders. Touching each ear to the corresponding shoulder assesses lateral bending, and putting the head back can check extension.

The Chest

Because examination of the chest (the thorax) involves everything within the thoracic cage (ribs, sternum, and thoracic vertebrae), the chest examination involves both the front and the back of the patient, and the patient's back is sometimes referred to as the posterior chest.

Have the patient expose her chest so that you can see the entire chest. It is not necessary to remove a female patient's bra. Proceed in an orderly fashion, comparing side with side by inspection, palpation, percussion, and auscultation. When doing so, try to visualize mentally the underlying lobes of the lungs and the chest cavity (Figure 21-17).

Observe the thorax and the movement of the ventilations, noting rate, rhythm, depth, and effort of breathing. Check the patient for cyanosis, and listen without a stethoscope to the patient's breathing. Observe the shape of the chest. When examining the chest, note any deformities, asymmetry, or abnormal shape (Figure 21-18) such as barrel chest, flail chest, pigeon chest (pectus carinatum), or funnel chest (pectus excavatum). Also note any curvature of the spine such as humpback (kyphosis) or scoliosis. Also keep in mind the question of whether the patient has retractions or any impairment of respiratory movement.

Next palpate the patient's chest, noting any tender areas, such as the point tenderness of a rib injury. Look closely at the patient's respiratory expansion. Percussion is best done on the posterior chest by tapping bilateral locations and noting any area of abnormal percussion sounds such as dullness, resonance, or hyperresonance. Dullness can be heard in patients with conditions such as atelectasis, consolidation or a pneumonia, pleural effusion, pulmonary edema, or bronchiectasis. Resonance

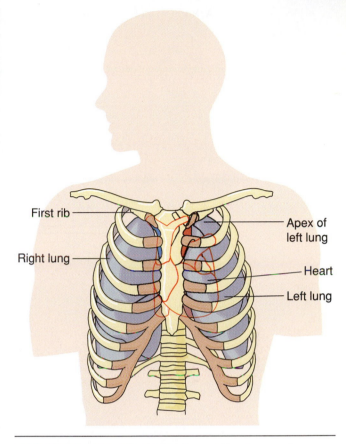

FIGURE 21-17 Note how the thoracic cage protects the heart and lungs. Visualize mentally the lobes of the lungs and the location of the heart in the chest.

can be heard in a normal healthy adult or in patients with a condition such as bronchitis, congestive heart failure, or bronchiectasis. Hyperresonance can be heard in patients with emphysema, pneumothorax, or asthma. Determine the level of the diaphragm and the diaphragmatic excursion by tapping the chest and comparing the hollow (chest) and dull (abdomen) sounds above and below the diaphragm and then having the patient take a deep breath and hold it for a moment to compare the location, as shown in Figure 21-19. Next auscultate for lung sounds, noting the vesicular, bronchovesicular, bronchial, and tracheal sounds.

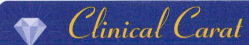

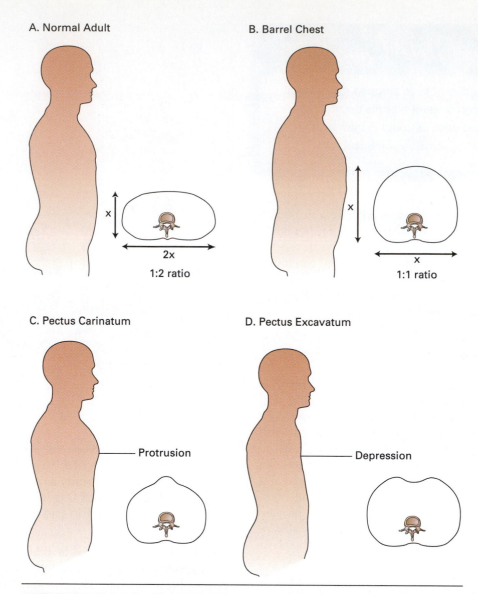

A. Normal Adult

x

2x

1:2 ratio

B. Barrel Chest

x

x

1:1 ratio

C. Pectus Carinatum

Protrusion

D. Pectus Excavatum

Depression

FIGURE 21-18 Chest configurations.

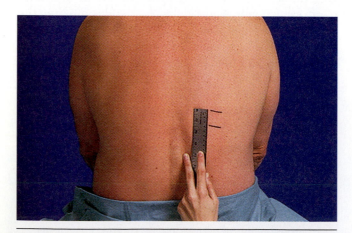

FIGURE 21-19 Diaphragmatic excursion is normally 3 to 5 cm. The level of the diaphragm is thoracic vertebra 12 on inspiration and thoracic vertebra 10 on expiration.

The vesicular sounds are heard over the lower airways; bronchovesicular sounds are heard in the center of the chest or the area of the bronchioles; bronchial sounds are heard over the bronchioles; and tracheal sounds are heard over the neck and trachea. The characteristics of normal breath sounds are illustrated in Table 21-2.

Assess for breath sounds in the medical patient by positioning the patient in an upright position such as the Fowler's position for easy access. Of course, if the patient must stay supine for a medical reason, such as spinal immobilization or syncope from hypotension, the EMS provider will need to work around the patient's position. If the patient is bedridden, it may be necessary to roll the patient onto her side to auscultate the posterior chest. Ask the patient to take deep breaths through her mouth and avoid talking or coughing if possible. Auscultation is always done by comparing the level of

TABLE 21-2
Characteristics of Normal Breath Sounds

Breath Sound	Pitch	Intensity	Quality	Relative Duration of Inspiratory and Expiratory Phases	Location
Bronchial	High	Loud	Blowing/hollow	I < E	Trachea
Bronchovesicular	Moderate	Moderate	Combination of bronchial and vesicular	I = E	Between scapulae, first and second intercostal spaces lateral to the sternum
Vesicular	Low	Soft	Gentle rustling/ breezy	I > E	Peripheral lung

From Estes, M. E. Z. (2002). *Health assessment and physical examination* (2nd ed.). Clifton Park, NY: Delmar Learning.

the chest on the right with the same level of the chest on the left. It would be inappropriate to try to compare the bronchial sounds on the right with the vesicular sounds on the right. Whenever possible, the stethoscope should be placed in direct contact with the skin. Do not listen to the shirt! Place the stethoscope directly on the skin. Listening through clothing decreases the ability to hear and may create false noises from rubbing on the clothing.

On the anterior chest, begin at the second intercostal space in the midclavicular line. Listen and compare the two sides. Next listen at the fourth intercostal space between the sternum and the midclavicular line bilaterally, and last listen at the fifth intercostal space (nipple level) and the midaxillary line bilaterally (Figure 21-20). Listen on the back between the shoulder blades, comparing the right with the left and moving from the

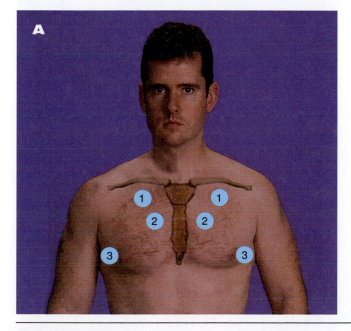
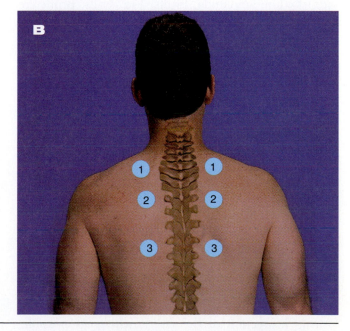

FIGURE 21-20 The location for listening to breath sounds on the (**A**) chest and (**B**) back.

top to the bottom. Begin at the level of cervical vertebra 7 (apices of the lungs) to the level of thoracic vertebra 10 (bases of the lungs). At the bases, move out laterally and listen at the level of ribs 7 and 8. On the anterior chest, lung sounds are best heard at the second intercostal midclavicular line and the fifth intercostal midaxillary line. On many patients, the fourth intercostal area adipose tissue creates a barrier for listening. Also heart tones on the left chest are often louder in this area, making it difficult to hear the lung sounds.

Although it may be possible to listen to breath sounds on the back of a trauma patient, it is most common to listen on the anterior chest. Trauma patients are often managed in the supine position to maintain the integrity of the spine. To listen for bronchial breath sounds, place the diaphragm of the stethoscope on the chest over the intercostal space at the midclavicular line on one side of the chest. Then repeat and compare with the other side. To listen for vesicular breath sounds, place the diaphragm over the fifth anterior axillary line and midaxillary line and repeat bilaterally. Adventitious sounds are abnormal breath sounds. The characteristics of adventitious breath sounds are compared in Table 21-3.

The Cardiovascular System

Examination of the cardiovascular system involves assessing the arterial pulses, blood pressure, jugular venous pressure and pulsation, and the heart. Note the presence of surgical scars on the chest, which may indicate coronary artery bypass graft (CABG), an internal pacemaker, or an implanted defibrillator. The arterial pulses are assessed at numerous locations (Figure 21-21) for rate, rhythm, amplitude, bruits, and thrills. Bruits are blowing sounds heard on auscultation caused by turbulent blood flow past an obstruction in the artery. Thrills are the vibrations from turbulent blood flow. They often feel like the purring of a cat. The blood pressure measurement and normal ranges are discussed in detail in Chapter 6. The EMS provider should observe the jugular venous pressure and jugular vein pulsation. Assess for jugular venous distension (JVD). The presence of JVD indicates back pressure in the systemic venous system commonly due to acute or chronic heart failure. This sign is commonly due to left heart failure, pulmonary edema, and cor pulmonale (right heart failure). However, if the patient is hypovolemic, this sign will not be present. To properly assess for the presence of JVD, the EMS provider should place the patient's head in a neutral position and elevate the torso approximately 45 degrees (semi-Fowler's position).

The key cardiac landmarks the EMS provider should be familiar with are shown in Figure 21-22. During inspection of the chest, whenever possible,

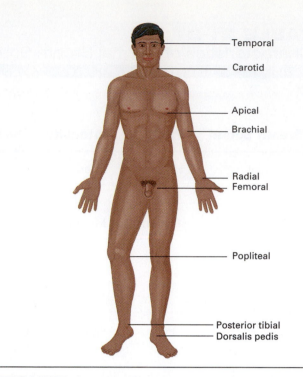

FIGURE 21-21 The arterial pulse sites.

make sure the room is warm, and the patient should be supine if she can tolerate the position. Otherwise have the patient keep the position of comfort, usually semi-Fowler's position. Expose only as much of the patient's chest as is needed to do the assessment.

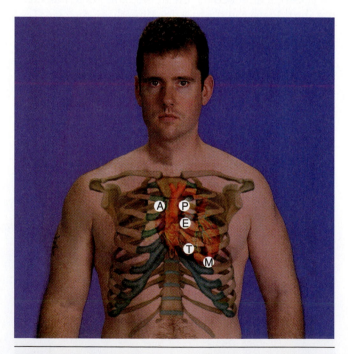

FIGURE 21-22 The cardiac landmarks: A, aortic area; P, pulmonic area; E, Erb's point; T, tricuspid area; M, mitral area.

TABLE 21-3
Characteristics of Adventitious Breath Sounds

Breath Sound	Respiratory Phase	Timing	Description	Clear with Cough	Etiology	Conditions
Fine crackle (rale)	Predominantly inspiration	Discontinuous	Dry, high-pitched crackling, popping, short duration; roll hair near your ears between your fingers to simulate this sound	No	Air passing through moisture in small airways that suddenly reinflate	Chronic obstructive pulmonary disease (COPD), congestive heart failure (CHF), pneumonia, pulmonary fibrosis, atelectasis
Coarse crackle (coarse rale)	Predominantly inspiration	Discontinuous	Moist, low-pitched crackling, gurgling; long duration	Possibly	Air passing through moisture in large airways that suddenly reinflate	Pneumonia, pulmonary edema, bronchitis, atelectasis
Sonorous wheeze (rhonchi)	Predominantly expiration	Continuous	Low pitched; snoring	Possibly	Narrowing of large airways or obstruction of bronchus	Asthma, bronchitis, airway edema, tumor, bronchiolar spasm, foreign body airway obstruction
Sibilant wheeze (wheeze)	Predominantly expiration	Continuous	High pitched; musical	Possibly	Narrowing of large airways or obstruction of bronchus	Asthma, chronic bronchitis, emphysema, tumor, foreign body airway obstruction
Pleural friction rub	Inspiration and expiration	Continuous	Creaking, grating	No	Inflamed parietal and visceral pleura; can occasionally be felt on thoracic wall as two pieces of dry leather rubbing against each other	Pleurisy, tuberculosis, pulmonary infarction, pneumonia, lung abscess
Stridor	Predominantly inspiration	Continuous	Crowing	No	Partial obstruction of the larynx or trachea	Croup, foreign body airway obstruction, large airway tumor

From Estes, M. E. Z. (2002). *Health assessment and physical examination* (2nd ed.). Clifton Park, NY: Delmar Learning.

Visual inspection of the aortic, pulmonic, midprecordial, and tricuspid areas should reveal no pulsations. The mitral area of about 50% of adults will normally show a pulsation at the point where the left ventricle is closest to the skin. This is called the point of maximal impulse (PMI), and its pulsations should correspond with the carotid pulse. Palpation goes hand in hand with inspection, and the EMS provider should systematically palpate each of the key areas for the presence of pulsations, thrills, and heaves (Figure 21-23). Heaves, or lifts, are described as a lifting of the cardiac area secondary to an increased workload and force on the left ventricular contraction. Palpation of the aortic, pulmonic, midprecordial, and tricuspid areas should reveal no pulsations, thrills, or heaves. Thrills and heaves are absent upon palpation of the mitral area of a healthy individual. In about half the adult population, an apical pulse may be felt as a light tap of about 1 to 2 cm in diameter. This impulse is also normally found and sometimes exaggerated in young patients. Lateral displacement of the PMI may indicate an enlarged heart, and the PMI may be displaced to the left during the third trimester of pregnancy or a right-sided tension pneumothorax.

To auscultate heart sounds, use the bell of the stethoscope. The diaphragm is designed to transmit high-frequency sounds, such as lung sounds, whereas the bell is used for the low-pitched sounds, such as heart sounds. When using the bell, rest it lightly on the skin; when pressed tightly against the skin it will act like a diaphragm and the low-pitched heart sounds will not be heard well. Place the bell of the stethoscope at the fifth intercostal space at the midclavicular line and listen to determine whether heart sounds are normal or abnormal. Normal heart sounds have two clear, distinct sounds, "lub-dub." Abnormal heart sounds or muffled or distant heart sounds may indicate the presence of fluid, as with a pericardial tamponade or hemothorax.

The two normal heart sounds to auscultate for are S1 and S2. S1 is the first heart sound and is produced by the closing of the atrioventricular valves (tricuspid and mitral) during ventricular contraction. The second heart sound, S2, is produced when the semilunar valves (pulmonic and aortic) close during ventricular diastole. Abnormal heart sounds are extra sounds. S3, or ventricular gallop, might be heard in CHF due to ventricular overload or failure, and S4, which is heard just before the S1 sound, is associated with an extra atrial contraction and decreased ventricular compliance.

Heart sounds are rarely evaluated in the prehospital phase for a couple of reasons. It is difficult to assess heart sounds in an uncontrolled environment and even under ideal conditions, and the results do not significantly change the patient's field management. Heart sounds are assessed by placing the bell of the stethoscope over the point of maximal impulse (PMI) on the left anterior chest at the fifth intercostal space at the midclavicular line. This location is referred to as the mitral area, and the S1, often described as the "lub" sound, can be heard loudest here. Both the aortic and pulmonic areas are locations where the S2, often described as the "dub" sound, can be heard. If time for listening is limited, some experts recommend simply listening at Erb's point, as it is often the best place to quickly hear the sounds of the four heart valves. A summation of the normal and abnormal heart sounds can be found in Figure 21-24.

Some abnormal heart sounds can be heard in the mitral and tricuspid areas (e.g., gallop sounds such as the S3, with its "ken-tuc-ky" sound, and the S4 with its "ten-nes-see" sound). Some patients may have a murmur or a pericardial friction rub, which are different sounds from the heart sounds already discussed. Murmurs of either the aortic or pulmonic valve are usually heard at Erb's point, which is the third intercostal space to the left of the sternum. Murmurs often sound like a whizzing noise and are not generally a significant problem for field concern. A murmur is a sound of longer duration that is produced by turbulent blood flow and may be caused by any of the following situations:

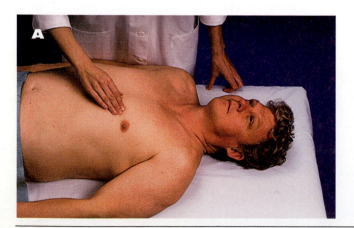
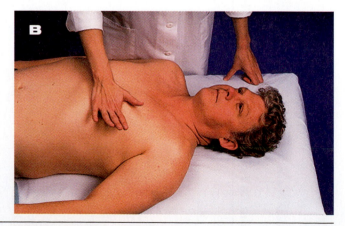

FIGURE 21-23 Palpating for (**A**) pulsations and (**B**) thrills.

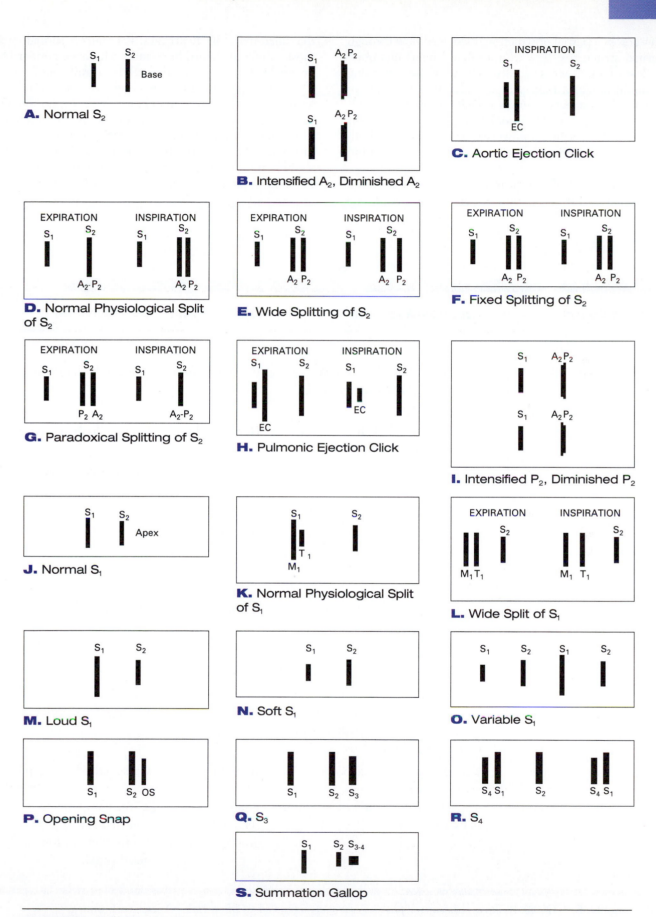

FIGURE 21-24 Summation of normal and abnormal heart sounds.

flow across a partial obstruction, increased flow through normal structures, flow into a dilated heart chamber, backward flow across faulty valves, or the shunting of blood out of a high-pressure chamber through an abnormal passageway, such as a small hole in the heart. It is beyond the scope of this book to describe all the details concerning murmurs; however, a summary of both murmurs and pericardial friction rubs can be found in Table 21-4.

The sound of a pericardial friction rub is due to inflamed visceral and parietal layers of the membrane that surrounds the heart, and it is never normal. It is most commonly heard in patients who have pericarditis or renal failure. A pericardial rub is a significant finding. The pericardial friction rub is a high-pitched, scratchy or grating sound that does not change with respiration. On the other hand, if a patient has a pleural rub, which is a lower-pitched sound, and the EMS provider needs to distinguish between the two sounds, the EMS provider should simply have the patient hold her breath for a moment. A pleural rub cannot be heard when the lungs are not moving.

TABLE 21-4
Murmurs and Pericardial Friction Rubs

Heart Sound	Location/Radiation	Quality/Pitch	Configuration
Systolic murmurs			
Aortic stenosis	Second right intercostal space (ICS); may radiate to neck or left sternal border	Harsh/medium	Crescendo/decrescendo
Pulmonic stenosis	Second or third left ICS; radiates toward shoulder and neck	Harsh/medium	Crescendo/decrescendo
Mitral regurgitation	Apex; fifth ICS, left midclavicular line; may radiate to left axilla and back	Blowing/high	Holosystolic/plateau
Tricuspid regurgitation	Lower left sternal border; may radiate to right sternum	Blowing/high	Holosystolic/plateau
Diastolic murmurs			
Aortic regurgitation	Second right ICS and Erb's point; may radiate to left or right sternal border	Blowing/high	Decrescendo
Pulmonic regurgitation	Second left ICS; may radiate to left lower sternal border	Blowing/high	Decrescendo
Mitral stenosis	Apex; fifth ICS, left midclavicular line; may get louder with patient on left side; does not radiate	Rumbling/low	Crescendo/decrescendo
Tricuspid stenosis	Fourth ICS, at sternal border	Rumbling/low	Crescendo/decrescendo
Pericardial friction rub	Third to fifth ICS, left of sternum; does not radiate	Leathery, scratchy, grating/high	Three components: ventricular systole, ventricular diastole, atrial systole

From Estes, M. E. Z. (2002). *Health assessment and physical examination* (2nd ed.). Clifton Park, NY: Delmar Learning.

The Abdomen

In the general assessment approach for the abdomen, keep in mind the following tips. Ideally, the patient should not have a full bladder. Make sure the patient is comfortable in a supine position, provided the medical condition allows it (e.g., a pulmonary edema patient needs to be sitting up). The normal abdomen should be soft, nontender, and without masses or bulges. Ask the obese patient whether this is the normal size of her belly or whether any distension or bloating is present. Ask the patient to point out the area of pain and leave that quadrant as the last to be examined. To begin, make sure hands and stethoscope are warm and that fingernails are short and trimmed. Approach the patient slowly and avoid any quick, unexpected movement. The EMS provider should be aware of the location of the abdominal organs and be able to visualize them in the mind during the examination (Figure 21-25).

Inspect each of the four quadrants of the abdomen, including the flanks, and note the appearance of the skin. Note any striae (stretch marks) or scars. The most common scars are from surgical procedures such as an appendectomy, a hysterectomy, or a cesarean section. Note any dilated veins, rashes and lesions, discoloration, or ascites. On the patient who has been bedridden, edema tends to develop in the sacral area. Look closely at the umbilicus for its contour and location. If there are any signs of inflammation, bulges at the flanks, or hernia, ask the patient about it. Observe the contour of the abdomen for bulges. The abdomen can be described using any of these terms: flat, rounded, scaphoid, or protuberant, as illustrated in Figure 21-26. Are any pulsations visible in the abdomen?

Bowel sounds are not usually auscultated in the prehospital setting because of noise and time constraints. To listen properly takes time (5 minutes to auscultate for accuracy of absent bowel sounds). When time permits, listen for the presence of bowel sounds. This assessment technique is performed before any palpation because physical manipulation can increase peristalsis; an increase in peristalsis increases bowel sounds, thus giving a false evaluation of bowel sounds. Changes in bowel sounds are most helpful in evaluating patients with possible peritoneal irritation or bowel obstruction regardless of the cause. During the comprehensive assessment, listen for bowel sounds in any person with acute abdominal distress or trauma.

For examination purposes, the abdomen is divided into four quadrants by imaginary lines running perpendicular through the umbilicus. These quadrants are labeled right upper quadrant (RUQ), left upper quadrant (LUQ), right lower quadrant (RLQ), and left lower quadrant (LLQ). Auscultate for the presence or absence of bowel sounds in each quadrant. Normal bowel sounds occur irregularly from 5 to 30 times a minute. The significant finding of listening for bowel sounds is the absence of sounds, and this should be noted. Absent

Right upper quadrant	Left upper quadrant
RUQ	LUQ
Right lower quadrant	Left lower quadrant
RLQ	LLQ

FIGURE 21-25 The locations of the abdominal organs.

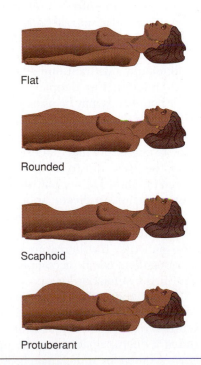

Flat

Rounded

Scaphoid

Protuberant

FIGURE 21-26 Configurations of the abdomen.

bowel sounds indicate obstruction, inflammation of the peritoneum (**peritonitis**), or a twisted and paralyzed bowel (**paralytic ileus**).

Listen to bowel sounds by placing the diaphragm lightly on the abdomen beginning in the RLQ. Listen for the frequency and character of the sounds. It usually takes approximately 3 to 5 minutes in a quadrant to conclude that the bowel sounds are absent. Next move on to the RUQ then to the LUQ and finally the LLQ, as illustrated in Figure 21-27. The bowel sounds will be heard as intermittent (normally 5 to 30 times per minute) gurgling sounds in each of the four quadrants. The sounds are the result of the movement of air and fluid throughout the gastrointestinal (GI) tract. Normally, bowel sounds are always present at the ileocecal valve area in the RLQ. Absent or hypoactive bowel sounds are abnormal and may indicate an obstruction. Hyperactive bowel sounds may indicate gastroenteritis, diarrhea, laxative use, or a subsiding ileus. Bruits can be auscultated by placing the bell of the stethoscope over the abdominal aorta, renal arteries, iliac arteries, and femoral arteries, as shown in Figure 21-28. The presence of any bruit is an abnormal finding and may be indicative of an abdominal aortic aneurysm or renal artery stenosis.

The abdomen should normally be soft and nontender. There should be no abnormal signs such as tenderness, masses, ascites, bloating, distension, rigidity, absent bowel sounds, or signs of incontinence. Light palpation may be used to assess most body parts; deep palpation is usually reserved for the abdomen. Light palpation is used to assess for softness, tenderness, large masses or deformities, and abnormal body temperature. To palpate the four quadrants of the abdomen using light palpation, use the pads of the fingers to gently depress each abdominal quadrant one at a time, about 1 cm (less than 1 inch). For deep palpation of the abdomen, one or both hands may be used to depress 2 to 3 inches in each abdominal quadrant. Often, two hands are used on an obese or muscular tense abdomen. Deep palpation is used to assess rebound tenderness, to appreciate the size of the liver, and to further evaluate any masses or enlarged organs. Do not palpate over pulsating masses (which could indicate abdominal aortic aneurysm) or areas where a bruit was found because plaque can be ruptured.

On some patients, the hepatojugular reflux is assessed. This assessment can be accomplished by placing the patient in the semi-Fowler's position with the head at a 30-degree angle. First observe the jugular veins to determine whether they are normal or distended. Next observe the jugular veins while simultaneously performing a deep palpation on the upper right quadrant of the abdomen for approximately 30 to 60 seconds. An increase of more than 1 cm in JVD may indicate right heart failure or fluid overload.

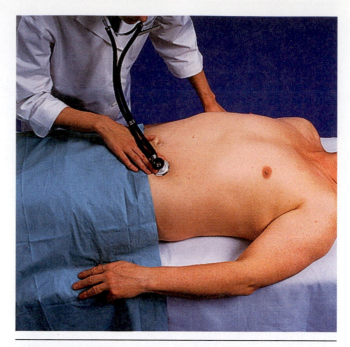

FIGURE 21-27 The technique of auscultation of the abdomen.

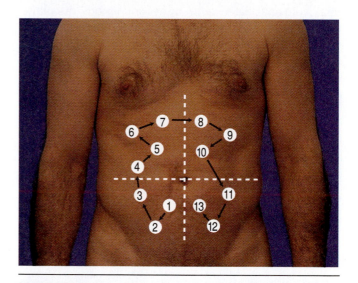

FIGURE 21-28 Stethoscope placement for auscultation of abdominal vasculature.

The External Genitalia

Examination of the external genitalia is usually not necessary unless a specific injury was sustained in that area or the female patient is in labor and crowning needs to be determined. In most cases, except for the woman in labor, this examination can be delayed until arrival in the emergency department. When examination of the external genitalia is necessary on a patient of either gender, it is preferable to use an EMS provider of the same sex or at the minimum to have an assistant of the same sex as the patient present during the examination. Keep in mind that this examination may be both awkward and uncomfortable for the patient, so explain why it is necessary and what is being done. The examination should include inspection for bleeding, bruises, lacerations, inflammation, discharge, swelling, and lesions.

An examination of the anus is rarely conducted in the field unless there is a serious soft-tissue injury or a foreign body. This examination can be accomplished with the patient in one of several positions. For most patients, the side-lying position is satisfactory. Drape the patient appropriately and inspect the sacrococcygeal and perineal areas for trauma, bleeding, lumps, ulcers, inflammations, rashes, and excoriations (raw, worn-down areas of skin). In the emergency department, patients are routinely tested for the presence of occult blood as part of the assessment.

Musculoskeletal Examination of the Upper Extremities

When examining the extremities, direct your attention to circulation and motor function as well as to structure. Assess general appearance, bodily proportions, pulses, skin turgor, and ease of movement. Pay particular attention to any limitations in the range of motion (ROM) and any unusual increase or decrease in the mobility of a joint. In general, assess for DCAP-BTLS as well as for signs of inflammation such as redness, increased heat localized to touch, or any decreased function. Take note of any pain, crepitation (crepitus), deficit of muscular strength, asymmetry, or muscular atrophy (shrinking due to lack of use as is the case when a cast has recently been removed).

When the patient is sitting up, examine the hands and wrists for range of motion. Ask the patient to make a fist with each hand. Then extend and spread the fin-

gers. Now have the patient flex and extend the wrists. With the palms down, move the hands in a lateral motion and then a medial motion. Inspect for DCAP-BTLS as well as for redness, nodules, and muscular atrophy. Palpate the medial and lateral aspect of each distal interphalangeal joint. Feel the proximal interphalangeal joint. Then squeeze the hand from each side between the thumb and fingers, compressing the metacarpophalangeal joints. Feel each wrist joint, and note any abnormality such as swelling, tenderness, or bogginess (Figure 21-29). Check for a radial and an ulnar pulse in each wrist. Note color, temperature, condition, and sensation of the fingers and nail beds.

Raynaud's disease is a vasospastic condition characterized by pain, pallor, and cyanosis (onycholysis) of both hands and sometimes both feet. Its cause is unknown, but it occurs almost exclusively in women. Severe cases may progress to small gangrenous ulcers on the fingers and permanent disability due to contractures and severe pain.

The elbow joints should be assessed for ROM by asking the patient to stand and bend, or flex, the elbow (Figure 21-30). Next have the patient straighten the elbow. With the patient holding her arm straight out, check supination by asking the patient to turn her palms up and pronation by having her turn her palms down. The EMS provider inspects the elbow joint by supporting the patient's forearm with his nondominant hand so that the elbow is flexed to about 70 degrees. The EMS provider next assesses for strength by taking his dominant hand and holding the patient's wrist and asking the patient to attempt to flex her elbow (pull it toward the chest) and attempt to extend her elbow (push it away from the body) while the EMS provider applies opposing resistance (Figure 21-31). Palpate the groove between the epicondyle and the olecranon process. Press on the lateral and medical epicondyle, noting any tenderness, swelling, or thickening.

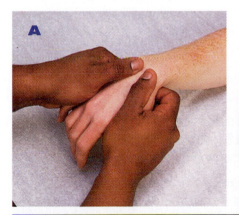
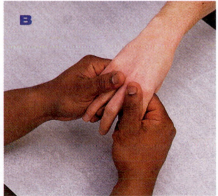
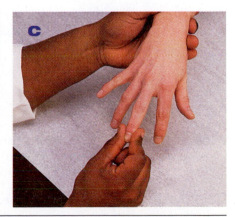

FIGURE 21-29 Palpating the (**A**) wrist, (**B**) metacarpophalangeal joints, (**C**) interphalangeal joint.

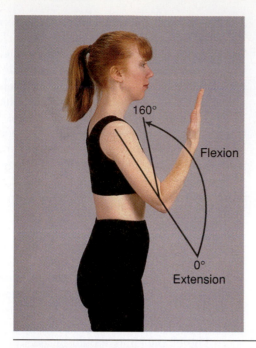
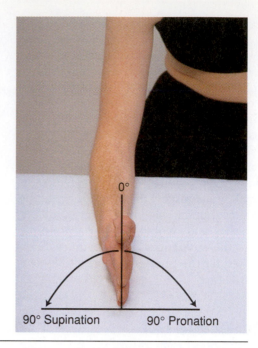

FIGURE 21-30 The range of motion of the elbow joint.

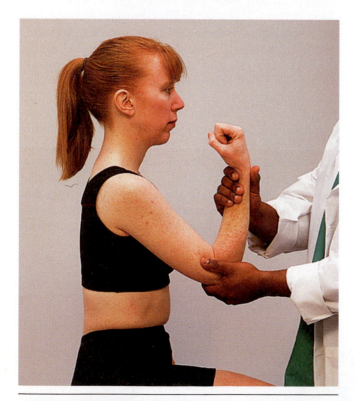

FIGURE 21-31 Testing for the muscle strength of the elbow joint.

The shoulders should be examined for size, shape, and symmetry with the patient in a standing position. Be sure to examine the anterior and the posterior. Check the range of motion of the shoulder joint. First, assess flexion by having the patient place her arms at her sides with her elbows extended and move her arms in an arc. Then have the patient move her arms backward in an arc to test for hyperextension. Next, have her place her arms at her sides with the elbows extended and move both arms out to the sides in an arc until the palms touch together overhead, as shown in Figure 21-32. To test for adduction, have the patient move one arm at a time in an arc toward the midline and cross it as far as possible. Test internal rotation by having the patient place both hands behind her back and reach up as if trying to touch the scapulae. Test external rotation by having the patient place both hands behind her head with the elbows flexed. Finally, ask the patient to shrug her shoulders with the EMS provider's hands on the shoulders to oppose the movement. This maneuver tests the joint strength as well as cranial nerve XI function. Cup both hands over the patient's shoulders and note any crepitation. Palpate over the following locations for tenderness and swelling: the sternoclavicular joint, the acromioclavicular joint, the subacromial area, and the bicipital groove.

Musculoskeletal Examination of the Lower Extremities

Inspect all of the surfaces of the ankle and feet. In addition to looking for DCAP-BTLS, also check for nodules, calluses, and corns. A callus is a thickening of the skin due to pressure. A corn is a conical area of thickened skin, which can be painful because it extends into the dermis.

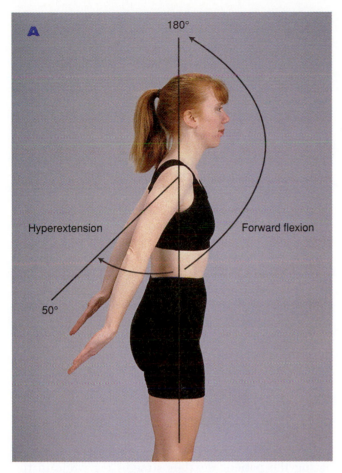

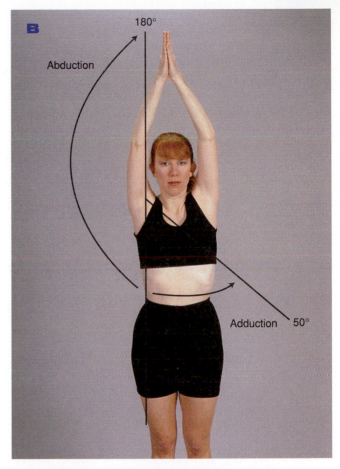

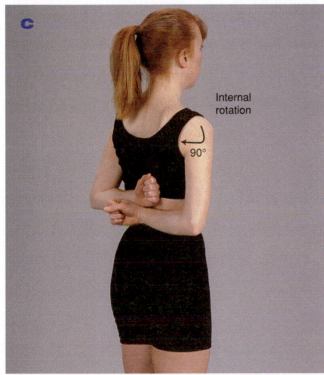

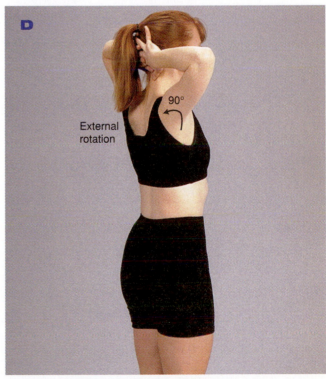

FIGURE 21-32 Testing the range of motion in the shoulder joint: (**A**) forward flexion and hyperextension, (**B**) abduction and adduction, (**C**) internal rotation, (**D**) external rotation.

Palpate for tenderness, bogginess, and swelling in the anterior aspects of each ankle joint (Figure 21-33). Also palpate the Achilles tendon and the metarsophalangeal joints. The strength of the ankle and foot should be assessed. To do this assessment, place one hand under the foot to support it and place the other hand against the toes and provide some resistance. Ask the patient to press her toes down against the resistance (plantar flexion). Then ask the patient to point her toes to her chest against the resistance (dorsiflexion).

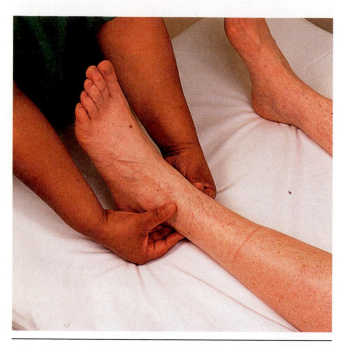

FIGURE 21-33 Palpation of the ankle.

Next test the ankle's ROM. Inspect dorsiflexion by asking the patient to point her toes toward her chest. Plantar flexion can be assessed by asking the patient to point her toes toward the floor by moving her ankle. Eversion is examined by having the patient turn the soles of her feet outward, and inversion is examined by having her turn the soles of her feet inward. Flexion can be observed by asking the patient to curl her toes toward the floor. To assess abduction, have the patient spread her toes, and to check adduction move the toes together. The range of motion of the ankle and foot is shown in Figure 21-34.

Next inspect the hips, looking closely for alignment and deformity. Observe for atrophy of the quadriceps, and palpate the hip joints, noting any thickening or swelling. To assess for the ROM of the hips, lay the patient supine. Assess the flexion by lifting one leg straight up with the knee straight. Then assess flexion with the knee flexed, and assess internal rotation and external rotation by bending the knee and swinging the leg from side to side as shown in Figure 21-35. To assess full external rotation, move the flexed leg laterally as the foot moves medially. Next, with the knee straight, swing the leg away from the midline to assess abduction and toward the midline to assess adduction. To assess hyperextension of the hip joint while the patient is in the prone position, have the patient lift her leg as far back as she can. The strength of the hip joint is assessed by having the patient flex her straight leg while in the supine position against the EMS provider's applying opposing resistance on the thigh. Then have the patient abduct her legs against the resistance on the outsides of the knees.

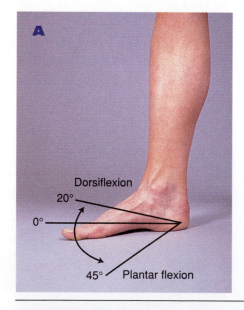

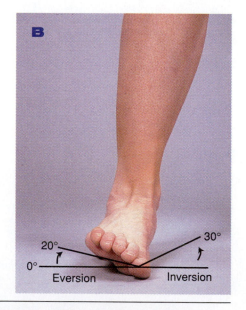

FIGURE 21-34 The range of motion of the ankle and foot: (**A**) plantar flexion and dorsiflexion, (**B**) eversion and inversion.

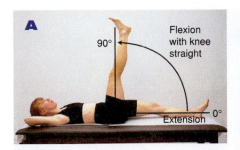
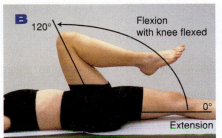
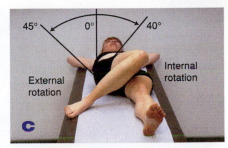
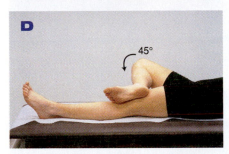
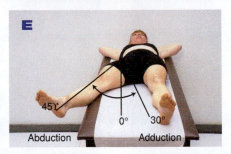
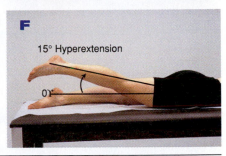

FIGURE 21-35 Assessing the range of motion of the hip joint: (**A**) flexion with the knee straight, (**B**) flexion with the knee flexed, (**C**) internal rotation and external rotation, (**D**) position of the leg for full external rotation, (**E**) abduction and adduction, (**F**) hyperextension.

Inspect the knees, looking closely for scarring, alignment, and deformity. Observe for any thickening or swelling. Palpate the knee and the tibiofemoral joint. The knee joint ROM is assessed by having the patient stand and bend or flex her knee. Then extend and hyperextend the knee as shown in Figure 21-36. The strength of the knee is assessed by having the patient sit down with her legs hanging off the edge of the table. The EMS provider places his nondominant hand under the patient's knee and his dominant hand over her ankle. He then asks the patient to bend and straighten her knee against the resistance.

The Spine

With the patient in the standing position, inspect the spine from side to side, noting the cervical, thoracic, and lumbar curves. Note any abnormal curvatures such as lordosis, kyphosis, or scoliosis.

The normal spine has a cervical concavity, a thoracic convexity, and a lumbar concavity, as shown in Figure 21-37. If you draw imaginary lines across the back from the shoulders, iliac crest, and gluteal fold, they should be level and symmetrical. Look for differences in the height of the shoulders or iliac crest.

The spine's ROM is measured with the patient in a standing position. Observe flexion by asking the patient to bend forward and touch her toes. Pay attention to the smoothness and symmetry of the movement. Assess lateral bending by asking the patient to bend

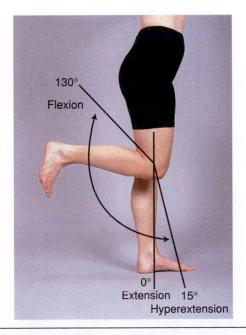

FIGURE 21-36 Assessing the flexion, extension, and hyperextension of the knee joint.

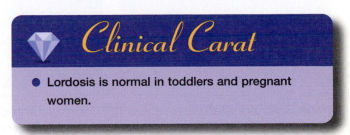

Clinical Carat

- Lordosis is normal in toddlers and pregnant women.

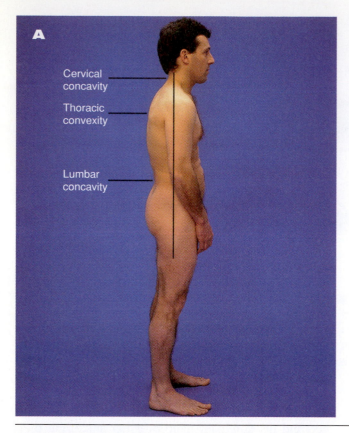

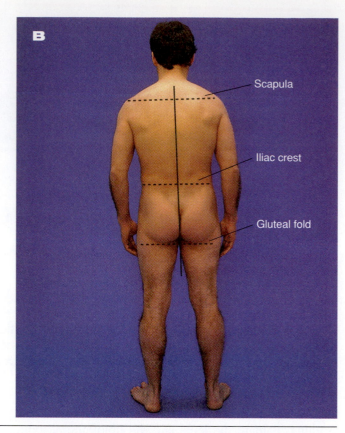

FIGURE 21-37 Alignment of the spinal landmarks: (**A**) lateral view, (**B**) posterior view.

sideways. The EMS provider stands behind the patient to assess extension by asking the patient to carefully bend backward toward him. He then asks the patient to twist her shoulders one way and then the other to assess rotation, as shown in Figure 21-38. Palpate the spinous process with the thumb to identify tender areas. Also palpate the paravertebral muscles for tense areas or muscular guarding. Any pain or tenderness found during ROM assessment could indicate muscle spasm, herniated disc, or problems with ligaments.

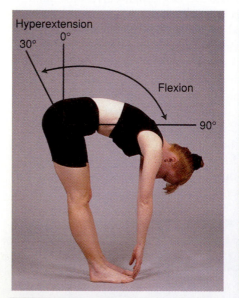

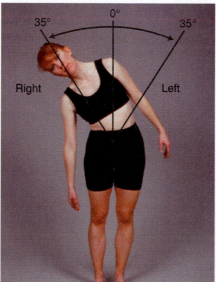

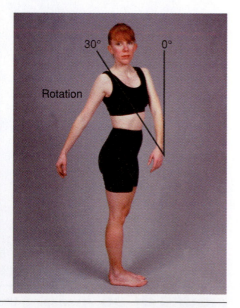

FIGURE 21-38 The range of motion of the spine: (**A**) flexion and hyperextension, (**B**) lateral bending, (**C**) rotation.

Geriatric Gem

- The water content of the intervertebral discs decreases with aging. This decrease results in a reduction of vertebral flexibility. Thinning of the discs, which results in decreased height, makes the geriatric patient prone to back pain and injury.

TABLE 21-5
Pitting Edema Four-Point Scale

+1:	0–¼ inch
+2	¼–½ inch
+3	½–1 inch
+4	>1 inch

The Peripheral Vascular System

The examination of the vascular system begins with an inspection from the fingertips to the shoulders, noting the size, symmetry, presence of swelling, venous pattern, color of the skin and nail beds, and texture of the skin. Palpate the radial pulse. If the EMS provider suspects arterial insufficiency, he should feel for the brachial pulse. Feel for epitrochlear nodes (medial epicondyle at the distal end of the humerus) and assess the legs. The patient should be lying down and appropriately draped. A successful examination cannot be completed with socks or stockings on. Inspect from the groin and buttocks to the feet, noting the size, symmetry, swelling, venous pattern and any venous enlargement, pigmentation, rashes, scars, ulcers, and color and texture of the skin. Palpate the superficial inguinal nodes and the pulses in order to assess arterial circulation. Be sure to assess the following pulses: femoral, popliteal, dorsalis pedis, and posterior tibial. When palpating, be sure to note the temperature of the feet and legs as well as the alterations in the arterial pulses, as discussed in Figure 21-39.

Patients should be assessed for peripheral edema. Edema is an abnormal accumulation of fluid that settles within the intracellular space of the body. With the help of gravity, the spaces where edema settles will be closest to the ground. For example, many people have edema in their feet, ankles, lower legs, arms, and hands because they are usually standing or sitting. When a patient is non-ambulatory or bedridden, edema tends to settle in the sacral area, although it may be present in the extremities. When edema is present unilaterally, consider poor circulation from deep vein thrombosis, recent leg surgery, or injury; bilateral edema is suggestive of heart failure.

Edema is rated as none present, mild, moderate, or severe on a four-point scale. First, observe whether there is edema, then note whether it is pitting. Assess for pitting by pressing your thumb or finger firmly into an area that appears to be edematous and then lifting it. The usual place to check is the dorsum of each foot, behind each medial malleolus, and over the shin. Note the depth of the indentation (pitting) on the skin and how long it takes the skin to return to normal. The deeper the indentation and the longer the skin takes to return to normal, the more severe the edema. Note whether pitting edema is absent. The four-point scale is shown in Table 21-5.

A tool used in the assessment of the peripheral vascular system is called a Doppler. The Doppler principle states that the intensity of sound waves changes as the source changes distance from the listener. For example, when an ambulance approaches, the siren gets louder, reaches a peak as it passes, and then decreases in intensity. A Doppler ultrasound device takes advantage of this principle by using fixed sound waves (the probe) to measure a moving target (flowing blood). Occasionally, the Doppler may be used to detect blood flow in the extremities where a pulse is difficult to obtain.

The Nervous System

The components of the neurological exam may be completed during other assessments. It is best to organize the findings into five categories: mental status and speech (discussed already), cranial nerves, the motor system, the sensory system, and the reflexes. The general approach includes a comparison between the right and left sides of the body for symmetrical findings. The techniques of examination of the cranial nerves include the following steps:

- Cranial nerve I. The olfactory nerve is responsible for the sense of smell. In the field, this is rarely tested. In the clinical setting, the patient would be asked to close her eyes and occlude one nostril. Substances such as tobacco, cloves, coffee, orange, peanut butter, or chocolate are used to assess the patient's sense of smell. Do not use noxious odors because they may stimulate the trigeminal nerve endings in the nasal mucosa.

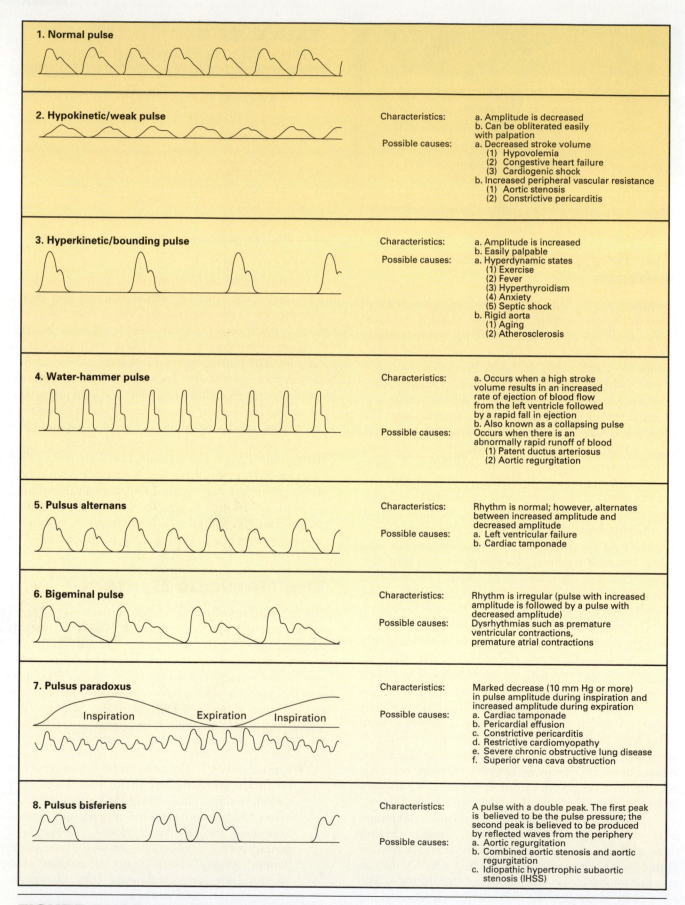

1. Normal pulse

2. Hypokinetic/weak pulse

Characteristics:
a. Amplitude is decreased
b. Can be obliterated easily
with palpation

Possible causes:
a. Decreased stroke volume
    (1) Hypovolemia
    (2) Congestive heart failure
    (3) Cardiogenic shock
b. Increased peripheral vascular resistance
    (1) Aortic stenosis
    (2) Constrictive pericarditis

3. Hyperkinetic/bounding pulse

Characteristics:
a. Amplitude is increased
b. Easily palpable

Possible causes:
a. Hyperdynamic states
    (1) Exercise
    (2) Fever
    (3) Hyperthyroidism
    (4) Anxiety
    (5) Septic shock
b. Rigid aorta
    (1) Aging
    (2) Atherosclerosis

4. Water-hammer pulse

Characteristics:
a. Occurs when a high stroke
volume results in an increased
rate of ejection of blood flow
from the left ventricle followed
by a rapid fall in ejection
b. Also known as a collapsing pulse

Possible causes:
Occurs when there is an
abnormally rapid runoff of blood
    (1) Patent ductus arteriosus
    (2) Aortic regurgitation

5. Pulsus alternans

Characteristics:
Rhythm is normal; however, alternates
between increased amplitude and
decreased amplitude

Possible causes:
a. Left ventricular failure
b. Cardiac tamponade

6. Bigeminal pulse

Characteristics:
Rhythm is irregular (pulse with increased
amplitude is followed by a pulse with
decreased amplitude)

Possible causes:
Dysrhythmias such as premature
ventricular contractions,
premature atrial contractions

7. Pulsus paradoxus

Inspiration   Expiration   Inspiration

Characteristics:
Marked decrease (10 mm Hg or more)
in pulse amplitude during inspiration and
increased amplitude during expiration

Possible causes:
a. Cardiac tamponade
b. Pericardial effusion
c. Constrictive pericarditis
d. Restrictive cardiomyopathy
e. Severe chronic obstructive lung disease
f. Superior vena cava obstruction

8. Pulsus bisferiens

Characteristics:
A pulse with a double peak. The first peak
is believed to be the pulse pressure; the
second peak is believed to be produced
by reflected waves from the periphery

Possible causes:
a. Aortic regurgitation
b. Combined aortic stenosis and aortic
regurgitation
c. Idiopathic hypertrophic subaortic
stenosis (IHSS)

FIGURE 21-39 Alterations in the arterial pulse.

- Cranial nerve II. The optic nerve is responsible for sight and is assessed by testing visual acuity, accommodation, and the field of vision.

- Cranial nerve III. The oculomotor nerve is partially responsible for movement of the eyes. Test the pupil response to light, the cardinal positions of gaze, and the consensual light reflex.

- Cranial nerve IV. The trochlear nerve is partially responsible for movement of the eyes. Test the cardinal positions of gaze and down and inward eye movement.

- Cranial nerve V. The trigeminal nerve is involved with facial sensation, speech, and chewing. Assess the patient's speech for aphasia, dysphasia, dysarthria, or drooling. Move the jaw from side to side against resistance. Palpate contraction of the masseter muscles while the patient bites down, and palpate the temporalis muscles as shown in Figure 21-40. Check for sensation by touching the forehead, cheeks, and jaw on each side for pain sensation.

- Cranial nerve VI. The abducens is partially responsible for movement of the eyes. Test the cardinal positions of gaze and lateral eye movement. Also note any presence of a nystagmus. A nystagmus is a rapid involuntary oscillation of the eyeballs, also seen in VIII evaluation.

- Cranial nerve VII. The facial nerve is responsible for facial movement. Inspect the face at rest and during conversation. Ask the patient to smile and show her upper and lower teeth, then frown and raise her eyebrows. Have the patient puff out both cheeks. Note symmetry, and observe for tics or abnormal movement. Ask the patient to close both eyes tightly and resist while the examiner uses the thumbs to gently open the lids. Test muscular strength by trying to open the patient's eyes, as shown in Figure 21-41. This test should not be done in the back of a moving ambulance.

- Cranial nerve VIII. The acoustic (vestibulocochlear) nerve handles hearing and balance. Assess for acute hearing loss and the presence of vertigo.

- Cranial nerve IX. The glossopharyngeal nerve is responsible for the gag reflex and the palate (taste). Cranial nerves IX and X are assessed together because of their overlap in function. Assess the gag reflex with a tongue depressor or ask the patient to swallow. Have the patient say "aah." Assess the patient's quality of speech and sensation and movement of the palate by checking to see whether the patient can produce guttural and palatal sounds such as the letters k, q, ch, b, and d.

- Cranial nerve X. The vagus nerve is responsible for the gag reflex, swallowing, and stimulation of parasympathetic tone on the heart (causing bradycardia). Assessment of the vagus was done along with cranial nerve IX.

- Cranial nerve XI. The spinal accessory nerve is responsible for the trapezius and sternocleidomastoid muscles (shoulder shrug and head turning). To assess this nerve, have the patient turn her head against resistance and shrug her shoulders against resistance, as shown in Figure 21-42.

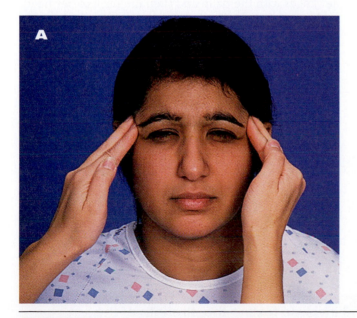 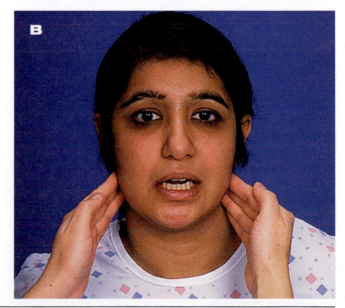

FIGURE 21-40 Assessment of the motor component of cranial nerve V involves the (**A**) temporalis muscles and the (**B**) masseter muscles.

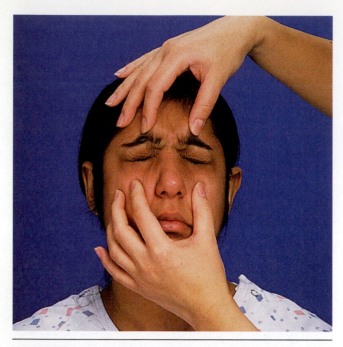

FIGURE 21-41 Assessing the motor component of cranial nerve VII by having the patient try to keep her eyes shut while the examiner tries to pull them open.

- Cranial nerve XII. The hypoglossal nerve is responsible for tongue movements, which are essential to speech clarity. Ask the patient to stick out her tongue and to say "la la la."

The motor system is evaluated by first observing body position and posture during movement and at rest. Look for involuntary movements such as extrapyramidal rigidity, which is an indication of a brain lesion. If there are any involuntary movements, note the quality, rate,

Clinical Carat

- Caution and gentle handling are taken with any patient with a painful injury or condition such as arthritis. Many of these motor tests are not performed if they cause further pain for the patient.

rhythm, and amplitude in relationship to the patient's posture and activity, tremors, tics, fatigue, or emotions. Compare the muscle bulk and contour of the muscles and feel the muscle tone for resistance to passive stretch.

Asking the patient to actively move against resistance can assess muscle strength. Normal muscle tone involves active movement against full resistance without evident fatigue. Watch for any of the following reactions that may occur when the EMS provider asks the patient to move against the resistance: no muscular contraction detected, a barely detectable flicker or trace of contraction, active movement of the body part with gravity eliminated, active movement against gravity, or active movement against gravity and some resistance.

Test for the movement of the following muscle motions in the upper extremities: flexion and extension of the arms, extension at the wrist, grip strength, and the opposition of the thumb. Test for the flexion, extension, abduction, and adduction movement of the muscles in the hips and knees.

Coordination is tested by having the patient demonstrate rapid alternating movements such as moving the hands from supination to pronation and patting her knees with the palm and then the back of her hand, as shown in Figure 21-43. Point-to-point movements are

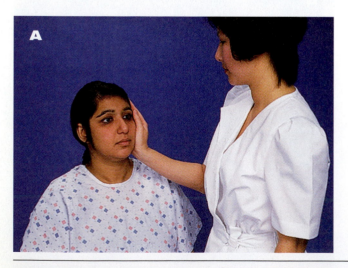

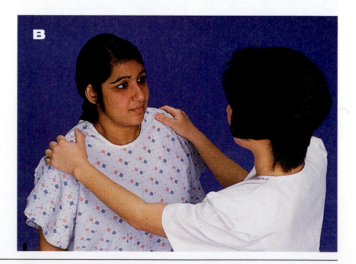

FIGURE 21-42 Assessment of cranial nerve XI involves testing the strength of the (A) sternocleidomastoid muscles and (B) the trapezius muscles.

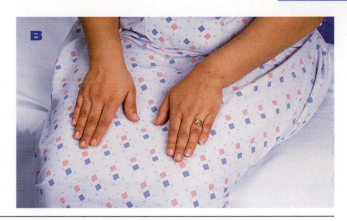

FIGURE 21-43 Assessment of coordination using rapid alternating hand movements from (**A**) supination to (**B**) pronation, patting the knees before turning the hands each time.

also a good way to assess coordination. With the patient's eyes closed, have the patient continue to rapidly alternate touching the index fingers to the nose and extending the arm away from the body as shown in Figure 21-44. Another useful test used to assess the patient's coordination is to have the patient lie supine and slide the heel of one foot along the front of the opposite leg just below the knee down to the shin. Then repeat this test on the opposite leg. Gait is assessed by noting any disturbances in equilibrium. The ability of the body to stand upright and maintain balance and coordination depends on the vestibular, cerebellar, and proprioceptive systems working correctly. Ask the patient to do the following simple tests to examine the gait: walk heel to toe, walk on the toes, walk on the heels, hop in place, do a shallow knee bend, and rise from a sitting position. Next perform the Romberg test, which involves having the patient stand erect with her feet together and arms at her sides. Do this with the patient's eyes open and then closed. The patient should be able to maintain balance with the eyes open or closed for 20 seconds with only a minimum of swaying.

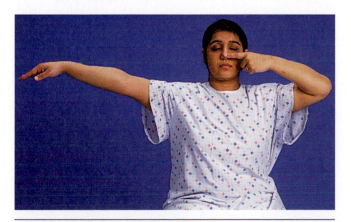

FIGURE 21-44 Assessment of coordination of the fingertip to nose touch.

Clinical Carat

- Some people normally walk with an abnormal gait (e.g., stroke patients or those with multiple sclerosis or Parkinson's disease). Be sure to ask the patient whether this is a new or an existing walking pattern.

Test for pronator drift by having the patient extend her arms out in front of her with the palms up for 20 seconds. There should be no downward drifting of either arm during this time period. The presence of a pronator drift may be an indication that the patient has sustained a stroke.

The deep tendon reflexes are assessed with a reflex hammer in the following locations: biceps, brachioradialis, triceps, patellar, and Achilles, as shown in Figure 21-45. The degree and speed of response of the muscles from the reflex hammer should be noted. The grading of deep tendon reflex appears in Table 21-6.

Finally, assess the sensory system by comparing areas on the two sides of the body. When testing pain, temperature, and touch, compare distal and proximal areas. Assessment of the sensation should be in relationship to the dermatomes and involve the patient's reaction to pain as well as to light touch. If areas are found that have an abnormal response to sensation, make very specific notes on their location. In these instances, it is useful to actually make marks on the patient to note the location of dermatomes that lack sensation. The normal response is that a patient is able to feel without seeing whether the examiner is touching the skin with a sharp or a dull object, such as the point or the eraser of a pencil.

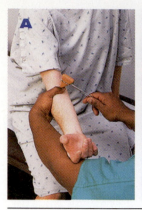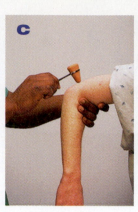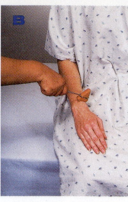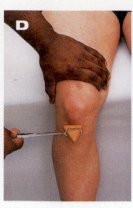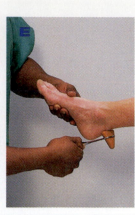

FIGURE 21-45 Assessment of the deep tendon reflexes in the following locations: (**A**) biceps, (**B**) brachioradialis, (**C**) triceps, (**D**) patellar, (**E**) Achilles.

TABLE 21-6
Grading of Deep Tendon Reflexes

0 (−):	absent
+ (1+):	present but diminished
++ (2+):	normal
+++ (3+):	mildly increased but not pathological
++++ (4+):	markedly hyperactive; clonus may be present

THE HEALTH ASSESSMENT

The history of the patient's health assessment is generally not obtained in the field owing to the lack of time. The patient history taken in the field by the EMS provider is a summary of the historical items relevant to today's complaint, known as the SAMPLE history (*s*ymptoms, *a*llergies, *m*edications, *p*ast (pertinent) medical history, *l*ast oral intake, and *e*vents leading up to this incident). This section discusses the additional information that constitutes the comprehensive patient history.

The patient history always includes the date and may also include the time, as is relevant. Next obtain identifying data on the patient such as the age, sex, race, birthplace, and occupation. The latter three items are good examples of information that is not included in a SAMPLE history. Questions the EMS provider should keep in mind include:

- Who called EMS (the patient herself or others)?
- Who was the source of the history (patient, family, friends, police, bystanders), and how reliable is the information?

The history may vary by the patient's memory, how well she trusts you as a health care provider, and her motivation. The EMS provider judges the reliability of the history at the end of the evaluation, not at the beginning.

Clearly, the chief complaint is the main part of the health history. The one or more symptoms that the patient is seeking medical care for are usually described in her own words (e.g., "My head hurts" or "I can't catch my breath"). The history of the present illness is designed to identify the chief complaint and provide a full, clear, chronological account of the signs and symptoms. The letters OPQRST are used to elaborate on the chief complaint: *o*nset; *p*rovocation; *q*uality; *r*egion, *r*adiation, relief, recurrence; *s*everity; and *t*ime.

The past medical history is a description of the following relevant information: general state of the patient's health, childhood illnesses, adult illnesses, psychiatric illnesses, accidents and injuries, major operations, and hospitalizations. The patient's health assessment is the EMS provider's best assessment of her current health status and focuses on the present state of health, environmental conditions, and the patient's personal habits. The following information will offer insight into the patient's state of health: current medications; allergies; use of tobacco, alcohol, or drugs and related substances; current diet; screening tests; immunizations; sleep patterns; exercise and leisure activities; environmental hazards; use of safety measures; family history; home situation; social status; significant others; daily life activities; important experiences; religious beliefs; and the patient's outlook. Finally ask the patient about each of the specific body systems (i.e., respiratory, cardiac, GI, urinary, reproductive, and neurological).

CONCLUSION

The comprehensive examination and health assessment has not traditionally been a part of the responsibilities of EMS providers in the field because it is often conducted on a stable patient in a clinical setting. Although this examination does not fit into the assessment algorithm we have used throughout this book, with the expanding scope of practice in some areas, as well as remote areas where the transportation times may be quite lengthy, your service medical director might decide to authorize this level of assessment. The information provided in this chapter is intended to give all EMS providers a better understanding of the areas that will ultimately be assessed in a comprehensive manner on many patients.

REVIEW QUESTIONS

1. The comprehensive examination involves using your senses to inspect and _____ as appropriate each body part or region.
   a. auscultate
   b. palpate
   c. percuss
   d. all of the above

2. Diseases or illnesses that cause an accumulation of fluid in the lungs will sound _____ upon percussion.
   a. brilliant
   b. hyporesonant
   c. resonant
   d. hyperresonant

3. A patient's insensitivity to unpleasant or painful stimuli due to a reduced level of consciousness from anesthetic or analgesia is called:
   a. coma.
   b. drowsiness.
   c. obtundation.
   d. stupor.

4. The types of speech impairments include each of the following except _____ disorders.
   a. CNS
   b. language
   c. articulation
   d. fluency

5. Difficulty in speaking is a speech disorder called:
   a. aphasia.
   b. dysphasia.
   c. dysarthria.
   d. dysphonia.

6. Fabricating events to cover memory gaps is known as:
   a. blocking.
   b. neologism.
   c. confabulation.
   d. circumlocution.

7. If the skin remains pinched or the natural contour returns slowly after pinching, this response is an indication of:
   a. increased turgor.
   b. poor hydration status.
   c. delayed capillary refill.
   d. increased perfusion to the area.

8. A swishing turbulent sound heard over an artery is known as:
   a. an occlusion.
   b. stenosis.
   c. a bruit.
   d. a thrill.

9. The S1 heart sound is best heard in the _____ area.
   a. tricuspid
   b. mitral
   c. aortic
   d. pulmonic

10. The cranial nerve that is responsible for the gag reflex and the palate for the sensation of taste is cranial nerve:
    a. VIII.
    b. V.
    c. IX.
    d. IV.

CRITICAL THINKING QUESTIONS

1. Explain when it may be appropriate to perform a comprehensive examination and health assessment. Is this commonly done in your service area? Determine any areas that you feel you need more information on, and discuss these areas with your service medical director.

2. Explain the variations that may be needed when doing a comprehensive examination of a pediatric patient, a geriatric patient, and a pregnant patient.

3. What additional information can you get from a comprehensive health assessment that may help in providing better care for the patient? Why is this information important?

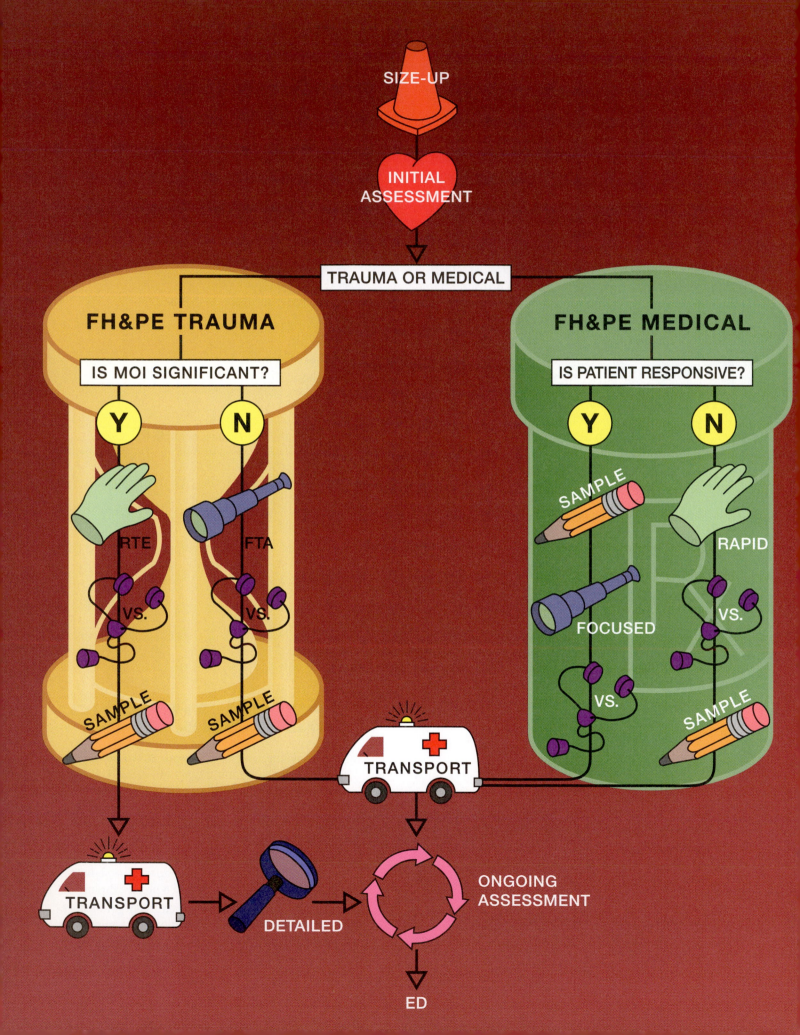

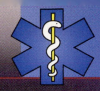

Chapter

22

Putting It All Together

OBJECTIVES

Upon completion of this chapter, the reader should be able to:

- Provide examples of an EMS provider's role in patient advocacy.
- Demonstrate how the patient assessment algorithm is an essential tool for the EMS provider to use in the field.

KEY TERMS

advocate

INTRODUCTION

How does one summarize the process of assessment aside from once again reviewing the assessment algorithm? The whole-part-whole method of teaching can be very effective. So far, this book has provided an overview of assessment (whole) and the specific details in assessment (part). This final chapter is designed to pull it all together (whole again!), using actual examples of practical applications in the field. Various chapters covered the aspects of assessment focused on specific patient medical complaints such as respiratory, cardiac, neurological, and other medical conditions. Other chapters discussed patient assessment for patients needing to have life-threatening conditions uncovered and managed as well as those for whom rapid transport would be essential. In the critical trauma patients, it would be an important decision to eliminate the time for detailed physical examination by doing it en route rather than on the scene. The comprehensive examination of a patient for whom time is not a critical factor and who can be assessed in a very detailed manner was also covered. Time was also spent on setting priorities for assessment and management of the patient. This chapter discusses patient advocacy and presents a series of cases to aid in understanding how the assessment algorithm can be applied in the field.

ADVOCACY

One important point the EMS provider will need to keep in mind is that of her role as a patient care **advocate**. It is the EMS provider's responsibility to advocate (to look out for) for the patient and the patient's needs. These days, emergency departments are usually overcrowded, and the EMS provider, who has spent the last 45 minutes assessing and managing the patient, must help the emergency department staff understand the urgency of the patient's needs by describing what was found and what was done at the scene. In the case of trauma, it may be necessary to impress upon them the speed of the impact, the damage to the vehicle, or the forces and energy involved in the collision. Some EMS providers have someone take Polaroid or digital photos to show the emergency department staff, such as those found in Figure 22-1. Consider the situation of a car crash victim who has a significant mechanism of injury (MOI) (Figure 22-2) yet miraculously sustains no obvious external injuries. This conscious and alert patient would arrive in the emergency department with oxygen, spinal immobilization, a precautionary IV line, and constant management for shock. Yet the potential still would exist for major internal injury due to the MOI, so it is helpful to paint a clear picture of the energy that was involved in the impact for the emergency department personnel.

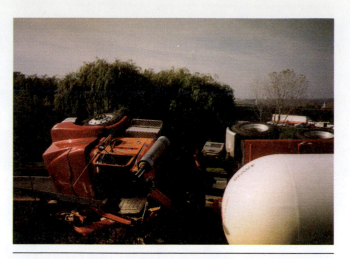

FIGURE 22-1 This photo was taken at the scene of a tanker collision to help the emergency department staff understand the mechanism of injury and degree of entrapment involved.

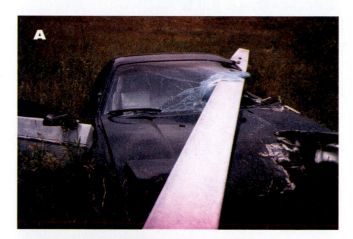

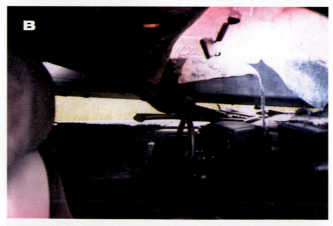

FIGURE 22-2 (**A**) This vehicle came to an abrupt stop when it struck a guardrail at a high rate of speed. (**B**) Notice the damage to the driver's area inside the vehicle.

With medical patients, prehospital interventions often provide dramatic improvements, which could rapidly deteriorate once in the emergency department if the EMS provider does not impress upon the staff the patient's initial condition. Examples include:

- A pulmonary edema patient who received oxygen, nitroglycerin, lasix, and morphine and whose breathing is improving

- A patient with a narcotic overdose who was found in respiratory arrest and was administered bag-valve-mask (BVM) ventilations and Narcan and is now awake

- A diabetic patient who was comatose or seizing who received intravenous dextrose and is now wide awake

- An asthmatic patient who was in severe respiratory distress who was evaluated, received oxygen and an albuterol and Atrovent treatment, was stabilized, and is now breathing more easily

Advocating for patients does not mean arguing with the triage nurse or emergency department physician; it just means making sure they understand what has been seen and learned about the patient. Of course the emergency department staff will have to prioritize the patient on the basis of the facility's available resources and what other patients they already are managing.

Patient Advocacy: A Lesson Learned the Hard Way

Sometimes, the first person to tell the patient's story can leave a lasting impression upon the hospital staff, an impression that can have a serious impact on the patient's care. This point is illustrated in the following story.

While working an evening shift on Medic Unit 185, my partner and I were dispatched to a shooting outside a movie theater in New York City's famed Times Square (Figure 22-3). At the time, which was pre–Mayor Rudy Giuliani, the crime rate was staggering, and most New Yorkers knew this section of the city as one of the most hectic and often dangerous. The non–New Yorkers know Times Square mainly from Dick Clark's New Year's Eve celebration.

Upon our arrival at the scene, the police told us that a male in his twenties had tried to rob the movie theater ticket seller at gunpoint, when an off-duty police officer who happened to be standing in the line intervened. The perpetrator took off on foot, and there was a rapid exchange of gunfire. To obtain cover, the off-duty officer dropped down on his belly behind a parked car. He shot one last time and struck the fleeing assailant in the buttocks.

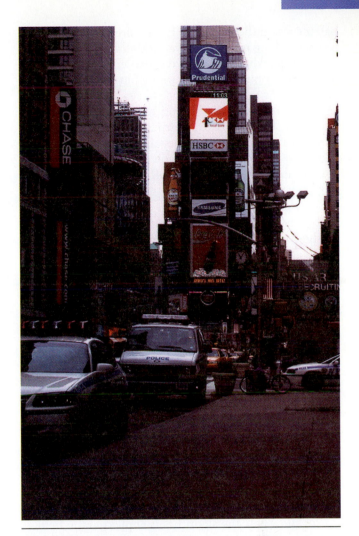

FIGURE 22-3 Times Square in New York City.

By the time we walked over to the patient, the police had surrounded him and secured his weapon, and he was lying on the cold pavement. With the scene secure, we began to evaluate the patient. His vitals were those of a patient with hypoperfusion, and there was no exit wound from the entry in his right buttock. He did have pulse, motor, and sensation (PMS) function in all four of his extremities and had no other apparent injury. The patient had no relevant past medical history but was thirsty, anxious, and very, very scared. We seemed to be the only ones at the scene taking him seriously; the police were all very amused by his shot in the butt! Fitting the criteria at that time for MAST/PASG, he received oxygen and had a large-bore IV inserted en route and the MAST/PASG inflated.

Just as we arrived at the emergency department, a police officer was exiting after "infecting" the emergency department staff with the hilarious story of the "kid who was shot in the ass." The staff were all laughing and said, "Just put him over there!" Trying to advocate for our patient was difficult; the staff had already decided this was something minor. Not wanting to argue, and having to leave quickly on another call, we emphasized that it was more serious and he was losing blood. Unfortunately our concerns fell on deaf ears.

It was a busy night, and we were off to another two calls, back to back, before transporting another patient to the same emergency department that we had taken the shooting victim. Upon our arrival, we found a very different greeting. The staff were no longer laughing; they were almost embarrassed and very concerned about what had happened to our shooting victim. Apparently, about 30 minutes after we left him there, he crashed and went into cardiac arrest. They ran a code on him only to end in asystole. The autopsy the next morning revealed that, owing to the angle of the trajectory, the bullet had struck the hip and fragments had veered downward, severing the femoral artery. The patient had bled to death while on the stretcher in the emergency department. We never seemed to have any problems getting that emergency department staff's attention after that unfortunate incident.

THE ASSESSMENT ALGORITHM IN ACTION

The assessment algorithm presented throughout this book provides a consistent step-by-step approach to assessment of a patient's chief complaint. The following stories show how the algorithm is applied in the field.

A Shiny New Mountain Bike

Let's take a look at a case of a child versus a truck and see how the assessment algorithm helps. For the purposes of this illustration, a few changes have been made to this story.

Having just received her new mountain bike for her birthday, Laura was anxious to try it out. The family loaded up all four bikes on the car's bike rack and drove up to Lake George, New York, to ride through the village and enjoy the sunny day. They parked the car just outside of the village, unloaded the bikes, donned their helmets, and began their ride down the long hill toward the lake. Mom was first, followed by the two kids, and then dad. This was Laura's first time on a bike with hand brakes, so she was not as experienced as she should have been. Suddenly, a rusty old truck made a quick turn from the roadway into a parking lot for the Lake George Diner. Laura saw the truck but was scared and froze for a moment. When she finally did apply the brakes, it was simply too little too late. The bike struck the side of the

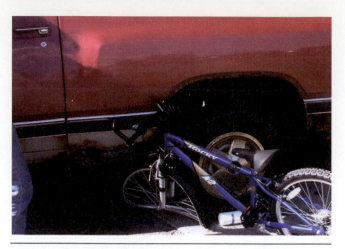

FIGURE 22-4 Laura's new mountain bike moments after the collision.

truck and went under the rear tire. Fortunately for Laura, the driver hit his brakes and stopped just short of crushing her under his rear wheels (Figure 22-4).

The sheriff and Lake George EMS were summoned immediately by cell phone as the child lay crying in pain. Dad quickly told the driver not to move the vehicle as he manually stabilized his daughter's head and neck and told her not to move. Because it was a very busy day for the sheriffs in town, the EMS unit arrived first and followed this course of action:

1. The scene size-up. The unit took body substance isolation (BSI) precautions and ensured that the traffic hazards were being controlled by some helpful bystanders and a few well-placed flares. They also determined there was one patient and that no rescue would be needed but an ALS unit would be helpful.

2. The initial assessment (IA). The IA revealed a general impression of an 11-year-old female conscious and in moderate distress needing spinal precautions due to the significant MOI. Evaluation of the MS-ABCs revealed no immediate threats to life, and the child was alert. Fortunately, she had been wearing a helmet and did not strike her head. She was prioritized as "potentially unstable" owing to the MOI, and oxygen (O_2) via nonrebreather mask was applied right away.

3. The rapid trauma examination. Being a trauma patient with a significant MOI, Laura warranted a rapid trauma examination (RTE), which revealed the following:
   • Head: no injuries
   • Neck: rule out an injury but no actual physical findings
   • Chest: no injuries

- Abdomen/pelvis: contusions to the right hip area, no injuries to the abdomen
- Extremities: right shoulder/humerus pain, positive PMS in all four extremities, possible right closed femur fracture (painful, swollen, deformed extremity)
- Back/buttocks: rule out spine injury by mechanism although no physical findings, abrasion to the right buttock

4. The baseline vital signs:

- Mental status (MS): alert to person, place, and day
- Respirations: 24 and regular
- Pulse: 110, thready, regular rate
- Blood pressure: 104/70
- Skin: pale, cool, and clammy

5. The SAMPLE history. This was obtained by interviewing both the patient and her father. It revealed the following:

- S: pain upon movement in right and left shoulder, no pain in the belly
- A: no known drug allergies
- M: no meds except vitamins
- P: no relevant past medical history
- L: breakfast 3 hours ago
- E: riding bike into side of truck, she remembers the entire incident

6. The detailed physical examination. Because she was a high-priority patient, the EMS unit decided to do the detailed physical examination en route to the hospital. Meanwhile, full spinal immobilization was applied; a Sager traction splint was rapidly applied; and the arm was immobilized to her side on the long backboard. The EMS personnel were on the scene for only about 9 minutes before transporting.

7. Transport. En route to the hospital, the pulse oximeter read 99%, and additional sets of vital signs were taken every 5 minutes. The splints and immobilization were reevaluated and a large-bore IV was inserted. An ongoing assessment (OA) and detailed physical examination (DPE) were also conducted during transport. The hospital emergency department was notified, and Laura was kept warm and comforted in a very caring manner.

Fortunately, what could have been a tragic day turned out to be only a hard lesson learned about biking with hand brakes and the next 6 weeks of the summer on crutches. Had it not been for the excellent assessment, rapid prioritizing, and management skills of the respond-ing EMS providers, who followed the assessment algorithm used throughout this book, the end of this story could easily have been tragic!

A New Garden

Spring had arrived and so had the warm weather. Nick was eager to get out in the garden and plant the early vegetables for the season. Nick had prepared the soil and started the seeds inside weeks before, so he was ready. He spent all morning in the hot sun working in the garden, just as he had done so many seasons before. Nick enjoyed gardening and would often lose track of time just as he had this day. It was early afternoon when he noticed that something was wrong. When Nick stood up, he was dizzy; he suddenly become very warm and headed inside to get some water and to rest. Just before reaching the back door, he collapsed to the ground. Bill and Joan, his neighbors, were outside in the yard next door and saw Nick drop to the ground. They came running over to see what was wrong. Nick was pale but breathing, so Bill tried to wake Nick while Joan used her cell phone to call 911.

Nick came around and told Bill he felt heaviness in his chest and also felt weak. Bill helped him out of the sun into the house just as the ambulance was arriving. As Joan led the paramedics to Nick, she explained what she had witnessed in the yard. The EMS providers took the following steps:

1. The scene size-up. Arriving at a single-family residence and waved in by a calm but concerned woman, the EMS providers determined there was just one patient while taking BSI precautions and ensuring scene safety.

2. The initial assessment. The general impression of a 64-year-old male who was clutching his chest and looking very sick (Figure 22-5) was rapidly

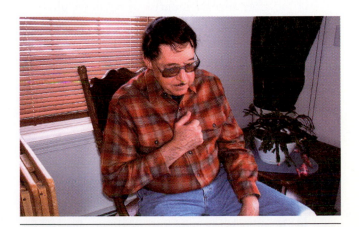

FIGURE 22-5 Nick clutching his chest in pain after being helped into the house by his neighbor.

formulated. The MS-ABCs were evaluated and found to be unstable. Nick was alert and able to describe his chest pain and said that he was having difficulty breathing. His pulse was irregular, and he was extremely sweaty. He was prioritized as "unstable" owing to his cardiac symptoms and was put on oxygen via non-rebreather mask, and a cardiac monitor was quickly attached.

3. The focused history. Because Nick was alert and answering questions reasonably, a focused history using OPQRST and SAMPLE was quickly obtained by the crew leader, while his partner obtained baseline vital signs. The OPQRST revealed:

   - O: while working outside in the garden suddenly began to feel sick and tried to come inside to rest
   - P: physical exertion for several hours before the event
   - Q: heaviness in the center of the chest
   - R: the pain is centered in the chest and the left arm is becoming numb
   - S: worst pain ever, on a scale of 1 to 10 he described it as a 10
   - T: nearly 15 minutes since the syncopal event

   The SAMPLE history revealed the following :

   - S: chest pain, difficulty breathing, and signs of poor circulation
   - A: no known drug allergies
   - M: Lipitor for cholesterol, Accupril for blood pressure, folic acid, vitamins C and E, and one aspirin daily
   - P: one-pack-a-day smoker for 24 years
   - L: light breakfast at 8 A.M.
   - E: performing several hours of physical labor after several months of reduced physical activity

4. The baseline vital signs:
   - MS: alert to person, place, and day but focused on his pain
   - Respirations: 26 and regular
   - Pulse: 56 and irregular
   - BP: 94/58
   - Skin: pale, warm, and moist

5. The focused physical examination. This had been begun on the cardiothoracic system when the patient suddenly became unresponsive. The crew leader quickly assessed for breathing, checked for a pulse, and found none. His partner looked at the cardiac monitor, and the rhythm was ventricular fibrillation. Defibrillation paddles were quickly

applied, and the patient was shocked once. The ECG changed to sinus rhythm on the cardiac monitor. The crew leader checked once again for a pulse, and this time the patient had a pulse. Respirations returned spontaneously and were assessed to be shallow but improving. A blood pressure was obtained, and Nick opened his eyes and asked "What happened?"

6. Transport. Because Nick was a high-priority patient, an IV was quickly started and transportation begun. En route, dysrhythmia-stabilizing medications were administered and the hospital was notified. A rapid physical examination revealed the following:
   - Head: no injuries
   - Neck: flat neck veins
   - Chest: no surgical scars, no injuries
   - Abdomen: overweight, no tenderness or distension, no ascites, no surgical scars
   - Extremities: no injuries, positive PMS in all four extremities without any neurological or motor deficits, no edema
   - Back/buttocks: no injuries

7. The ongoing assessment. En route to the hospital, a 12-lead ECG reading was obtained and showed abnormal tracings. Blood glucose was normal at 118 mg/dL. Pulse oximetry read 100%, and serial vital signs were taken every 5 minutes. Early notification to the hospital had prepared the emergency department personnel, and upon arrival the patient was rapidly assessed and moved to the cardiac catheterization unit.

Luckily for Nick, his neighbors saw him collapse and called EMS right away. The skillful assessment, rapid recognition of a life-threatening dysrhythmia, rapid defibrillation, quality prioritizing and management skills, and early notification to the emergency department all made for a successful outcome for Nick. He spent a short time in the emergency department and then was taken right up to the cardiac catherization unit. Nick received angioplasty followed by bypass surgery that same day. Since then, he has made a full recovery and now has a second chance to enjoy life, his family, and his garden.

Bobcat on the Run

While Medic ambulance 621 was returning from the hospital, the dispatcher put out a call for a traumatic cardiac arrest. "A 36-year-old male involved in a tractor accident is in cardiac arrest" came over the speaker. The EMS crew acknowledged the dispatch, confirmed that the fire department was dispatched, and then switched on the emergency lights and sirens. Five minutes later they arrived at a nursery and garden center. Down a driveway approximately 40 yards from the road a crowd was gathered around a small backhoe called a Bobcat (Figure 22-6). Two men from the crowd ran up to the arriving ambulance and explained that the operator of the Bobcat was slumped over inside the compartment and that the backhoe had been going around in circles with the loader up in the air for several minutes until one of the men was able to jump aboard and shut down the engine.

Police and fire apparatus had arrived just before the ambulance, and other units arrived soon after. Two officers were handling crowd control and getting information about the accident. George and Sandra, the first two paramedics on the scene, proceeded with the following course of action:

1. **The scene size-up.** People from the crowd were attempting to pull the patient out of the tractor, which was on uneven ground with the loader up in the air. George stated that the scene was unsafe for everyone near the machinery, and, with the help of the police officers, directed everyone to get back from the tractor while Sandra found someone who could operate the loader. George had bystanders help chock the wheels with concrete blocks and support the shovel end of the loader with a large log. More EMS personnel arrived as the tractor was stabilized.

2. **The initial assessment.** The MOI was not immediately evident, the tractor did not over turn, and there did not appear to be any obvious crush injuries. Sandra reached into the compartment to check the patient. The general impression was that of a young man who was unresponsive, not breathing, and pulseless; there was blood visibly

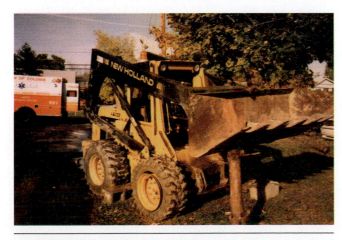

FIGURE 22-6 The Bobcat can be extremely dangerous when the safety cage has been removed.

draining from his mouth and ears. A backboard was quickly lifted up to the edge of the operator compartment, and the patient was rapidly extricated, placed on a backboard, and moved to the ground safely away from the tractor.

3. Manual stabilization of the head was maintained while Sandra performed evaluation of the ABCs, which revealed the following:

   - Airway: Full of blood and small white particles. The mouth and upper airway were suctioned clear and an oral airway was inserted.

   - Breathing: The patient was not breathing. Ventilation by bag-valve-mask was begun while one paramedic prepared to intubate.

   - Simultaneously another pulse check confirmed pulselessness, and chest compressions where begun immediately. The patient's shirt was cut away, and a cardiac monitor was attached. Asystole was the rhythm verified in three leads. The patient was rapidly intubated and moved to the ambulance for further evaluation and rapid transport to the regional trauma center.

   - Once in the ambulance, the patient was resuctioned because the mouth was once again filled with blood and tiny white particles. An IV line was started en route to the hospital, and advanced cardiac life support (ACLS) medications were administered following the asystole algorithm.

5. The rapid trauma examination. Because this was a high-priority patient, the crew decided to perform the rapid trauma examination en route to the hospital. The following was revealed:

   - Head: under the hair, scalp wounds were found on both sides of the head in the shape of two parallel lines, blood continued to seep from the ears

   - Neck: no obvious trauma or deformities

   - Chest: no injuries or scars

   - Abdomen: no injuries or scars, abdominal distension slowly became apparent during transport

   - Pelvis: stable without crepitation on palpation

   - Extremities: no obvious injuries

   - Back/buttocks: no obvious injuries

6. No one on the scene was able to provide a history of what had happened to the patient. The employer knew of no medical conditions, but family had been notified of the accident and would meet the ambulance at the emergency department. The hospital was given early notification of the incoming patient by the paramedic

supervisor on the scene just as the ambulance left the scene.

7. The ongoing assessment. This was limited to evaluation of the ABCs. The placement of the endotracheal tube was continuously reassessed, as were the hand placement and effectiveness of CPR. A second IV line was established before arrival at the emergency department, and a total of 3 liters of fluid had been administered along with the appropriate ACLS medications.

8. By the time they arrived at the emergency department, the ECG rhythm had never changed and the patient's condition had not improved. The patient's family, the police, and an environmental conservation (ENCON) officer arrived at the hospital shortly after the EMS crew. The ENCON officer was able to explain that the cause of accident began with the removal of the safety cage from the operator compartment of the backhoe. The loader has a hinge arm in the rear of the tractor, which raises and lowers the shovel. When the safety cage is removed, the operator is able to stick his head out of the compartment. The operator's head, for whatever reason, was out of the compartment and became crushed by the arm as it was lowering the shovel. This type of accident had happened six times in the past year. During cleanup, it was discovered that the small white particles in the suction container were pieces of brain matter that had bled out into the airway from the cracks in the skull.

Unfortunately for this patient and his family, the outcome was fatal. Even though there was a high potential for injury to people at the scene, no one else was injured. The EMS providers had done an exceptional job, from performing the scene size-up and making the scene safe to making the right priority decisions and providing the best care possible in a timely manner.

CONCLUSION

We hope you, the EMS provider, feel comfortable applying the assessment tools we have tried to convey in this book. They will work for you if you practice them often and follow the algorithm we have followed. We know they work because we see them work every day with our patients and the patients of the many students who have learned to follow this format and apply it in the field.

Thanks for your dedication to helping ill or injured people! You are the real heroes of the twenty-first century. We'll see you in the streets. Bob & Kirsten.

REVIEW QUESTIONS

1. A patient who presents with difficulty breathing of a medical nature should be assessed with the:

   a. scene size-up.

   b. initial assessment.

   c. focused history and physical examination.

   d. all of the above.

2. A patient who presents with a twisted ankle and who did not fall or strike his head should be assessed with all of the following except:

   a. scene size-up.

   b. detailed physical examination.

   c. initial assessment.

   d. FH&PE.

3. An EMS provider's looking out for the needs of the patient is called:

   a. being a patient care advocate.

   b. excessive management.

   c. due regard.

   d. a pertinent negative.

4. One way to help the emergency department staff understand the MOI that was involved in a crash is to:

   a. draw a diagram.

   b. take a Polaroid or digital photo.

   c. tell them more than once.

   d. none of the above.

5. An example of a medical patient for whom it is essential that the EMS provider impress upon the emergency department staff the patient's initial condition would be the:

   a. narcotic overdose patient who received Narcan in the field.

   b. the patient with an allergic reaction who denies any wheezing.

   c. a male who has had lower abdominal cramps for the past 6 hours.

   d. a female who is having labor pains but not yet crowning.

6. What is a key lesson in the case of the male shot in Times Square?

   a. Always take each patient's MOI very seriously.

   b. Sometimes a first impression can be very wrong.

   c. It is the EMS providers' responsibility to advocate for their patients.

   d. All of the above

7. Why was it necessary to conduct the RTE on the child who struck a truck while riding her bike?

   a. All patients should receive an RTE.

   b. All children should receive an RTE.

   c. She had a significant MOI.

   d. She was responsive.

8. If the patient is not responsive, from whom or how can the SAMPLE history be obtained?

   a. from the bystanders

   b. from a family member

   c. by searching for a Medic Alert bracelet

   d. all of the above

9. What was the importance of asking Nick about allergies when he was having his chest pain?

   a. If he had an irregular heartbeat, the medics might need to give him a medication.

   b. His chest pain could have been from an allergy to a medication.

   c. He will be going to surgery upon arrival at the hospital.

   d. He may be allergic to oxygen.

10. Nick's physical examination, based on his chief complaint, should focus on:

   a. abdominal sounds.

   b. lung sounds and pedal edema.

   c. the presence of chest trauma.

   d. strength in both hands.

Appendices

APPENDIX A: ASSESSMENT POCKET TOOL

Printing Instructions: Use this page as the template for these handy cards. Print or copy onto card stock, trim edges, and fold down the middle, leaving the back of card blank.

FOLD

PATIENT PROFILE
(If you need more room, use back of card.)

Age: _____ Sex: _____ CC: _____

General Impression:

Initial Assessment

Mental Status: [ ] A   [ ] V   [ ] P   [ ] U

A: _____

B: _____

C: _____

Priority/Status: [ ] C   [ ] U   [ ] P   [ ] S

Trauma (MOI) or Medical (NOI) _____

Lung Sounds _____ Skin CTC _____ Pupils _____

Baseline Vitals

RR _____ HR _____ BP _____ Temp _____

Focused History (elaborate on CC)

O _____

P _____

Q _____

R _____

S _____

T _____

S _____

A _____

M _____

P _____

L _____

E _____

Diagnostic Tools

SpO_2 _____ %   ECG _____

Glucose _____ mg/dL $EtCO_2$ _____ %

Focused Physical Exam
Significant Findings

Trauma _____

Respiratory _____

Cardiac _____

Neurological _____

Abdominal _____

Behavioral _____

Obstetric _____

GCS _____

Working Diagnosis _____

Treatment Plan _____

_____

_____

_____

_____

_____

_____

_____

_____

_____

_____

Principles of Patient Assessment in EMS, Delmar Learning

APPENDIX B: ABBREVIATIONS

AAA abdominal aortic aneurysm

AAL anterior axillary line

AAP American Academy of Pediatrics

ABC airway, breathing, and circulation

ABCD airway, breathing, circulation, defibrillation

abd abdomen/abdominal

AC antecubital fossa

ACE angiotensin-converting enzyme

ACEP American College of Emergency Physicians

ACH acetylcholine

ACLS advanced cardiac life support

ACS acute coronary syndrome; American College of Surgeons

ACTH adrenocorticotropic hormone

AD affective disorder

ADA Americans with Disabilities Act

AED automated external defibrillator

AEIOUTIPS alcohol; epilepsy, endocrine, exocrine, electrolytes; infection; overdose; uremia; trauma, temperature; insulin; psychosis; stroke, shock, space-occupying lesion, subarachnoid bleed

AF atrial fibrillation

AHA American Heart Association

AICD automated implanted cardiac defibrillator

AIDS acquired immunodeficiency syndrome

AL anterior-left lateral

ALS advanced life support; amyotrophic lateral sclerosis

ALTE acute life-threatening event

AMA against medical advice

AMI acute myocardial infarction

AMP adenosine monophosphate

AMS altered mental status; acute mountain sickness

ANS autonomic nervous system

ANSI American National Standards Institute

A/O alert and oriented

AOI apnea of infancy

AOP apnea of prematurity

AP anterior-posterior

APCO Association of Public Safety Communications Officials

APE acute pulmonary edema

APGAR appearance (color), pulse, grimace (reflex), activity (muscle tone), respirations

ARDS adult respiratory distress syndrome

ASA aspirin

ASL American Sign Language

ATLS advanced trauma life support

ATP adenosine triphosphate

ATV automatic transport ventilator

AV atrioventricular

AVPU alert, verbally responsive, painful response, unresponsive

BAC blood alcohol content

BCLS basic cardiac life support

BiPAP biphasic positive airway pressure

BLS basic life support

BM bowel movement

BP blood pressure

bpm beats per minute; breaths per minute

BS blood sugar; bowel sounds

BSA body surface area

BSI body substance isolation

BTLS basic trauma life support

BTS brady-tachy syndrome

BVM bag-valve-mask

CA cancer

Ca calcium

CAAMS Commission on Accreditation of Air Medical Services

CABG coronary artery bypass graft

CAD computer-aided dispatch; coronary artery disease; carotid artery disease

CAMP cyclic adenosine monophosphate

CAT computed axial tomography

CBF cerebral blood flow

CBT core body temperature

CC chief complaint

C-collar cervical collar

CCU critical care unit

CDC Centers for Disease Control and Prevention

CE continuing education

CEVO certified emergency vehicle operator

CFR Code of Federal Regulations

CHD coronary heart disease

CHF congestive heart failure

CISD critical incident stress debriefing

CISM critical incident stress management

CK-MB creatine kinase-muscle, brain

CI chloride

CMV cytomegalovirus

CN cranial nerve

CNS central nervous system

CO carbon monoxide; cardiac output

CO₂ carbon dioxide

CONTOMS Counter Narcotic and Terrorism Operational Medical Support

COPD chronic obstructive pulmonary disease

COT Committee on Trauma

CP chest pain

CPAP continuous positive airway pressure

CPR cardiopulmonary resuscitation

CQI continuous quality improvement

CRF chronic renal failure

CRT cardiac rescue technician

CSF cerebrospinal fluid

C-spine cervical spine

CT computed tomography

CTC color, temperature, and condition of skin; critical trauma care

CUPS critical, unstable, potentially unstable, stable

CVA cerebrovascular accident

CVC central venous catheter

CVP central venous pressure

DAI diffuse axonal injury

DAN Divers Alert Network

D&C dilation and curettage

DCAP-BTLS deformities, contusions, abrasions, penetrations or punctures, burns, tenderness, lacerations, swelling

DCI decompression illness

DDC defensive driving course

DEA Drug Enforcement Agency

DES diethystilbestrol

DIC disseminated intravascular coagulation

Dig digoxin

DKA diabetic ketoacidosis

DLS dispatch life support

DMD Duchenne's muscular dystrophy

DNA deoxyribonucleic acid

DNAR do not attempt resuscitation

DNR do not resuscitate

DOA dead on arrival

DOB date of birth

DOT Department of Transportation

DPE detailed physical examination

DPL diagnostic peritoneal lavage

DPT diphtheria, pertussis, tetanus

DTs delirium tremens

DVR demand-valve resuscitator

DVT deep vein thrombosis

Dx diagnosis

ECF extracellular fluid

ECG or EKG electrocardiogram

ED emergency department

EDD estimated due date

EEG electroencephalogram

EENT eyes, ears, nose, throat

EGTA esophageal-gastric tube airway

EID esophageal intubation detector

EIF emergency information form

EJ external jugular

EMD emergency medical dispatch

EMS emergency medical services

EMS-C emergency medical services for children

EMSS emergency medical services system

EMT-B emergency medical technician–basic

EMT-I emergency medical technician–intermediate

EMT-P emergency medical technician–paramedic

EOA esophageal obturator airway

EOM extraocular muscle

EPA Environmental Protection Agency

EPI epinephrine

ER emergency room

ERE emergency response employee

ET endotracheal; endotracheal tube

ETA estimated time of arrival

ETC esophageal tracheal combitube

EtCO₂ end-tidal carbon dioxide

EtOH ethyl alcohol

EVOC Emergency Vehicle Operator Course

FAS fetal alcohol syndrome

Fax facsimile

FBAO foreign body airway obstruction

FCC Federal Communications Commission

FD fire department

Fe iron

FEMA Federal Emergency Management Agency

FH&PE focused history and physical examination

FHR fetal heart rate

FHS follicle-stimulating hormone

FHTs fetal heart tones

FiO₂ fraction of inspired oxygen

FLSA Fair Labor Standards Act

FMLA Family and Medical Leave Act

FOIA Freedom of Information Act

FOIL Freedom of Information Law

FU follow up

FUO fever of unknown origin

Fx fracture

GAS general adaptation syndrome

GCS Glasgow Coma Scale

GI gastrointestinal

GSW gunshot wound

gtt/gtts drip/drops

GU genitourinary

GYN gynecology

HACE high-altitude cerebral edema

HAPE high-altitude pulmonary edema

HAV hepatitis A virus

hazmat hazardous material

Hb hemoglobin

HBV hepatitis B virus

Hct hematocrit

HCV hepatitis C virus

HDL high-density lipoprotein

HDV hepatitis D virus

HEENT head, eyes, ears, nose, throat

HELP heat escape–lessening position

HEPA high-efficiency particulate air

HEV hepatitis E virus

HF heart failure

H&H hemoglobin and hematocrit

HHNC hyperosmolar hyperglycemia nonketotic coma

HIV human immunodeficiency virus

HMO health maintenance organization

H₂O water

HPI history of the present illness

HPV human papilloma virus

HR heart rate

HTN hypertension

Hx history

IA initial assessment

IBS irritable bowel syndrome

IC incident commander

ICF intracellular fluid

ICS incident command system

ICHD Intersociety Committee on Heart Disease

ICP intracranial pressure

ICU intensive care unit

ID identification

IgE immunoglobulin

IM intramuscular

IMS incident management system

IO intraosseous

IPPB intermittent positive-pressure breathing

IQ intelligence quotient

IRB institutional review board

ISP Internet service provider

IUD intrauterine device

IV intravenous

IVP intravenous medication push

IVPB IV piggyback

JVD jugular venous distension

K potassium

KCl potassium chloride

KE kinetic energy

KED Kendrick extrication device

KVO keep vein open

LAPSS Los Angeles Prehospital Stroke Screen
LDL low-density lipoprotein
LEA law enforcement agency
LLQ left lower quadrant
LMA laryngeal mask airway
LMP last menstrual period
LOC level of consciousness
LPN licensed practical nurse
LR lactated Ringer's
LUQ left upper quadrant
LZ landing zone

MAL midaxillary line
MAP mean arterial pressure
MAST/PASG military antishock trousers/pneumatic antishock garment
MCI multiple-casualty incident
MD muscular dystrophy; medical doctor
MDI metered-dose inhaler
MI myocardial infarction
MMR measles, mumps, rubella
MODS multiple organ dysfunction syndrome
MOI mechanism of injury
MRI magnetic resonance imaging
MS mental status; musculoskeletal
MS-ABC mental status, airway, breathing, and circulation
MVA motor vehicle accident
MVC motor vehicle crash

N$_2$ nitrogen
Na sodium
NAERG *North American Emergency Response Guidebook*
NAID nonsteroidal anti-inflammatory drugs
NALS neonatal advanced life support
NFNA National Flight Nurses Association
NFPA National Fire Protection Agency; National Flight Paramedics Association
NG nasogastric
NHTSA National Highway Traffic Safety Administration
NIOSH National Institute of Occupational Safety and Health

NKA no known allergies
NOI nature of the illness
NPA nasopharyngeal airway
NPO nothing by mouth
NRB non-rebreather
NREMT National Registry of Emergency Medical Technicians
NS normal saline
NSR normal sinus rhythm
NTG nitroglycerin
N/V nausea and vomiting

O$_2$ oxygen
OA ongoing assessment
OB-GYN obstetrics and gynecology
OD overdose
OG orogastric
OPA oropharyngeal airway
OPQRST onset; provocation; quality; region, radiation, relief, recurrence; severity; time
OR operating room
OSHA Occupational Safety and Health Administration
OTC over the counter

P pulse
PA physician assistant
PAC premature atrial contraction
PaCO$_2$ partial pressure of carbon dioxide in arterial blood
PAD public access defibrillation
PALS pediatric advanced life support
PAR primary area of responsibility
PAT paroxysmal atrial tachycardia
PCC Poison Control Center
PCO$_2$ partial pressure of carbon dioxide
PCP phencyclidine
PCR prehospital care report
PDA personal digital assistant
PE physical examination; pulmonary embolism; pulmonary edema
PEA pulseless electrical activity
PEEP positive end-expiratory pressure
PERRLA *p*upils *e*qually *r*ound, *r*eactive to *l*ight and *a*ccommodation

PFD personal flotation device

pH potential of hydrogen

PHTLS Prehospital Trauma Life Support

PIAA personal injury auto accident

PICC peripherally inserted central catheter

PID pelvic inflammatory disease

PKU phenylketonuria

PMH past medical history

PMI point of maximal impulse

PMS pulse, motor, and sensation; premenstrual syndrome

PND paroxysmal nocturnal dyspnea

PNI psychoneuroimmunology

PNS peripheral nervous system

PO per os (by mouth)

PO$_2$ partial pressure of oxygen

PPE personal protective equipment

PPV positive pressure ventilation

PR per rectum

PSAP public safety access point

PSVT paroxysmal supraventricular tachycardia

Pt patient

PTL pharyngeotracheal lumen

PTSD posttraumatic stress disorder

PTU propylthiouracil

PVC premature ventricular contraction

QA quality assurance

QI quality insurance

RAD radiation absorbed dose

RAS reticular activating system

RBC red blood cell

REM roentgen equivalent in man

RIBA recombinant immunoblot assay

RL Ringer's lactate

RLQ right lower quadrant

RMA refusal of medical assistance

RN registered nurse

ROM range of motion

RPE rapid physical examination

RR respiratory rate

RSI rapid sequence induction

RTE rapid trauma examination

RTPA recombinant tissue plasminogen activator

RTS rapid trauma score

RUQ right upper quadrant

RV right ventricular

RX prescription

SA sinoatrial

SABA supplied-air breathing apparatus

SAMPLE signs and symptoms, allergies, medications, pertinent past medical history, last oral intake, events leading up to this incident

SAR search and rescue

SARA Superfund Amendments and Reauthorization Act

SBS shaken baby syndrome

SCBA self-contained breathing apparatus

SCI spinal cord injury

SCIWORA spinal cord injury without radiographic abnormalities

SIDS sudden infant death syndrome

SL sublingual

SOB shortness of breath

SOP standard operating procedure

SpO$_2$ oxygen saturation of arterial blood measured by pulse oximetry

SQ or SC subcutaneous

SRS supplemental restraint system

SSKI supersaturated solution of potassium iodide

SSM system status management

SSS sick sinus syndrome

START simple triage and rapid treatment

STD sexually transmitted disease

SUDS single unit diagnostic study

SUX succinylcholine

SV stroke volume

SVN small-volume nebulizer

SVR systemic vascular resistance

SVT supraventricular tachycardia

TB tuberculosis

TBI traumatic brain injury

TCP transcutaneous pacer

TEMS Tactical Emergency Medical Support

TIA transient ischemic attack

TKO to keep open
TLCV translaryngeal cannula ventilation
TMJ temporomandibular joint
TOT turned over to
TPA tissue plasminogen activator

UHF ultra-high frequency
ULQ upper left quadrant
URI upper respiratory infection
URQ upper right quadrant
USFPA U.S. Fire Protection Administration
UTI urinary tract infection

VAD vascular access device
VD venereal disease
VF ventricular fibrillation
VHF very high frequency
VS vital signs
VSD ventricular septal defect
V&T vehicle and traffic
VT ventricular tachycardia

WBC white blood cell

APPENDIX C: SKILLS SHEETS FOR FOCUSED ASSESSMENTS

Focused Respiratory Assessment Skills Sheet

	Yes	No
Scene Safety and BSI		
INITIAL ASSESSMENT DID THE STUDENT DEMONSTRATE THE FOLLOWING?		
Assess MS using AVPU		
Assess airway / gag reflex when unresponsive		
Assess respiratory rate, depth, pattern and describe abnormal patterns Assess the patient's effort to speak Listen to lung sounds / Recognize adventitious sounds Recognize level of distress as mild, moderate, or severe		
Assess circulatory status: Recognize abnormal vital signs		
Determine priority		
HISTORY TAKING DID THE STUDENT OBTAIN THE FOLLOWING?		
Obtain SAMPLE history		
Obtain OPQRST information		
FOCUSED EXAMINATION DID THE STUDENT EVALUATE THE FOLLOWING?		
Assess skin CTC / Note the presence of edema—central or peripheral		
Assess for JVD		
Listen to heart sounds / Recognize abnormal heart sounds		
Examine the chest—look, listen, feel, percuss / Note fremitus, abnormal chest size, barrel chest cx, trauma, presence of surgical scars, pacemakers, AICD, transdermal patches		
Assess extremities / Note the presence of peripheral edema or clubbing		
Diagnostic Tools Obtain SpO_2		
Obtain ECG		
Obtain temperature		
Obtain $EtCO_2$		
Peak flow meter		

Focused Cardiac Assessment Skills Sheet

	Yes	No
Scene Safety and BSI		
INITIAL ASSESSMENT DID THE STUDENT DEMONSTRATE THE FOLLOWING?		
Assess MS using AVPU		
Assess airway / gag reflex when unresponsive		
Assess respiratory rate, depth, pattern and describe abnormal patterns Assess the patient's effort to speak Listen to lung sounds / Recognize adventitious sounds Recognize level of distress as mild, moderate, or severe		
Assess circulatory status: Recognize abnormal vital signs and pattern of heart failure or cardiogenic shock		
Determine priority		
HISTORY TAKING DID THE STUDENT OBTAIN THE FOLLOWING?		
Obtain SAMPLE history		
Obtain OPQRST information		
FOCUSED EXAMINATION DID THE STUDENT EVALUATE THE FOLLOWING?		
Assess skin CTC / Note the presence of edema—central or peripheral		
Assess for JVD		
Examine the chest and abdomen / Note the presence of surgical scars, pacemakers, AICD, transdermal patches		
Listen to heart tones		
Identify location of PMI / Note any shift of PMI		
Assess extremities / Note the presence of peripheral edema and surgical scars		
Diagnostic Tools		
Obtain ECG/12-Lead		
Obtain SpO_2		
Obtain $EtCO_2$		

Focused Neurological Assessment Skills Sheet

	Yes	No
Scene Safety and BSI		
INITIAL ASSESSMENT DID THE STUDENT DEMONSTRATE THE FOLLOWING?		
Assess MS using AVPU		
Assess airway / gag reflex when unresponsive		
Assess respiratory rate, depth, pattern and describe abnormal patterns Listen to lung sounds / Recognize adventitious sounds		
Assess circulatory status: Recognize vital sign changes and patterns of Rising ICP = ↑BP, ↓PR, changing respiratory pattern Neurogenic shock = ↓BP, normal or ↓PR, ↓RR		
Determine priority		
HISTORY TAKING DID THE STUDENT OBTAIN THE FOLLOWING?		
Obtain SAMPLE history		
Obtain OPQRST information		
FOCUSED EXAMINATION DID THE STUDENT EVALUATE THE FOLLOWING?		
Assess MS using GCS and by evaluating affect, behavior, cognition, and memory (short- and long-term recall)		
CN II, III: Assess visual acuity, accommodation, field of vision		
CN III, IV, VI: Assess EOMs, consensual light reflex		
CN V, VII: Assess speech, facial movement and sensations (smile, frown, show teeth, move jaw against resistance)		
CN VIII: Recognize acute hearing loss		
CN IX, X: Recognize intact or absent gag reflex, assess uvula		
CN XI: Assess shoulder shrug		
CN XII: Assess protruded tongue for symmetry		
MOTOR SENSATION: Upper extremities—Assess grip strength and pronator drift, finger-to-nose touching, or index finger to index finger with eyes closed Lower extremities—Observe gait, push and pull feet against resistance		
SENSORY SENSATION: Assess sensitivity—sharp vs. dull. When the patient is unresponsive, test deep pain response		
REFLEXES: Plantar reflex, withdrawing from pain stimulus, gag reflex, flexion, extension, or no response		

(continues)

Focused Neurological Assessment Skills Sheet *(continued)*

Diagnostic tools		
Obtain glucose level		
Obtain SpO_2		
Obtain ECG		
Obtain temperature		
Obtain $EtCO_2$		

Focused Abdominal Assessment Skills Sheet

	Yes	No
Scene Safety and BSI		
INITIAL ASSESSMENT DID THE STUDENT DEMONSTRATE THE FOLLOWING?		
Assess MS using AVPU		
Assess airway / gag reflex when unresponsive		
Assess respiratory rate, depth, pattern and describe abnormal patterns Listen to lung sounds / Recognize adventitious sounds		
Assess circulatory status: Recognize abnormal vital signs or shock		
Determine priority		
HISTORY TAKING DID THE STUDENT OBTAIN THE FOLLOWING?		
Obtain SAMPLE history		
Obtain OPQRST information		
FOCUSED EXAMINATION DID THE STUDENT EVALUATE THE FOLLOWING?		
Assess skin CTC		
Assess for JVD		
Examine the chest / Note the presence of surgical scars, pacemakers, AICD, transdermal patches		
Examine the abdomen / Auscultate prior to palpation Note the presence of surgical scars, ascites, distension, rigidity, pulsations, masses, tenderness—generalized vs. localized, rebound		
Assess extremities / Note unilateral or bilateral pulse deficits		
Diagnostic tools		
Obtain ECG		
Obtain SpO_2		
Temperature		

Focused Mental Status (Behavioral) Assessment Skills Sheet

	Yes	No
Scene Safety and BSI		
DID THE STUDENT DEMONSTRATE THE FOLLOWING?		
Ensure personal safety at all times / Wait for police on scene		
Ensure crew safety at all times		
Keep patient safety a priority		
Check for weapons		
Recognize a criminal situation		
INITIAL ASSESSMENT		
DID THE STUDENT DEMONSTRATE THE FOLLOWING?		
Assess ABCs and correct life-threats the same as for any other patient		
Establish baseline vital signs		
Determine priority		
HISTORY TAKING		
DID THE STUDENT IDENTIFY THE FOLLOWING?		
Any psychosocial stress factors		
The number of patients involved		
Any previous or similar episodes		
Additional risk factors		
Obtain SAMPLE history		
Obtain OPQRST information		
EXAMINATION		
DID THE STUDENT DEMONSTRATE THE FOLLOWING?		
Assess patient presentation: affect/behavior using verbal and nonverbal cues		
Assess the patient's orientation and long- and short-term memory		
Recognize speech characteristics; clarity, intonation, content, pace, word choice		
Assess hygiene/appropriate dress		
Consider patient's judgment to be reasonable for the situation / Screen for suicidal/violent thoughts		
Diagnostic tools		
Obtain ECG		
Obtain SpO_2		
Obtain glucose level		

Focused Obstetric Assessment Skills Sheet

	Yes	No
Scene Safety and BSI		
INITIAL ASSESSMENT DID THE STUDENT DEMONSTRATE THE FOLLOWING?		
Assess MS using AVPU		
Assess airway / gag reflex when unresponsive		
Recall the normal vital sign changes that occur throughout pregnancy		
Assess respiratory rate, depth, and pattern and describe abnormal patterns / Respiratory rate is usually normal or slightly increased Listen to lung sounds / Recognize adventitious sounds		
Assess HR / Note that resting heart rate is increased 15 to 20 bpm throughout pregnancy		
Assess BP / Note that normal decrease by 10 to 15 mm Hg during the second trimester and a return to normal in the third trimester Note hypertension as being abnormal and a significant finding in pregnancy		
Determine priority		
HISTORY TAKING DID THE STUDENT OBTAIN THE FOLLOWING?		
Obtain obstetric history • Date of last menstrual period (LMP) • Current week of gestation (38 to 42 is term) / Estimated due date (EDD) • Number of fetuses / Is the fetus in an abnormal position? • Has there been any preterm labor or false labor (Braxton Hicks contractions)? • Prior pregnancies: Gravida—total number of pregnancies / Parity—total number of births • Duration of each prior gestation / Number of preterm pregnancies • Any prior abortions or miscarriages? How many and were they spontaneous or elective? • Type of prior delivery—vaginal (spontaneous or induced) or cesarean section (use of force or vacuum extraction, episiotomy or laceration) • Complications during pregnancy (hypertension, gestational diabetes) • Length of labor(s), precipitous delivery (labor and delivery in less than 3 hours)		
Obtain SAMPLE history		
Obtain OPQRST information		
FOCUSED EXAMINATION DID THE STUDENT EVALUATE THE FOLLOWING?		
Let the patient keep a position of comfort and provide reassurance during examination		
Assess lung sounds / Note that the costal angle may feel wider / Note that abnormal heart sounds may be heard and are normal during pregnancy		

(continues)

Focused Obstetric Assessment Skills Sheet *(continued)*

Assess the abdomen for tenderness, guarding, and rebound tenderness		
Assess skin CTC / Note the presence of generalized edema (signs of preeclampsia)		
Note orthostatic changes / postural hypotension in third trimester		
Assess external genitalia for signs of imminent delivery, crowning, bleeding, cord or limb presentation		
FETAL ASSESSMENT DID THE STUDENT EVALUATE THE FOLLOWING?		
Fundal height		
Fetal heart rate		
Fetal movement / Contractions—timed, length, and regularity		

APPENDIX D: PRACTICAL EVALUATION SKILL SHEETS

These two assessment practical skill sheets are only a part of the National Registry of Emergency Medical Technicians' (NREMT) Advanced Level Practical Examination for the 1998 EMT-Paramedic National Standard Curriculum. These skill sheets should not be used as a substitute during an NREMT Advanced Level Practical Examination. The NREMT representative will provide the actual testing sheets to be used which are color coded. The sheets were designed to be used as a standardized evaluation instrument for determining an individual's competency for an identified psychomotor skill.

National Registry of Emergency Medical Technicians
Advanced Level Practical Examination

PATIENT ASSESSMENT - TRAUMA

Candidate: _____   Examiner: _____

Date: _____   Signature: _____

Scenario # _____

Time Start: _____ NOTE: Areas denoted by "**" may be integrated within sequence of Initial Assessment	Possible Points	Points Awarded
Takes or verbalizes body substance isolation precautions	1	
SCENE SIZE-UP		
Determines the scene/situation is safe	1	
Determines the mechanism of injury/nature of illness	1	
Determines the number of patients	1	
Requests additional help if necessary	1	
Considers stabilization of spine	1	
INITIAL ASSESSMENT/RESUSCITATION		
Verbalizes general impression of the patient	1	
Determines responsiveness/level of consciousness	1	
Determines chief complaint/apparent life-threats	1	
Airway -Opens and assesses airway (1 point) -Inserts adjunct as indicated (1 point)	2	
Breathing -Assess breathing (1 point) -Assures adequate ventilation (1 point) -Initiates appropriate oxygen therapy (1 point) -Manages any injury which may compromise breathing/ventilation (1 point)	4	
Circulation -Checks pulse (1point) -Assess skin [either skin color, temperature, or condition] (1 point) -Assesses for and controls major bleeding if present (1 point) -Initiates shock management (1 point)	4	
Identifies priority patients/makes transport decision	1	
FOCUSED HISTORY AND PHYSICAL EXAMINATION/RAPID TRAUMA ASSESSMENT		
Selects appropriate assessment	1	
Obtains, or directs assistant to obtain, baseline vital signs	1	
Obtains SAMPLE history	1	
DETAILED PHYSICAL EXAMINATION		
Head -Inspects mouth**, nose**, and assesses facial area (1 point) -Inspects and palpates scalp and ears (1 point) -Assesses eyes for PERRL** (1 point)	3	
Neck** -Checks position of trachea (1 point) -Checks jugular veins (1 point) -Palpates cervical spine (1 point)	3	
Chest** -Inspects chest (1 point) -Palpates chest (1 point) -Auscultates chest (1 point)	3	
Abdomen/pelvis** -Inspects and palpates abdomen (1 point) -Assesses pelvis (1 point) -Verbalizes assessment of genitalia/perineum as needed (1 point)	3	
Lower extremities** -Inspects, palpates, and assesses motor, sensory, and distal circulatory functions (1 point/leg)	2	
Upper extremities -Inspects, palpates, and assesses motor, sensory, and distal circulatory functions (1 point/arm)	2	
Posterior thorax, lumbar, and buttocks** -Inspects and palpates posterior thorax (1 point) -Inspects and palpates lumbar and buttocks area (1 point)	2	
Manages secondary injuries and wounds appropriately	1	
Performs ongoing assessment	1	

Time End: _____   **TOTAL**   43

CRITICAL CRITERIA

_____ Failure to initiate or call for transport of the patient within 10 minute time limit
_____ Failure to take or verbalize body substance isolation precautions
_____ Failure to determine scene safety
_____ Failure to assess for and provide spinal protection when indicated
_____ Failure to voice and ultimately provide high concentration of oxygen
_____ Failure to assess/provide adequate ventilation
_____ Failure to find or appropriately manage problems associated with airway, breathing, hemorrhage or shock [hypoperfusion]
_____ Failure to differentiate patient's need for immediate transportation versus continued assessment/treatment at the scene
_____ Does other detailed/focused history or physical exam before assessing/treating threats to airway, breathing, and circulation
_____ Orders a dangerous or inappropriate intervention

You must factually document your rationale for checking any of the above critical items on the reverse side of this form.

p301/8-003k

National Registry of Emergency Medical Technicians
Advanced Level Practical Examination

PATIENT ASSESSMENT - MEDICAL

Candidate: _____   Examiner: _____

Date: _____   Signature: _____

Scenario: _____

	Possible Points	Points Awarded
Time Start: _____		
Takes or verbalizes body substance isolation precautions	1	
SCENE SIZE-UP		
Determines the scene/situation is safe	1	
Determines the mechanism of injury/nature of illness	1	
Determines the number of patients	1	
Requests additional help if necessary	1	
Considers stabilization of spine	1	
INITIAL ASSESSMENT		
Verbalizes general impression of the patient	1	
Determines responsiveness/level of consciousness	1	
Determines chief complaint/apparent life-threats	1	
Assesses airway and breathing	3	
-Assessment (1 point)		
-Assures adequate ventilation (1 point)		
-Initiates appropriate oxygen therapy (1 point)		
Assesses circulation	3	
-Assesses/controls major bleeding (1 point) -Assesses skin [either skin color, temperature, or condition] (1 point)		
-Assesses pulse (1 point)		
Identifies priority patients/makes transport decision	1	
FOCUSED HISTORY AND PHYSICAL EXAMINATION/RAPID ASSESSMENT		
History of present illness	8	
-Onset (1 point) -Severity (1 point)		
-Provocation (1 point) -Time (1 point)		
-Quality (1 point) -Clarifying questions of associated signs and symptoms as related to OPQRST (2 points)		
-Radiation (1 point)		
Past medical history	5	
-Allergies (1 point) -Past pertinent history (1 point) -Events leading to present illness (1 point)		
-Medications (1 point) -Last oral intake (1 point)		
Performs focused physical examination [assess affected body part/system or, if indicated, completes rapid assessment]	5	
-Cardiovascular -Neurological -Integumentary -Reproductive		
-Pulmonary -Musculoskeletal -GI/GU -Psychological/Social		
Vital signs	5	
-Pulse (1 point) -Respiratory rate and quality (1 point each)		
-Blood pressure (1 point) -AVPU (1 point)		
Diagnostics [must include application of ECG monitor for dyspnea and chest pain]	2	
States field impression of patient	1	
Verbalizes treatment plan for patient and calls for appropriate intervention(s)	1	
Transport decision re-evaluated	1	
ON-GOING ASSESSMENT		
Repeats initial assessment	1	
Repeats vital signs	1	
Evaluates response to treatments	1	
Repeats focused assessment regarding patient complaint or injuries	1	
Time End: _____		
CRITICAL CRITERIA **TOTAL**	48	

_____ Failure to initiate or call for transport of the patient within 15 minute time limit

_____ Failure to take or verbalize body substance isolation precautions

_____ Failure to determine scene safety before approaching patient

_____ Failure to voice and ultimately provide appropriate oxygen therapy

_____ Failure to assess/provide adequate ventilation

_____ Failure to find or appropriately manage problems associated with airway, breathing, hemorrhage or shock [hypoperfusion]

_____ Failure to differentiate patient's need for immediate transportation versus continued assessment and treatment at the scene

_____ Does other detailed or focused history or physical examination before assessing and treating threats to airway, breathing, and circulation

_____ Failure to determine the patient's primary problem

_____ Orders a dangerous or inappropriate intervention

_____ Failure to provide for spinal protection when indicated

You must factually document your rationale for checking any of the above critical items on the reverse side of this form.

p302/8-003k

APPENDIX E: EMERGENCY INFORMATION FORM FOR CHILDREN WITH SPECIAL NEEDS

Emergency Information Form for Children With Special Needs

American College of
Emergency Physicians®

American Academy
of Pediatrics

| Date form completed By Whom | Revised | Initials |
| | Revised | Initials |

Last name:

Name:	Birth date:	Nickname:
Home Address:	Home/Work Phone:	
Parent/Guardian:	Emergency Contact Names & Relationship:	
Signature/Consent*:		
Primary Language:	Phone Number(s):	

Physicians:

Primary care physician:	Emergency Phone:
	Fax:
Current Specialty physician: Specialty:	Emergency Phone:
	Fax:
Current Specialty physician: Specialty:	Emergency Phone:
	Fax:
Anticipated Primary ED:	Pharmacy:
Anticipated Tertiary Care Center:	

Diagnoses/Past Procedures/Physical Exam:

1.

Baseline physical findings:

2.

3.

Baseline vital signs:

4.

Synopsis:

Baseline neurological status:

*Consent for release of this form to health care providers

(Reprinted with permission of the American College of Emergency Physicians)

Diagnoses/Past Procedures/Physical Exam continued:

Medications:

1.

2.

3.

4.

5.

6.

Significant baseline ancillary findings (lab, x-ray, ECG):

Prostheses/Appliances/Advanced Technology Devices:

Management Data:

Allergies: Medications/Foods to be avoided   and why:

1.

2.

3.

Procedures to be avoided   and why:

1.

2.

3.

Immunizations

Dates						Dates					
DPT						Hep B					
OPV						Varicella					
MMR						TB status					
HIB						Other					

Antibiotic prophylaxis: Indication: Medication and dose:

Common Presenting Problems/Findings With Specific Suggested Managements

Problem	Suggested Diagnostic Studies	Treatment Considerations

Comments on child, family, or other specific medical issues:

Physician/Provider Signature: **Print Name:**

APPENDIX F: ANSWER KEY TO REVIEW QUESTIONS

Chapter 1
1. b
2. c
3. b
4. c
5. b
6. a
7. d
8. b
9. b
10. a

Chapter 2
1. d
2. c
3. c
4. b
5. d
6. c
7. a
8. b
9. a
10. b

Chapter 3
1. c
2. d
3. c
4. b
5. a
6. d
7. b
8. a
9. b
10. d

Chapter 4
1. c
2. d
3. b
4. c
5. b
6. b
7. c
8. d
9. a
10. c

Chapter 5
1. b
2. b
3. c
4. a
5. d
6. b
7. b
8. d
9. a
10. c

Chapter 6
1. b
2. d
3. c
4. c
5. c
6. d
7. c
8. c
9. b
10. d

Chapter 7
1. c
2. b
3. d
4. b
5. c
6. b
7. c
8. a
9. b
10. d

Chapter 8
1. c
2. d
3. b
4. a
5. c
6. b
7. c
8. d
9. c
10. c

Chapter 9
1. b
2. d
3. a
4. b
5. d
6. c
7. d
8. a
9. c
10. b

Chapter 10

1. c
2. d
3. b
4. d
5. a
6. c
7. a
8. c
9. d
10. b

Chapter 11

1. c
2. b
3. c
4. d
5. b
6. a
7. d
8. c
9. b
10. a

Chapter 12

1. b
2. c
3. d
4. c
5. d
6. a
7. c
8. a
9. c
10. b

Chapter 13

1. c
2. d
3. a
4. d
5. b
6. c
7. a
8. b
9. c
10. d

Chapter 14

1. b
2. a
3. b
4. c
5. d
6. b
7. a
8. d
9. c
10. c

Chapter 15

1. c
2. a
3. b
4. c
5. a
6. b
7. d
8. a
9. b
10. a

Chapter 16

1. c
2. d
3. a
4. b
5. c
6. d
7. a
8. c
9. b
10. d

Chapter 17

1. c
2. b
3. d
4. b
5. b
6. c
7. c
8. d
9. d
10. c

Chapter 18

1. c
2. b
3. a
4. c
5. b
6. d
7. d
8. b
9. b
10. b

Chapter 19

1. b
2. a
3. d
4. c
5. c
6. b
7. b
8. c
9. a
10. d

Chapter 20

1. c
2. d
3. a
4. d
5. b
6. d
7. c
8. a
9. d
10. b

Chapter 21

1. d
2. b
3. c
4. a
5. b
6. c
7. b
8. c
9. b
10. c

Chapter 22

1. d
2. b
3. a
4. b
5. a
6. d
7. c
8. d
9. a
10. c

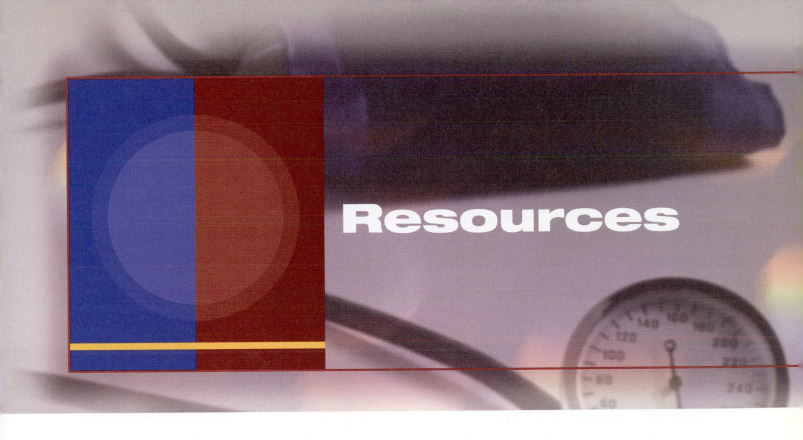

Resources

Abrams, W., & Berkow, R. (Eds.). (1990). *The Merck manual of geriatrics*. Rahway, NJ: Merck Sharp & Dohme Research Laboratories.

American Cancer Society. (2001, April 9). *What causes cancer?* [On-line]. Available: http://www.cancer.org.

American College of Emergency Physicians. (1997, April 29). Emergency care guidelines. *Annals of Emergency Medicine, 4*, 564–571.

American College of Emergency Physicians, Tintinalli, J., Rothstein, R., & Krome, R. (Eds.). (1992). *Emergency medicine: A comprehensive study guide* (3rd ed.). New York: McGraw-Hill.

American Diabetes Association. (2002, August). *Diabetes and seniors* [On-line]. Available: http://www.diabetes.org.

American Psychiatric Association. (1994). *Diagnostic and statistical manual of mental disorders: DSM-IV*. Washington, DC: American Psychiatric Association.

American Psychiatric Association. (1997). *Mental illnesses: An overview* [On-line]. Available: http://www.psych.org/public_info/overview.cfm.

Anderson, D. (1994). *Dorland's illustrated medical dictionary* (28th ed.). Philadelphia: Saunders.

Bates, B. (1995). *A guide to physical examination and history taking* (6th ed.). Philadelphia: Lippincott.

Brown, E. (1998). *Basic concepts in pathology: A student's survival guide*. New York: McGraw-Hill.

Campbell, J. (1998). *Basic trauma life support* (2nd ed.). Upper Saddle River, NJ: Prentice Hall.

Centers for Disease Control and Prevention. (1999, Fall). *Preventing the diseases of aging*. Chronic Disease Notes and Reports, 12(3) 1–3.

Centers for Disease Control and Prevention, National Center for Health Statistics. (1995, Feb. 1). *Injury-related visits to hospital emergency departments: United States, 1992* [On-line]. Available: http://www.cdc.gov/nchs/releases/95facts/fs_ad261.htm.

Centers for Disease Control and Prevention, National Center for Injury Prevention and Control. http://www.cdc.gov/ncipc/ncipchm.htm

Champion, H. R. (1989). A revision of the trauma score. *Journal of Trauma, 29*(5), 623.

Cleveland Clinic. (2000). *High blood pressure* [On-line]. Available: http://my.webmd.com/condition_center/cvd.

Committee on Trauma. (1997). Shock. In Committee on Trauma, American College of Surgeons, *Advanced trauma life support for doctors*. Chicago: American College of Surgeons.

Cummins, R., & Hazinski, M. (Eds.). (2000, August 22). Guidelines 2000 for cardiopulmonary resuscitation and emergency cardiovascular care. *Circulation, 102*(8) (American Heart Association Suppl.).

Eichelberger, M., Pratsch, G., Ball, J., & Clark, J. (1992). *Pediatric emergencies*. Upper Saddle River, NJ: Prentice Hall.

Elling, B. (1989, January). Expanding the primary survey of a trauma patient. *Emergency Medical Services, 18*(1), 33–40.

Elling, B. (1989, January). The primary survey: Another perspective. *Emergency, 21*(1), 12.

Elling, B. (1989, March). Waging war on trauma. *Emergency, 21*(3), 36–39.

Elling, B. (1992, February). Patient assessment. In *Pulse: Emergency Medical Update* [video series]. Carrollton, TX: Primedia.

Elling, B. (1992, May). Assessing lung sounds. In *Pulse: Emergency Medical Update* [video series]. Carrollton, TX: Primedia.

Elling, B. (1992, November). Assessment based approach to the patient with chest pain. In *Pulse: Emergency Medical Update* [video series]. Carrollton, TX: Primedia.

Elling, B. (1993, May). Assessment approach to the acute abdomen. In *Pulse: Emergency Medical Update* [video series]. Carrollton, TX: Primedia.

Elling, B. (1993, August). Assessment approach to the patient with syncopy. In *Pulse: Emergency Medical Update* [video series]. Carrollton, TX: Primedia.

Elling, B. (1993, October). Assessment approach to the patient with dyspnea. In *Pulse: Emergency Medical Update* [video series]. Carrollton, TX: Primedia.

Elling, B. (1998, April). *The assessment tool: Designed to assist New York State's CICs and CLIs teaching EMT-Basic.* Albany, NY: New York State Emergency Medical Services Bureau.

Elling, B. (2002, May). *Pocket reference for the EMT-B and first responder* (2nd ed.). Upper Saddle River, NJ: Prentice Hall.

Elling, B., & Elling, K. (2001). *The paramedic review.* Clifton Park, NY: Delmar Learning.

Elling, B., Elling, K., & Rothenberg, M. (2001). *Why-driven EMS enrichment.* Clifton Park, NY: Delmar Learning.

Estes, M. E. Z. (2002). *Health assessment and physical examination* (2nd ed.). Clifton Park, NY: Delmar Learning.

Fultin, G., Tunik, M., Cooper, A., Markenson, D. Treiber, M., Phillips, R., & Karpeles, T. (1998). *Teaching resource for instructors of prehospital pediatrics.* New York: Center for Pediatric Emergency Medicine.

Ghajar, G. (2000). *Guidelines for prehospital management of traumatic brain injury.* New York: Brain Trauma Foundation.

Gray, H. (1977). *Gray's anatomy* (16th ed.). London: Bounty Books.

Guyton, A. (1986). *Textbook of medical physiology* (7th ed.). Philadelphia: Saunders.

Heide, E. A. (1989). *Disaster response: Principles of preparation and coordination.* St. Louis, MO: Mosby.

Henry, M., & Stapleton, E. (1992). *EMT prehospital care.* Philadelphia: Saunders.

Hubble, M., & Hubble, J. (2002). *Principles of advanced trauma care.* Clifton Park, NY: Delmar Learning.

Huszar, R. (1994). *Basic dysrhythmias* (2nd ed.). St. Louis, MO: Mosby Year-Book.

Kidwell, C. S., Sauer, J. L., Schubert, G. B., Eckstein, M., & Starkman, S. (1998). Design and retrospective analysis of the Los Angeles Prehospital Stroke Screen (LAPSS). *Prehospital Emergency Care, 2,* 267–273.

Kidwell, C. S., Starkman, S., Eckstein, M., Weems, K., & Sauer, J. L. (2000). Identifying stroke in the field: Prospective validation of the Los Angeles Prehospital Stroke Screen (LAPSS). *Stroke, 31,* 71–76.

Kposowa, A. (2000, March). National longitudinal mortality study on suicide. *Journal of Epidemiology and Community Health, 54*(4), 254–261.

Limmer, D., Elling, B., & O'Keefe, M. (2002). *Essentials of emergency care: A refresher for the practicing EMT-B* (3rd ed.). Upper Saddle River, NJ: Prentice Hall.

Limmer, D., O'Keefe, M., Grant, H., Murray, R., & Bergeron, J. (2001). *Emergency care* (9th ed.). Upper Saddle River, NJ: Prentice Hall Publishers.

Luckman, J. (2000). *Transcultural comminication in health care.* Clifton Park, NY: Delmar Learning.

Manisclaco, P. (2002). *Understanding terrorism and managing the consequences.* Upper Saddle River, NJ: Prentice Hall.

Martini, F. (1998). *Fundamentals of anatomy and physiology* (4th ed.). Upper Saddle River, NJ: Prentice Hall.

Mitchell, J., & Bray, G. (1990). *Emergency services stress.* Upper Saddle River, NJ: Prentice Hall.

National Safety Council. (2000). *Accident facts.* Itasca, IL: author.

Prehospital Trauma Life Support Committee of the National Association of Emergency Medical Technicians In Cooperation with the Committee on Trauma of The American College of Surgeons. (1999). *PHTLS: Basic and advanced prehospital trauma life support* (4th ed.). St. Louis, MO: Mosby.

Peters, K. D., Kochanek, K. D., & Murphy, S. L. (1998). Deaths: Final data for 1996. *National Vital Statistics Reports, 47*(9). Hyattsville, MD: National Center for Health Statistics.

Rothenberg, M. (2001). *Pathophysiology: A plain English approach.* Eau Claire, WI: PESI HealthCare.

Saltrones, M., Elling, B., & Politis, J. (1995, March). *Basic skills video series* (seven videos and instructor guides for the EMT-B instructor). Seattle, WA: Emergency Medical Update.

Stoy, W., & Margolis, G. (1997, March). *Intermediate: National standard curriculum.* Washington, DC: U.S. Government Printing Office.

Stoy, W., & Margolis, G. (1997, March). *Paramedic: National standard curriculum.* Washington, DC: U.S. Government Printing Office.

Thibodeau, G., & Patton, K. (Eds.). (1999). *Anthony's textbook of anatomy and physiology* (16th ed.). St. Louis, MO: Mosby.

U.S. Consumer Product Safety Commission. (2002). *Home safety checklist for older consumers* (CPSC Document 701) [On-line]. Available: http://www.cpsc.gov/cpscpub/pubs/701.html.

Venes, D., & Thomas, C. (Eds.). (2001). *Tabor's cyclopedic medical dictionary* (19th ed.). Philadelphia: F. A. Davis.

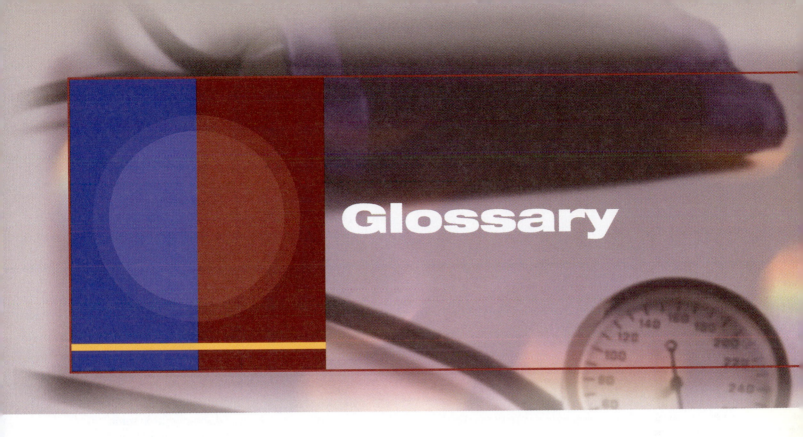

Glossary

abrasion Damage to the outermost layer of skin due to shearing forces.

absence seizure A type of seizure in which the patient stares off into space or seems to be daydreaming; common in children; once called petit mal.

accommodation The ability of the lenses of the eyes to adjust to focus on objects at different distances.

acuity Clarity or sharpness of vision.

acute coronary syndrome (ACS) A broad category of cardiovascular disorders associated with coronary atherosclerosis that may develop a spectrum of clinical syndromes representing varying degrees of coronary artery occlusion. Those syndromes include unstable angina, non-Q wave MI, Q wave MI, and sudden cardiac death.

acute life-threatening event (ALTE) An event that is a combination of apnea, choking, gagging, and change in skin color and muscle tone and is not a sleep disorder.

acute pulmonary edema (APE) A rapid onset of fluid in the alveoli and interstitial tissue of the lungs.

adventitious Abnormal.

advocate Someone who looks out for the needs of others who are not in a position to look out for themselves for various reasons, such as ignorance, incapacity, underage, or misfortune; also to look out for another.

AEIOUTIPS The mnemonic used to remember the many possible reasons a person may experience an altered mental state; *a*lcohol, *e*pilepsy, *i*nfection, *o*verdose, *u*remia, *t*rauma, *i*nsulin, *p*sychosis, *s*troke.

affect The emotional mind-set prompting an expressed emotion or behavior.

agonal respirations Dying breaths; irregular and progressively slowing gasps of air.

allergy A reaction from the body after an exposure to a foreign substance.

altered mental status (AMS) The mental status of a patient whose level of consciousness is anything other than alert (knows his name, where he is, and the day of the week).

American Sign Language (ASL) A communication technique in which the hands and arms are used to sign words or phrases for individuals who are deaf or hard of hearing.

Americans with Disabilities Act (ADA) Federal legislation that regulates the rights of individuals with disabilities to ensure these individuals have access to equipment and information that can improve their ability to function and interact.

amputation Loss of a limb or other body part.

anaphylaxis The most severe type of reaction to an allergen, involving cardiovascular collapse.

anemia of pregnancy An increase in the total blood volume that occurs during pregnancy without a proportionate increase in hemoglobin, creating a dilution effect.

angioedema Cutaneous swelling that most often affects the face, neck, head, and upper airways.

anisocoria Unequal pupils. Normal in a small percentage of the population or may indicate a central nervous system disease.

APGAR scoring system A well-accepted assessment scoring system for newborns that assigns a rating of 0, 1, or 2 to each of the following signs: color, pulse, reflex, muscle tone, and respirations. The APGAR score (Table 17-6) is measured at 1 minute and 5 minutes after birth.

aphasia A defect or loss of the ability to either say or comprehend words. The person may have difficulty reading, writing, speaking, or understanding the speech of others.

apnea A cessation of breathing.

ascites An abnormal accumulation of fluid in the peritoneal cavity.

aspirate To inhale vomitus, blood, or other secretions into the lungs.

assessment card A pocket-sized card designed to prompt the EMS provider as to the key questions to ask the patient for the prehospital patient assessment and to document assessment findings and vital signs; also known as a patient profile.

asthma A form of reversible obstructive lung disease. A multifactorial hypersensitivity reaction causing constriction of the bronchioles and difficulty breathing.

ataxia An abnormal gait that appears wobbly and unsteady as when one is intoxicated or heavily medicated.

atelectasis Collapse of lung tissue.

aura A sensation (e.g., color, lights) experienced just before a seizure.

AVPU An abbreviation for the mini-neuro exam used by the EMS provider during the initial assessment of a patient: *a*lert, *v*erbally responsive, *p*ainful response, *u*nresponsive.

avulsion Loose or torn tissue.

Babinski's reflex An abnormal response of dorsiflexion of the big toe and fanning of all the toes when the outer surface of the sole is firmly stroked from the heel to the toe; indicates a disturbance in the motor response in the central nervous system.

baseline The first set of a patient's vital signs measured.

Biot's respirations An irregular but cyclic pattern of increased and decreased rate and depth of breathing with periods of apnea.

body language The expression of thoughts or emotions by means of posture or gestures.

body surface area (BSA) The amount of skin surface on the body; used to measure the area burned on a person's body.

bradypnea Slow breathing.

Braxton Hicks Contractions that are irregular and inconsistent; also called false labor.

bronchiolitis A viral infection of the bronchioles that causes swelling of the lower airways.

bruit A swishing turbulent sound heard over the arteries that indicates blockage of blood flow.

capnography A measurement of the level of carbon dioxide exhaled by the patient.

capnometer A device that has a digital readout of end-tidal carbon dioxide.

cardiomegaly An increase in heart size for any number of reasons.

carotid artery disease (CAD) Deterioration in the carotid artery as a result of blockage or breakdown in the vessel that can result in inadequate blood flow and blood supply to the organs of the body.

carpopedal spasms Spasmodic contractions of the hands, wrists, feet, and ankles associated with alkalosis and hypocapnia.

cerebrospinal fluid (CSF) A clear body fluid, manufactured in the ventricles of the brain, that bathes the brain and spinal cord.

cerebrovascular accident (CVA) A stroke in which there is an interruption of blood flow to an area of the brain caused by an embolus, hemorrhage, or thrombus.

Cheyne-Stokes respirations A rhythmic pattern of gradually increased and decreased rate and depth of breathing with periods of apnea.

chief complaint (CC) The reason EMS was called; best told in the patient's own words.

chloasoma Mild darkening on the face that sometimes develops during pregnancy; also called the mask of pregnancy.

chronic obstructive pulmonary disease (COPD) A form of obstructive lung disease (emphysema, chronic bronchitis, aspestosis, black lung) that is progressive and irreversible.

Cincinnati Prehospital Stroke Scale A prehospital ministroke assessment tool.

clarification A communication technique in which the EMS provider asks the patient for more information to determine whether his interpretation is accurate.

closed question A type of question that requires only a yes or no response or a one- or two-word response; also known as a direct question.

communication process The process by which a sender encodes a message to be decoded by an intended receiver, who in turn provides feedback.

comprehensive examination and health assessment An examination of the body as a whole.

conjugate gaze The normal position of the eyes.

consensual light reflex Constriction of both pupils when a light is shone into one eye; a normal response.

contrecoup An injury to the brain that develops on the opposite side of the point of impact.

contusion A closed soft-tissue injury in which cells are damaged and blood vessels are torn.

converge To move closer together; normal movement of the eyes as an object comes closer to the face.

coup An injury to the brain that develops directly beneath the point of impact.

coup-contrecoup A type of head injury that results when the head is struck on one side and the force of the impact causes injury to the side that was struck as well as to the opposite side.

crackles A sound similar to that made by the crumpling up of a candy wrapper, usually heard on expiration; also called rales.

cranial nerves The 12 pairs of nerves that come directly out of the brain that innervate mostly the head and face and control sensory and motor functions.

crepitation The sound or sensation of broken bone ends grating on each other.

crisis An internal experience that can create reactions such as severe anxiety, panic, paranoia, or some other brief psychotic event.

croup A viral respiratory infection often caused by other types of infection, such as an ear infection, causing swelling of the vocal cords, trachea, and upper airway tissues and thereby a partial obstruction of the airway.

crushing injury A closed soft-tissue injury resulting in organ rupture and severe fractures from a crushing force.

Cullen's sign Ecchymosis in the periumbilical region (around the belly button), indicating internal bleeding.

cultural diversity The traits and characteristics common among a particular group of people, such as lifestyle, language, traditions, beliefs, and behavior patterns, passed from one generation to the next that vary from the traits and characteristics of another group of people.

CUPS A system used in EMS to prioritize patients by severity of presenting problem: *c*ritical, *u*nstable, *p*otentially unstable, *s*table.

Cushing's triad Three assessment findings that, when displayed together, indicate increasing intracranial pressure (ICP): rising blood pressure, decreasing pulse rate, and changes in the respiratory pattern.

DCAP-BTLS A mnemonic for assessment points in the examination of soft tissue: *d*eformities, *c*ontusions, *a*brasions, *p*enetrations or *p*unctures, *b*urns, *t*enderness, *l*acerations, and *s*welling.

decerebrate A form of neurological posturing characterized by the patient's stiffly extending both the arms and legs and retracting the head.

decode To interpret a message.

decorticate A form of neurological posturing characterized by the patient's flexing the upper extremities to the torso, or core of the body, while extending the lower extremities.

degloving Type of open soft-tissue injury in which the epidermis is removed.

delusion A false personal belief or idea that is portrayed as true.

dermatomes The areas on the surface of the body that are innervated by afferent fibers from one spinal root.

detailed physical examination (DPE) A component of the patient assessment, to be conducted on trauma patients who have significant MOI; this should be done only while en route to the hospital.

developmentally disabled Term used to describe an individual with impaired or insufficient development of the brain resulting in an inability to learn at the usual rate.

diabetic ketoacidosis (DKA) During hypoglycemia, the inability of patients with diabetes to metabolize fat.

diagnosis The identification of a specific disease or condition; usually made after the medical team has evaluated the entire situation.

diastolic The residual blood pressure in the arterial system as the left ventricle relaxes.

diffuse axonal injury (DAI) Injury to brain tissues that results from rapid acceleration or deceleration on the brain.

diplopia Double vision.

diverge To move apart; normal movement of the eyes as they focus on a distant object.

dysarthria An abnormal articulation of speech due to disturbances in muscle control.

dysphagia Difficulty swallowing.

dysphasia Abnormal speech due to lack of coordination and failure to arrange words in the proper order.

dysphonia Discomfort when speaking due to laryngeal disease.

dyspnea Difficulty breathing.

dysuria Difficulty urinating.

emergency doctrine The type of consent given for emergency intervention for a patient who is physically or mentally unable to provide expressed consent; also called implied consent. This type of consent remains in effect for as long as the patient requires lifesaving treatments.

emergency information form (EIF) A form containing standardized information about special needs children, designed to be helpful to emergency personnel inside and outside of the hospital setting.

empathy A sensitivity to and an understanding of another person's feelings.

encode To determine what terms to use to convey a message.

end-tidal carbon dioxide (EtCO$_2$) The concentration of carbon dioxide (CO$_2$) in the exhaled gas at the end of the exhalation.

epidural hematoma An injury to the brain that involves an arterial tear resulting in increased intracranial pressure.

epiglottitis A rare life-threatening infection causing severe inflammation and swelling of the epiglottis.

escharotomy A surgical incision into necrotic tissue of a burn to expand the tissue and decrease ischemia from a circumferential burn.

eupnea Normal breathing.

exacerbation An increase in the seriousness of a disease or disorder.

extraocular muscles (EOMs) Muscles that produce movement of the eyes.

extravasate Escape of fluid, such as blood from a vessel into the surrounding tissues.

facilitation The method in which EMS providers speak and use posture and actions to encourage the patient to say more.

feedback   A receiver's response to a message.

festination   An abnormal gait that appears uneven and hurried as seen in Parkinson's patients.

fetal heart rate (FHR)   The heart rate of a fetus.

fetal heart tones (FHTs)   The heartbeats of a fetus.

Fick principle   Oxygen transport principle that states that adequate cellular perfusion requires that four components be present and working: an adequate oxygen supply, oxygen exchange in the lungs, the circulation of oxygen to the cells, and an adequate number of red blood cells.

field impression   A working diagnosis to determine the cause of a patient's condition.

field of vision   Peripheral vision.

first responder awareness level   Level at which an EMS provider is trained to recognize a hazardous materials incident, back off, and call for help.

first responder operations level   Level at which an EMS provider is trained to perform risk assessment, to select and don appropriate personal protective equipment, and to contain the scene and carry out basic decontamination procedures.

flail segment   A section of the rib cage that has two or more ribs broken in two or more places, creating a paradoxical movement of the broken section as the patient breathes; also called flail chest.

fluid wave test   A special procedure that is performed on the abdomen to test for ascites.

focal head injury   Injury to the brain tissues resulting in lesions.

focused history and physical examination (FH&PE)   A component of patient assessment that varies depending on whether the patient has a medical or a trauma complaint. If trauma, the mechanism of injury is determined, vital signs are taken, and a SAMPLE history is taken; if medical, the nature of the illness is determined, vital signs are taken, and a history of the present illness is determined on the basis of OPQRST.

foreign body airway obstruction (FBAO)   The blockage of the upper airways due to the inhalation of objects such as a large bolus of meat, a coin, or a balloon.

frequent flier   A colloquial term or buzzword for a person who relies on EMS services for care and treatment on a very regular basis.

fundus   The top of the uterus.

general impression   The EMS provider's first impression of the patient to determine the priority of care, taking into consideration the environment and the patient's chief complaint.

generalized seizure   A type of seizure that involves the entire brain and is classified as complete motor seizure, absence seizure, or atonic seizure; once called grand mal.

Glasgow Coma Scale (GCS)   An objective measure of eye opening, verbal response, and motor response, with a numerical score from 3 to 15; used to establish priority for head-injured patients.

Global Med-Net   A medical information service with a toll-free phone number EMS providers can call to obtain a patient's complete medical profile using the patient's member identification number.

golden hour   The optimum limit of 1 hour between time of injury and surgery at the hospital.

gravida   The total number of pregnancies a woman has had.

Grey Turner's sign   Ecchymosis in the flanks and periumbilical areas that is a late sign indicating internal bleeding.

grunting   A sound that results from breathing out against a partially obstructed epiglottis.

guarding   A particular position of comfort to protect a body part from pain.

hallucination   A perception, visual or auditory, of something that is not actually present.

hazardous material (hazmat)   Any substance that can cause injury or death to an individual who has been exposed to the substance.

HEENT   An acronym for *h*ead, *e*yes, *e*ars, *n*ose, and *t*hroat.

hematoma   A collection of blood beneath the skin.

hemoglobin and hematocrit (H&H)   Hemoglobin is the part of the red blood cell that contains iron and carries oxygen to the lungs and tissues. Hematocrit is the percentage of the whole volume of blood contributed by cells.

hemoptysis   Coughing up blood from the respiratory tract.

history of the present illness (HPI)   Specific patient information about the current illness or condition.

hypercapnia   An abnormally high concentration of carbon dioxide in the blood.

hypercarbia   Carbon dioxide retention.

hyperventilation   A respiratory rate greater than that required for normal body function.

hyphema   Bleeding into the anterior chamber of the eye.

hypocapnia   An abnormally low concentration of carbon dioxide in the blood.

hypoventilation   Irregular and shallow breathing.

hypoxia   Inadequate oxygenation of the blood cells.

ictal phase   The period during a seizure attack.

illusions   Misperceptions of actual existing stimuli by any sense.

impaled object   An object that has pierced and become fixed in the skin and tissues.

incident command system (ICS)   See IMS.

incident management system (IMS)   A system of organization and administration involving all emergency service providers that focuses on the three critical components of large-incident management: command, control, and communications.

incision   A clean break in the skin, usually made by a knife.

index of suspicion Injury patterns associated with specific mechanisms of injury from which the EMS provider can anticipate the potential for shock or other problems.

initial assessment (IA) The second component of patient assessment; an orderly and sequential examination with correction of life threats and determination of the patient's priority.

kinesthetic Refers to the sense of body position.

Kussmaul's respirations Air hunger.

laceration A break in the skin; can be deep or superficial and usually has uneven edges.

linea nigra Darkened line that runs midline from the umbilicus down to the pubic bone during pregnancy.

loaded bumper A shock-absorbing bumper on a motor vehicle that has been compressed and can release suddenly without warning.

Los Angeles Prehospital Stroke Screen (LAPSS) A prehospital ministroke assessment tool.

McBurney's point A landmark on the abdomen associated with the late pain of appendicitis; an imaginary triangle on the anterior lower right quadrant, from the navel out to the right superior iliac spine.

mechanism of injury (MOI) The instrument or event that results in harm to the patient.

Medic Alert Foundation An organization that maintains a 24-hour emergency response center with a toll-free phone number EMS providers can call to obtain information on patients who wear medical identification necklaces or bracelets with an identifiable symbol (Medic Alert).

melena Blood in stool.

mental status (MS) Determination of whether a patient is alert and oriented.

message The points being conveyed by a sender to a receiver.

minute volume The amount of gas inspired in a minute.

multiparous Term used to describe a woman who has given birth.

nasal flaring Widening of the nostrils during breathing.

nature of the illness (NOI) The condition or chief complaint of the patient.

neonatal sepsis Severe overwhelming infection in a neonate (birth to 1 month).

neurogenic shock A form of shock, often called fainting or syncope, due to disorders of the nervous system with an absence of sympathetic response. Three assessment findings that, when displayed together, indicate neurogenic shock are decreasing blood pressure, decreasing pulse rate, and decreasing respiratory rate.

North American Emergency Response Guidebook (NAERG) A book that provides responders instructions and information on how to handle the first 30 minutes of a hazmat spill.

nulliparous Term used to describe a woman who has never given birth.

nystagmus A fine motor twitching of the eyeball, normal during extreme lateral gaze but not in any other position.

objective information Data representing the clinical signs that can be observed and measured by the examiner such as the pulse, respiratory rate, and blood pressure.

ongoing assessment (OA) The last component of patient assessment, which is conducted en route to the hospital. The OA involves reassessing vital signs and interventions, repeating the initial assessment as necessary, and reprioritizing the patient.

opacification The forming of cataract cloudiness, impairing vision.

open-ended question A type of question that requires a narrative form of response.

ophthalmoscope A tool used by health care personnel to perform a detailed examination of the eye.

OPQRST An elaboration of the chief complaint such as pain or difficulty breathing: *o*nset; *p*rovocation; *q*uality; *r*egion, *r*adiation, *r*elief, *r*ecurrence; *s*everity; *t*ime.

orthopnea The abnormal condition in which a patient must sit or stand to breathe comfortably.

orthostatic changes An increase in heart rate and a decrease in blood pressure when a patient rises from a supine or sitting position.

otorrhea A discharge from the ear.

otoscope A tool used by health personnel to perform a detailed examination of the ear.

paradoxical motion Seen when a free-floating section of the rib cage moves in the opposite direction of the rest of the rib cage during respirations.

paralytic ileus A twisted and paralyzed bowel.

paraverbal cues Tone and volume of voice, speed of talking, and inflection, used to convey meaning through speech.

parity The total number of births a woman has had.

paroxysmal nocturnal dyspnea (PND) A form of transient pulmonary edema that wakes the patient during the night with severe shortness of breath; associated with heart failure.

partial seizure A type of seizure that occurs only in a particular area of the brain, so the patient remains conscious and effects are apparent only in a specific area of the body.

patient assessment The methodical process by which a patient's condition is evaluated.

patient profile See assessment card.

peak flow A measurement of how rapidly a patient can exhale.

penetration A break in the skin due to an object's being forced into and tearing the skin and internal organs.

perfusion Blood flow to the tissues of the body.

peritonitis Inflammation of the peritoneum.

PERRLA An acronym for documenting normal findings with the eyes: *pupils equally round, reactive to light and accommodation.*

personal protective equipment (PPE) Items that can be worn to protect the EMS provider from harm from bodily fluids or hazardous substances, such as disposable gloves, eye shields or goggles, masks, and gowns.

pertinent negatives Symptoms the patient does not have that may be relevant to the case (e.g., a patient struck his head but did not lose consciousness).

piloerection A reflexive response to cold; also known as goose pimples.

plantar reflex A reflex that is assessed on both conscious and unconscious patients with suspected spinal cord injury. With the end of a capped pen, a light stroke is drawn up the lateral side of the sole of the foot and across the ball of the foot, like an upside-down letter J. The normal response is plantar flexion of the toes and foot.

platinum 10 minutes The optimum limit of 10 minutes at the scene with a critical trauma patient; used in both Montana's and New York State's Critical Trauma Care courses.

pleural friction rub A grating sound in the chest caused by inflamed pleural surfaces.

pleurisy Inflammation of the lining of the lungs.

pleuritic pain Pain caused by any condition that causes inflammation in the lung or heart that extends to the pleural surfaces of the lung.

pneumonia An inflammation of the lungs commonly caused by bacteria, a virus, or other pathogens.

pneumothorax A collection of air or gas in the pleural space of the chest causing one or both lungs to collapse.

point of maximal impulse (PMI) The point on the chest where the impulse of the left ventricle is felt most strongly.

polypharmacy The administering or taking of many medications concurrently, often for the same condition.

positive findings Information obtained in the focused history and physical examination that is clearly relevant to the chief complaint.

post-ictal The third phase of a seizure, during which the patient is extremely exhausted and confused while slowly regaining consciousness.

prehospital care report (PCR) A report that should be completed on every call; an accurate and thorough documentation of the assessment findings and field management of the patient.

pre-ictal phase The period before a seizure attack.

presbycusis Normal hearing loss that occurs with aging.

preterm labor True labor that occurs before 38 weeks' gestation.

pronator drift A test used to assess focal weakness. The patient is asked to extend both arms out in front of him with palms up while both eyes are closed. If one arm "drifts" lower or the palm turns down, this is considered a deficit.

proprioception The perceptions concerning movements and position of the body.

psychosis A serious mental disorder characterized by a loss of contact with reality.

pulmonary embolism (PE) A serious condition caused by a foreign body (e.g., a clot) that lodges in the pulmonary capillary bed.

pulse oximetry A technique used to measure the percentage of hemoglobin saturated with oxygen.

pulsus differens A condition in which the pulses on either side of the body are unequal.

puncture A break in the skin as a result of an object's being forced into the skin.

pursed-lip breathing Exhaling past partially closed lips to build up air pressure in the lungs.

rales See crackles.

range of motion (ROM) The area and span of motion of the joints.

rapid physical examination (RPE) A systematic quick examination of the major body sections (head, neck, chest, abdomen, pelvis, back, buttocks, and extremities) for injuries, conducted on the medical patient who is not responsive (i.e., hypoglycemia, hypothermia, or post-ictal state).

rapid trauma assessment (RTE) A quick head-to-toe assessment conducted on a trauma patient with significant mechanism of injury involving the major body sections (head, neck, chest, abdomen, pelvis, back, buttocks, and extremities).

rapid trauma examination (RTE) A systematic quick examination of the major body sections (head, neck, chest, abdomen, pelvis, back, buttocks, and extremities) for injuries.

referred pain Pain that originates from one area of the body that is also sensed in another area.

reflection A communication technique in which the EMS provider repeats the patient's words to encourage further discussion.

retraction A pulling in of skin in the suprasternal, subclavicular, and intercostal areas during inhalation.

revised trauma score (RTS) A numerical grading system used for triage and to predict patient outcomes, developed by Howard Champion, MD; also known as the trauma score; *see also* trauma score.

rhonchi Rattling noises in the upper airways caused by mucus or other secretions; singular, rhoncus.

rotavirus A virus that causes acute gastroenteritis in children.

rubberneckers Individuals who pose a traffic hazard when passing the scene of an accident so they can get a look at the damage and rescue taking place.

rule out Process by which a diagnosis is made in the cardiac care unit in order to determine a definitive diagnosis.

S1   A normal heart sound; the first sound heard, which is produced by the atrioventricular valves.

S2   A normal heart sound; the second sound heard, which is produced by the semilunar valves.

SAMPLE history   An acronym for the information needed to assess and manage today's incident or complaint: *s*igns and symptoms, *a*llergies, *m*edications, *p*ertinent past medical history, *l*ast oral intake, *e*vents leading up to this incident.

scaphoid abdomen   A sinking, or concave, shape to the abdomen.

scene size-up   The first component of patient assessment, which involves determining whether the location, or environment, is safe for the responders and the patient.

semantics   The study of the meanings in language.

serial vital signs   All measurements after, or comparisons against, the baseline measurements.

sign   A finding that can be measured accurately by hand or with a measuring device such as a sphygmomanometer (blood pressure cuff), oximeter, or thermometer.

silent myocardial infarction (MI)   An MI with atypical signs and symptoms.

sinus arrhythmia   A cardiac rhythm typical in children and healthy adults characterized by a regular rate that increases and decreases rhythmically with breathing.

skin color, temperature, and condition (CTC)   Assessment the EMS provider can do to determine circulatory status.

somatic pain   Pain caused by irritation of pain fibers in the parietal peritoneum; tends to be localized to the area of pathology.

spastic hemiparesis   An abnormal gait with unilateral weakness and foot dragging.

START   An acronym for *s*imple *t*riage *a*nd *r*apid *t*reatment; a system used to triage patients in a multiple-casualty incident.

steppage   An abnormal gait in which the person appears to be walking up steps when on an even surface.

Stokes-Adams syndrome   Syncope or convulsions caused by complete heart block and a pulse rate of 40 or less.

striae   Atrophic lines or streaks from a rapid or prolonged stretching of the skin.

stridor   A high-pitched sound associated with upper airway obstruction.

subcutaneous emphysema   Air bubbles under the skin resulting from a pneumothorax; sometimes exhibits as crackling like Rice Krispies or the sensation of plastic packaging bubbles.

subdural hematoma   An injury to the brain resulting in bleeding from the rupture of bridging vessels between the cortex and dura mater.

subjective information   Data obtained from the patient and commonly referred to as the symptoms; this cannot be measured by the EMS provider.

sudden infant death syndrome (SIDS)   The sudden unexplained death of an infant in the first year of life.

supine hypotension   A drop in blood pressure that occurs during the third trimester of pregnancy if the mother is supine because the weight of the fetus lies on the inferior vena cava.

sympathy   An expression of sorrow for another's loss, grief, or misfortune; implies having feelings and emotions similar to or shared with another person.

symphysis pubis   The area of the anterior pelvis where the two pubic bones grow together.

symptom   A subjective finding that the patient tells the EMS provider.

syncope   Fainting.

systolic   The peak blood pressure in the arterial system as the left ventricle contracts.

tachypnea   Rapid, shallow breathing.

tactile fremitus   A vibration of the chest wall during breathing that can be felt by the examiner, often associated with inflammation, infection, or congestion.

technical terminology   Language or professional jargon that has meaning only for the medical community or professional group.

tension pneumothorax   A life-threatening condition resulting from air or gas trapped in the pleural space of the chest and causing collapse of one or both lungs, movement of the mediastinum, and a dramatic decrease in cardiac output.

tenting   Characteristic of skin that has poor turgor or a connective tissue disease; the skin remains in a tent position when pinched and does not return to normal.

tilt test   A test used to assess heart rate and blood pressure for orthostatic changes when a patient rises up from a lying position.

transient ischemic attack (TIA)   A temporary interruption of blood flow to an area of the brain; may be a precursor to a major cerebrovascular accident.

trauma center   A hospital that has the capability of caring for the acutely injured patient.

trauma score   An assessment tool that assigns a numerical value to represent the extent of injury on the basis of respiratory rate and chest expansion, capillary refill, and blood pressure ranges; also known as the revised trauma score.

traumatic brain injury (TBI)   A blunt or penetrating injury to the brain.

trending   Changes over time observed by the comparison of multiple sets of vital signs and/or assessments to establish a diagnostic picture of the patient's status.

triage   A French word that means "to sort."

trimester   One of the 3-month segments of pregnancy.

tripod position   A sitting position often assumed by patients who are having difficulty breathing; leaning forward, with elbows outward and hands on knees.

true labor Persistent, regular contractions.

tunnel vision The making of judgments or determinations on the basis of history and past experiences with an individual or an event.

tympany A drumlike sound.

up triaging A concept used in medicine that means that if a patient's presenting problem could be either more or less serious, the patient should be managed as having the more serious of the two possibilities until the patient's condition has been absolutely determined.

Vial of Life A rolled piece of paper with pertinent medical information about the patient that is kept in a plastic tube similar to a prescription drug container. Patients are often told to keep this in their refrigerator for ease of EMS providers locating them.

visceral pain Pain caused by the stretching of nerve fibers surrounding either solid or hollow organs in the abdomen; this type of pain is often poorly localized and diffuse.

vital signs Pulse, blood pressure, and respirations, often considered the starting point for assessment and a gauge of a person's health status.

Waddell's triad An injury pattern seen in children that involves the legs, chest, and head.

wheezing A continuous whistling sound caused by narrowing of the lower airways, usually heard at the end of exhalation.

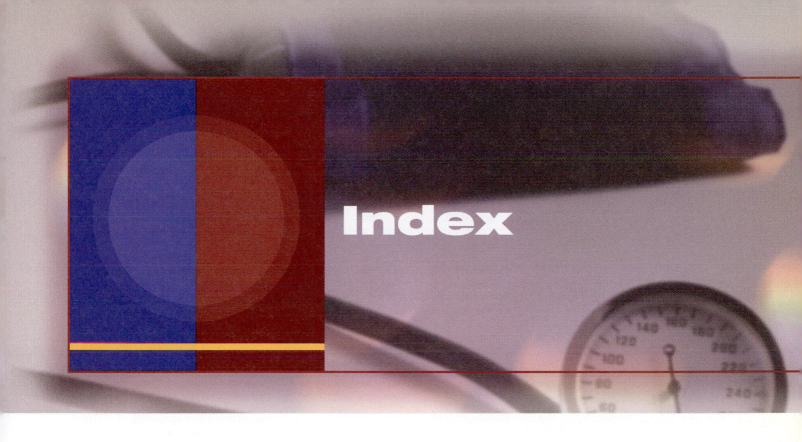

Index